Q0004382
£9.50.

Barrett's Esophagus and
Esophageal Adenocarcinoma

To my parents; my brother, Sandeep; and my wife, Priyanka, for their constant support and love. PS

To my loving wife Linda, who accepts and encourages my professional mistress Barrett's esophagus, and to my sons Rob and Steve, who share the focus of my attention with my interest in Barrett's esophagus. RES

Barrett's Esophagus and Esophageal Adenocarcinoma

EDITED BY

Prateek Sharma, MD
Associate Professor of Medicine
University of Kansas School of Medicine and
Veterans Affairs Medical Center
Kansas City, Kansas

Richard Sampliner, MD
Chief of Gastroenterology
Southern Arizona VA Health Care System
Professor of Medicine
University of Arizona Health Sciences Center
Tuscon, Arizona

SECOND EDITION

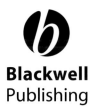

Blackwell
Publishing

Blackwell Publishing, Inc., 350 Main Street, Malden, Massachusetts 02148-5020, USA
Blackwell Publishing Ltd, 9600 Garsington Road, Oxford OX4 2DQ, UK
Blackwell Publishing Asia Pty Ltd, 550 Swanston Street, Carlton, Victoria 3053, Australia

First published 2001
Second edition 2006

Library of Congress Cataloging-in-Publication Data

Barrett's esophagus and esophageal adenocarcinoma / edited by Prateek Sharma, Richard Sampliner. – 2nd ed.
    p. ; cm.
  Includes bibliographical references and index.
  ISBN-13: 978-1-4051-2786-8 (alk. paper)
  ISBN-10: 1-4051-2786-4 (alk. paper)
  1. Esophagus–Cancer. 2. Esophagus–Precancerous conditions. 3. Adenocarcinoma.
  [DNLM: 1. Barrett Esophagus. 2. Adenocarcinoma. 3. Esophageal Neoplasms. WI 250 B27415 2006 I. Sharma, Prateek. II. Sampliner, Richard E.

  RC280.E8B37 2006
  616.99′432–dc22

                               2005030969

A catalogue record for this title is available from the British Library

Set in 9 on 12 pt Meridien by SNP Best-set Typesetter Ltd., Hong Kong
Printed and bound in India by Replika Press PVT Ltd.

Commissioning Editor: Alison Brown
Development Editor: Helen Harvey
Production Controller: Kate Charman

For further information on Blackwell Publishing, visit our website:
http://www.blackwellpublishing.com

The publisher's policy is to use permanent paper from mills that operate a sustainable forestry policy, and which has been manufactured from pulp processed using acid-free and elementary chlorine-free practices. Furthermore, the publisher ensures that the text paper and cover board used have met acceptable environmental accreditation standards.

Notice: The indications and dosages of all the drugs in this book have been recommended in the medical literature and conform to the practices of the general community. The medications described do not necessarily have specific approval by the Food and Drug Administration for use in the diseases and dosages for which they are recommended. The package insert for each drug should be consulted for use and dosage as approved by the FDA. Because standards for usage change, it is advisable to keep abreast of revised recommendations, particularly those concerning new drugs.

Contents

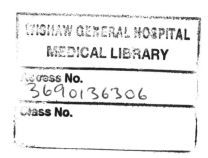

Color plate section falls between pp.148–9.

List of Contributors

Ajay Bansal, MD
Assistant Professor of Medicine
University of Kansas School of Medicine
and
Veterans Affairs Medical Center
4801 E. Linwood Blvd
Kansas City, MO 64128-2295, USA

Jacques J. G. H. M. Bergman, MD, PhD
Department of Gastroenterology and
Hepatology
Academic Medical Center
Meibergdreef 9
1105 AZ, Amsterdam
The Netherlands

Navtej S. Buttar, MD
Assistant Professor of Medicine
Mayo Clinic and Foundation
Rochester, MN 55905, USA

Alan J. Cameron, MD, FRCP
Emeritus Professor of Medicine
Division of Gastroenterology and
Hepatology
Mayo Clinic
2727 Merrihills Drive SW
Rochester, Minnesota 55902, USA

Nicholas J. Clemons, PhD
Oesophageal Group
Cancer Cell Unit
Hutchison-MRC Centre
Hills Road
Cambridge CB2 2XZ, UK

Jacques Deviere, MD, PhD
Department of Gastroenterology and
Hepatopancreatology
ULB –Hôpital Erasme
Route de Lennik 808
B –1070 Brussels, Belgium

Christian Ell, MD, PhD
Professor of Medicine
Head, Department of Internal
Medicine 2
HSK Wiesbaden
Ludwig-Erhard-Strasse 100
65199 Wiesbaden
Germany

Gary W. Falk, MD
Professor of Medicine
Cleveland Clinic Lerner College of
Medicine of Case Western Reserve
University
Department of Gastroenterology and
Hepatology
Cleveland Clinic Foundation
9500 Euclid Avenue
Cleveland, OH 44195, USA

Michael J. G. Farthing, DSc (Med), MD, FRCP, FMed Sci
Professor of Medicine
St George's University of London
Cranmer Terrace
London SW17 0RE, UK

Linda A. Feagins, MD
Gastroenterology Fellow
University of Texas Southwestern
Division of Gastroenterology MC#111B1
Dallas VA Medical Center
4500 S. Lancaster Road
Dallas, TX 75216, USA

M. Brian Fennerty, MD
Professor of Medicine
Section Chief, Division of
Gastroenterology
Oregon Health Sciences University
3181 SW Sam Jackson Park Road
Mail Code PV310
Portland, OR 97239-3098, USA

Rebecca C. Fitzgerald, MACantab, MD, MRCP
Oesophageal Group
Cancer Cell Unit
Hutchison-MRC Centre
Hills Road
Cambridge CB2 2XZ, UK

Paul Fockens, MD, PhD
Department of Gastroenterdogy and
Hepatology
Academic Medical Center
Meibergdreef 9
1105 AZ, Amsterdam
The Netherlands

Gregory G. Ginsberg, MD
Professor of Medicine
Director of Endoscopic Services
University of Pennsylvania Medical
   School
3 Rardin, GI Division
3400 Spruce Street
Philadelphia, PA 19104, USA

John R. Goldblum, MD
Department of Anatomic Pathology
Cleveland Clinic Foundation
9500 Euclid Avenue
Cleveland, OH 44195, USA

John M. Inadomi, MD
University of California, San Francisco
San Francisco General Hospital
1001 Porrero Avenue, 3D5
San Francisco, CA 94110, USA

**Janusz Jankowski, MBChB, MSc,
   MD, PhD, FRCP (Edin, Lond)**
Professor of Gastroenterological
   Oncology
Senior Clinical Research Fellow
Department of Clinical Pharmacology
Woodstock Road
Oxford University
Radcliffe Infirmary
Oxford OX3 6HE, UK

Ann Marie Joyce, MD
Instructor of Medicine
University of Pennsylvania Medical
   School
3 Rardin, GI Division
3400 Spruce Street
Philadelphia, PA 19104, USA

Peter J. Kahrilas, MD
Gilbert H. Marquardt Professor of
   Medicine
Northwestern University
Feinberg School of Medicine
Division of Gastroenterology
Department of Medicine
676 N. St. Clair Street, Suite 1400
Chicago, IL 60611, USA

Mohammed A. Kara, MD
Department of Gastroenterology and
   Hepatology
Academic Medical Center
Meibergdreef 9
1105 AZ, Amsterdam
The Netherlands

Ernst J. Kuipers, MD
Department of Gastroenterology and
   Hepatology
Erasmus MC University Medical Center
PO Box 2040
3000 CA Rotterdam
The Netherlands

Jesper Lagergren, MD, PhD
Unit of Esophageal and Gastric Research
Department of Molecular Medicine and
   Surgery
Karolinska Institute, 17176
Stockholm
Sweden

Dave R. Lal, MD
Senior Fellow and Acting Instructor
Center for Videoendoscopic Surgery &
   Swallowing Center
University of Washington School of
   Medicine
1959 NE Pacific Street, Box 356410
Seattle, WA 98195-6410, USA

Peter Malfertheiner, MD
Department of Gastroenterology,
   Hepatology and Infection
Otto-von-Guericke University
Leipziger Strasse 44
D39120 Magdeburg
Germany

Andrea May, MD, PhD
Assistant Professor
Attending Physician
HSK Wiesbaden
Ludwig-Erhard-Strasse 100
65199 Wiesbaden, Germany

Joel E. Mendelin, MD
Department of Anatomic Pathology
Cleveland Clinic Foundation
9500 Euclid Avenue
Cleveland, OH 44195, USA

Brant K. Oelschlager, MD
Director, Center for Videoendoscopic
   Surgery
Director, Swallowing Center
Assistant Professor, Department of
   Surgery
University of Washington School of
   Medicine
1959 NE Pacific Street, Box 356410
Seattle, WA 98195-6410, USA

Roy C. Orlando, MD
Professor of Medicine and Adjunct
   Professor of Physiology
Chief of Gastroenterology and
   Hepatology
Tulane University Health Sciences
   Center
1430 Tulane Avenue (SL-35)
New Orleans, LA 70112, USA

John E. Pandolfino
Assistant Professor of Medicine
Northwestern University
Feinberg School of Medicine
Division of Gastroenterology
Department of Medicine
676 N. St. Clair Street, Suite 1400
Chicago, IL 60611, USA

Oliver Pech, MD
Department of Internal Medicine 2
HSK Wiesbaden
Ludwig-Erhard-Strasse 100
65199 Wiesbaden, Germany

Ulrich Peitz, MD, PhD
Senior Physician
Department of Gastroenterology,
   Hepatology and Infection
Otto-von-Guericke University
Leipziger Strasse 44
D39120 Magdeburg
Germany

Joel E. Richter, MD, FACP, MACG
Department of Medicine
Temple University School of Medicine
3041 N. Broad Street
800 Parkinson Pavillion
Philadelphia, PA 19140, USA

Joel H. Rubenstein, MD, MSC
Division of Gastroenterology
Department of Medicine
University of Michigan
Ann Arbor, MI 48105, USA

Richard E. Sampliner, MD
Chief of Gastroenterology
Southern Arizona VA Health Care
   System
Professor of Medicine
University of Arizona Health Sciences
   Center
3601 S 6th Avenue
Section of Gastroenterology (111G-1)
Tuscon, AZ 85723, USA

Prateek Sharma, MD
Associate Professor of Medicine
University of Kansas School of Medicine
    and
Veterans Affairs Medical Center
4801 E. Linwood Blvd
Kansas City, MO 64128-2295, USA

Rhonda F. Souza, MD
Associate Professor of Medicine
University of Texas Southwestern
Division of Gastroenterology
MC # 111 B1
Dallas VA Medical Center
4500 S. Lancaster Road
Dallas, TX 75216, USA

Stuart Jon Spechler, MD
Chief, Division of Gastroenterology
Dallas VA Medical Center
4500 South Lancaster Road
Dallas, Texas 75216, USA

Jacques Van Dam, MD, PhD
Professor of Medicine
Stanford University School of Medicine
Clinical Chief and Director of Edoscopy
Division of Gastroenterology and
    Hepatology
Stanford University Medical Center
Room H-1138
300 Pasteur Drive
Stanford, CA 94305, USA

Shyam Varadarajulu, MD
Department of Medicine
Division of Gastroenterology and
    Hepatology
University of Alabama at Birmingham
Birmingham, Alabama, USA

Michael B. Wallace, MD, MPH
Associate Professor of Medicine
Director of Endoscopic Research
Mayo Clinic
4500 San Pablo Road
Jacksonville, FL 32224, USA

Kenneth K. Wang, MD
Associate Professor of Medicine
Mayo Clinic
200 First Street SW
Alfred M430
Rochester, MN 55905, USA

Thomas D. Wang, MD, PhD
Clinical Instructor
Division of Gastroentrology and
    Hepatology
Stanford University School of Medicine
318 Campus Drive, Room E-150
Stanford, CA 94305-5427, USA

C. Mel Wilcox, MD
Department of Medicine
Division of Gastroenterology and
    Hepatology
633 ZRB, University of Alabama at
    Birmingham
Birmingham, AL 35294, USA

Stephan M. Wildi, MD
Department of Gastroenterology and
    Hepatology
University Hospital of Zürich
Switzerland

Edyta Zagorowicz, MBCh B, MD
Department of Gastroenterology
Institute of Oncology
5 Roentgen St
02-781 #Warsaw
Poland

Preface to the Second Edition

Barrett's esophagus is the premalignant lesion for adenocarcinoma of the esophagus. The incidence of adenocarcinoma of the esophagus continues to increase, especially in Caucasian males. Since the 2001 edition there has been a rapid expansion in the field of Barrett's esophagus and esophageal adenocarcinoma. Improved detection of neoplasia has been helped by the availability of imaging modalities such as high resolution endoscopy, narrow band imaging, and confocal microscopy. There have also been advances in the endoscopic therapeutic modalities for treating high grade dysplasia and early esophageal adenocarcinoma.

However, many uncertainties about Barrett's remain: the specific cause or causes of metaplasia and the development of neoplasia, the risk of cancer for individual patients, the role and specifics of screening and surveillance, and the ideal clinical management. In the face of these unknowns, on a daily basis, the clinician must still make decisions about each patient. The chapters in this book provide the clinician, the teacher, and the investigator with the latest evidence and information about the topical issues in Barrett's esophagus research and the latest approaches to patient management.

This edition also has updated chapters pertaining to the epidemiology, pathogenesis, diagnosis, staging, treatment, and management of these lesions. New chapters on emerging techniques including high resolution endoscopy, spectroscopy, confocal imaging and optical coherence tomography highlight the leading edge of technology research and development. Additional chapters deal with the controversial management of high grade dysplasia, the expanding role of endoscopic resection and the nascent field of chemoprevention.

Many questions remain unanswered in the field of Barrett's esophagus and continued investigation by both clinical and basic researchers will help enlighten us further as we continue our quest towards understanding this common but incompletely understood disease. We have assembled a highly distinguished group of investigators who present state of the art on the relevant topics of clinical importance in this field. Each chapter included in this book provides a comprehensive discussion of important issues, focusing on new and evolving concepts with regards to this premalignant lesion.

We hope that the collective efforts of all the authors and the editors have succeeded in achieving our goal of providing an educational reference for researchers and clinicians alike, and we wish to thank all the contributors for providing uniformly outstanding and detailed reviews. It is our hope that this book will provide further insights into our understanding and treatment of patients with Barrett's esophagus and esophageal adenocarcinoma.

Our work was greatly facilitated by the expert assistance of Mary Mackison and Lisa Camargo. Without their efforts this book would not have been possible, and we are indebted to them. We also wish to express our gratitude to our colleagues at Blackwell Publishing.

Prateek Sharma
Richard E. Sampliner
2006

CHAPTER 1

Definition and Diagnosis of Barrett's Esophagus

Ajay Bansal and Prateek Sharma

Introduction

Diagnosis of Barrett's esophagus is important to identify the subpopulation with gastroesophageal reflux disease (GERD) that not only has an altered quality of life but also is at an increased risk for esophageal adenocarcinoma as compared to the general population. Approximately 10–15% of patients with chronic GERD are diagnosed with Barrett's esophagus, a premalignant lesion for esophageal adenocarcinoma [1,2] This subgroup with Barrett's esophagus may benefit from regular surveillance to identify progression to dysplasia prior to the development of adenocarcinoma. Adenocarcinoma of the esophagus has risen almost fivefold in incidence over the past 20 years in the USA [3–6]. It now accounts for more than 50% of all esophageal cancers in this country [7].

The definition of Barrett's esophagus has evolved from endoscopic findings alone to the use of esophageal manometry and finally now to include a combination of endoscopic and histological findings in the distal esophagus. Novel endoscopic methods including magnification endoscopy, chromoendoscopy, narrow band imaging etc., are being extensively studied to assist in the endoscopic diagnosis of Barrett's esophagus but the studies are far from being conclusive. Application of newer molecular markers like cdx-2, muc-2 and sucrase isomaltase for confirming the intestinal origin of the metaplastic epithelium is being reported. In addition, use of special stains like Alcian blue in biopsies obtained from endoscopically suspected Barrett's esophagus has increased the histologic accuracy of confirming intestinal metaplasia.

Definition

The American Gastroenterological Association workshop in Chicago defined Barrett's esophagus as the displacement of the squamocolumnar junction (SCJ) proximal to the gastroesophageal junction (GEJ) with the presence of intestinal metaplasia [8] (Plate 1.1a,b; color plate section falls between pp. 148–9). The definition of Barrett's esophagus has evolved over many years since the first description in 1950s by N. R. Barrett [9]. All three types of columnar epithelium—fundic mucosa, cardia mucosa and intestinal metaplasia can be detected in the columnar lined distal esophagus [10]. However, currently there is general consensus (although controversial) on using intestinal metaplasia and not the other two types of mucosae, as the histological marker for Barrett's esophagus [8]. The reason for including intestinal metaplasia in the definition as opposed to fundic or cardia mucosa is the observation that dysplasia or cancer is usually associated with the presence of intestinal metaplasia. A review of 14 cases of esophageal adenocarcinoma revealed that 12 (86%) occurred in columnar epithelium as defined by the presence of distinctive intestinal type mucosa (confirmed Barrett's esophagus) [11]. Hamilton and Smith studied biopsy specimens from 14 Barrett's esophagus patients with known dysplasia and 43 esophagectomy specimens from patients with resected adenocarcinoma [12]. They showed that dysplasia was associated with intestinal type mucosa in 11 patients and with cardia type mucosa in three of 14 patients. Also, in the same study, evaluation of 43 esophagectomy specimens revealed that adenocarcinoma most often occurred in Barrett's mucosa of

the intestinal type. Another study identified six patients with dysplastic Barrett's mucosa, four with
high-grade dysplasia, and showed that dysplasia
arose in five of six cases from foci of intestinal metaplasia [13]. Besides these studies, other investigators
have also demonstrated that intestinal metaplasia is
associated with an increased risk of malignancy
[14,15]. However, the exact malignant potential of
each of the epithelia type is yet to be confirmed in a
prospective follow-up study.

Endoscopic Recognition of Barrett's Esophagus

Landmarks

Normally, the SCJ should coincide with the GEJ,
which is evidenced by the proximal limit of the linear
gastric mucosal folds. The lack of this concurrence
and the proximal displacement of the SCJ indicate
the endoscopic presence of a columnar lined esophagus (i.e. endoscopic or suspected Barrett's esophagus). The GEJ is best visualized when the esophagus
is distended minimally to the point at which the
proximal ends of the gastric folds appear and
coincide with the pinch at the end of the tubular
esophagus [16] (Plate 1.1a,b; color plate section falls
between pp. 148–9). Once the GEJ is accurately
identified, the distance between the proximally displaced SCJ and the GEJ should be measured endoscopically and recorded as the length of the Barrett's
esophagus segment [17]. In many situations, the SCJ
and the GEJ may coincide for the major portion, but
there maybe tongues of columnar mucosa extending
for some distance above the GEJ raising a suspicion
for Barrett's esophagus.

The diagnosis of Barrett's esophagus in cases of
columnar appearing mucosa extending for greater
than 3 cm above the GEJ is usually straightforward
[18]—the chances of detecting intestinal metaplasia
in this situation are greater than 90% and the recognition of the columnar lined esophagus is usually not
an issue. The difficulty arises in two different situations. Firstly, there is presence of columnar mucosa
on endoscopy that is at least 2–3 cm in length but histology may show cardiac type mucosa. Secondly,
what appears to be a short area of columnar mucosa
in the distal esophagus or an irregular Z line can show

intestinal metaplasia which may actually represent
intestinal metaplasia of the anatomic gastric
cardia—i.e., cardia intestinal metaplasia (CIM) leading to misclassification of CIM as short segment
Barrett's esophagus. The role of the endoscopist in
defining the endoscopic extent of Barrett's esophagus
above the GEJ is thus critical, especially in the
latter situation as the pathologist will report only
intestinal metaplasia that could be either Barrett's
esophagus or CIM based on the exact location of the
biopsy. This is of importance as Barrett's esophagus
and CIM appear to be distinct entities with different
demographics, symptoms and dysplasia/cancer risk
[19]. Moreover, the presence of a large hiatal hernia,
ulcers/erosions, strictures etc., may prevent the accurate assessment of endoscopic Barrett's esophagus,
sometimes leading to the overdiagnosis of Barrett's
esophagus, especially in the situation of a hernia.

Endoscopic Classification of Barrett's Esophagus

A clinically relevant classification Barrett's esophagus based on the length on endoscopy has proposed
to classify the finding of intestinal metaplasia on
biopsies into three categories—long segment Barrett's esophagus, short segment Barrett's esophagus,
and CIM. Traditionally, long segement and short
segment Barrett's esophagus have been distinguished by the length of the endoscopic Barrett's
esophagus segment (≥3 cm or <3 cm respectively)
whereas CIM is diagnosed by the lack of any
esophageal columnar mucosa on endoscopy but the
presence of intestinal metaplasia, if biopsies are obtained below the GEJ. The "3 cm" rule for traditional
Barrett's esophagus was applied in 1970s to avoid an
overdiagnosis of Barrett's esophagus resulting from
either failure to recognize the tubularized portion of
a herniated stomach on endoscopy and, also, because it was felt that the "normal esophagus" could
have 1–2 cm of columnar mucosa in its distal portion
[20]. Thereafter, it was documented that even short
lengths of Barrett's esophagus may undergo progression to dysplasia as well as adenocarcinoma [21,22].
A prospective study showed that although there was
a non-significant trend towards increased cancer risk
by 1.7-fold for every 5 cm increase in the length of
Barrett's esophagus ($P = 0.06$), the length of Barrett's

esophagus was not significantly related to risk for adenocarcinoma ($P > 0.2$) [23]. In view of this, the classification of Barrett's esophagus into long (≥ 3 cm) and short (<3 cm) segments may be less relevant clinically.

On the other hand, CIM may have a lower risk of neoplastic progression. Sharma *et al.*, in a study of 78 patients with short segment Barrett's esophagus and 34 patients with CIM, reported that dysplasia developed in nine short segment Barrett's esophagus patients and one CIM patient, whereas adenocarcinoma developed in one patient in the short segment Barrett's esophagus group and none in the CIM group [19]. But this issue is far from settled at this time. In a review of 22 resected specimens of adenocarcinoma occuring within 2 cm of the GEJ and 22 matched control specimens of resected esophageal squamous carcinoma, CIM with high- or low-grade dysplasia was associated with 64% of adenocarcinoma compared to 5% of controls ($P < 0.001$) [24]. Moreover, the incidence of cardia adenocarcinoma has increased over the past 15 years [25] and longer follow-up studies are needed to define the exact neoplastic risk of CIM.

The Z-line appearance (ZAP) classification has been developed to describe the endoscopic extent of Barrett's esophagus with particular reference to short segment Barrett's esophagus [26]. However, this system also uses a threshold of 3 cm to distinguish between grade II and III Barrett's esophagus making it insufficiently precise to document progression or regression of Barrett's esophagus. A new grading system called the Prague C and M criteria for the endoscopic extent of Barrett's esophagus has recently been put forth [17]. This classification proposes to use the length of circumferential Barrett's esophagus (C) as well as the maximal length (M) including the length of tongues to accurately describe the extent of Barrett's esophagus. This grading system may be useful in clinical practice as well as in multicenter research studies to follow the length of Barrett's esophagus over time in the same patient. Intial validation studies have shown good interobserver agreement using the Prague C and M criteria but they still need to be validated prospectively with respect to further interobserver agreement, clinical relevance and patient outcomes [17].

Histologic Diagnosis of Barrett's Esophagus: the Goblet Cell

The current working definition of Barrett's esophagus necessitates histologic confirmation of intestinal metaplasia on biopsies from the columnar lined esophagus. The "goblet cell" deserves special mention as it is the *sine qua non* for intestinal metaplasia. It is an integral part of the normal small intestinal mucosa and metaplasia in the setting of Barrett's esophagus and is responsible for the secretion of mucus into the gut lumen. On H&E staining, goblet cells have a distended lateral border, compressed basal nucleus and basophilic apical cytoplasm. Goblet cells have acid mucins and stain intensely with Alcian blue (at pH 2.5) [27–29], making it easy to distinguish them from the foveolar cells of gastric type mucosa which stain with periodic acid–Schiff (PAS) but not Alcian blue. The staining with Alcian blue is extremely useful in distinguishing the intestinal metaplasia from cardia mucosa as occasionally some of the gastric cardiac cells may look like goblet cells on routine hematoxylin and eosin (H&E) staining [30]. This may prevent overdiagnosis of Barrett's esophagus and avoid unnecessary enrollment of patients into a surveillance program. Occasionally, Alcian blue may stain the cytoplasm of foveolar cells that are called "columnar blues." However, the distinction from typical goblet cells is usually straightforward as the histology of these columnar blues is distinct from the goblet cells. Also, columnar blues are often seen in groups while goblet cells usually are seen as solitary cells amongst the columnar epithelium.

In summary, despite the usefulness of Alcian blue staining, this technique is laborious, time consuming, and more expensive than routine H&E staining, preventing its wider applicability. At this time, typically, Alcian blue is used if the routine H&E staining is not convincing enough to diagnose the presence of intestinal metaplasia.

Impact of Length on the Diagnosis of Barrett's Esophagus

It is important to understand that intestinal metaplasia is a patchy disease. First and foremost, the conventional method of four quadrant biopsies from short lengths of the columnar lined esophagus (<3 cm) provides a histologic confirmation of Barrett's esophagus in approximately 35–45% of the patients [31]. Intestinal metaplasia is more often found when the endoscopic Barrett's esophagus segment is >3 cm rather than <3 cm (80% vs. 30%) [32,33]. Secondly, repeat biopsies in these patients may increase the yield of intestinal metaplasia by almost 20% [34].

A prospective study of 177 patients enrolled in a surveillance program showed that the detection of intestinal metaplasia increased markedly with increasing number of surveillance endoscopies, particularly in short segments of columnar mucosa [35]. The cumulative percentage of intestinal metaplasia in endoscopic lengths 1–2 cm and 3–4 cm increased from 30.5% and 44.8% to 63.6% and 88.9% respectively after six endoscopies. Intestinal metaplasia was detected in all patients with greater than 4 cm of the endoscopic Barrett's esophagus segment after 2–4 endoscopies. This raises some very important questions, especially if we define Barrett's esophagus as the presence of intestinal metaplasia. Are biopsies on a single endoscopy sufficiently sensitive to rule out Barrett's esophagus in all patients? Do patients develop new intestinal metaplasia within the endoscopic segment during follow-up? In fact, the increasing yield of intestinal metaplasia on subsequent biopsies may be inferred to suggest that the endoscopic presence of columnar appearing mucosa cannot be ignored even in absence of intestinal metaplasia on biopsies. Some investigators have suggested that repeat endoscopy be considered in patients with endoscopic Barrett's esophagus if the initial biopsies are negative, especially in the short segment of suspected Barrett's esophagus. This may especially be relevant in light of data that dysplasia and adenocarcinoma can be associated with short segment Barrett's esophagus [21,22]. However, clear recommendations are lacking, and further research in this area is surely needed.

Molecular Markers for the Diagnosis of Intestinal Metaplasia (Barrett's Esophagus)

The intestinal columnar cell, the histological marker of Barrett's esophagus, shares a common lineage with the small intestinal epithelial cell. This may represent a novel method to diagnose Barrett's esophagus as the small intestinal columnar cell has some unique molecular signatures. The ability to identify these molecular markers characteristic for the intestinal cell type of Barrett's esophagus thus offers great promise, and given that intestinal metaplasia is patchy, these markers may confirm the presence of Barrett's esophagus on random biopsies.

Cdx-2 is a transcription factor whose expression in normal tissues is restricted to intestinal type epithelium. In a study of 90 patients with suspected short segment Barrett's esophagus, (45 with and 45 without intestinal metaplasia), all intestinal metaplasia (100%) cells stained for cdx-2 in the goblet cell and adjacent columnar cells while only 38% of columnar tissue without intestinal metaplasia stained for cdx-2 [36]. Moreover, none of the 25 samples of gastric cardiac mucosa (controls) and none of the "columnar blues" stained for cdx-2. This suggests that cdx-2 staining to detect cells of intestinal origin may allow for a more accurate diagnosis of Barrett's esophagus and, perhaps, a newer molecular classification of the columnar lined distal esophagus could be envisioned in the future.

Another study correlated the expression of cdx-2 and muc-2 (a type of acid mucin specific to the goblet cell) in patients suspected to have intestinal metaplasia in the esophagus [37]. They reported that all patients with histologic intestinal metaplasia had cdx-2 protein and mRNA expression as opposed to none of the 26 patients with gastric metaplasia and the 40 reflux esophagitis patients without Barrett's esophagus. Interestingly, cdx-2 mRNA was also detected in the squamous mucosa of 30% of the Barrett's esophagus patients suggesting that cdx-2 transcription may play a role in development of Barrett's esophagus. If this is shown to be the case, it may help identify GERD patients predisposed to the development of Barrett's esophagus in the future. The detection of cdx-2 mRNA also correlated with the expression of goblet cell specific Muc-2 mRNA in Barrett's esophagus patients. Another study also showed that MUC-2 was expressed in goblet cells and occasionally in columnar cells but not in cardiac type mucosa, also suggesting that MUC-2 expression could be a useful tool for the accurate detection of intestinal metaplasia [37].

Is it possible to distinguish intestinal metaplasia in the esophagus from that in the stomach? The use of cytokeratins 7 and 20 in initial studies showed that the pattern of CK7/CK20 immunoreactivity was found in both long and short segment Barrett's esophagus but not in CIM [38,39]. Barrett's esophagus was characterized by superficial and deep CK7 staining and superficial band like CK20 staining in the areas of intestinal metaplasia. However, other studies have yielded conflicting results [40–42]. More prospective studies are needed to define the exact role of these biomarkers for the diagnosis of Barrett's esophagus.

Diagnosis of Barrett's Esophagus: the Future

The cost associated with standard upper endoscopy is one of the major limiting factors in its application for the diagnosis of Barrett's esophagus. Newer techniques may help overcome this barrier.

One such technique to diagnose esophageal pathology is capsule endoscopy. A feasibility study from Israel [43] showed that in 17 patients (five with normal findings and 12 patients with erosive esophagitis on upper endoscopy), capsule endoscopy was able to identify all the 12 patients with esophageal pathology on upper endoscopy. Our center is currently involved in a prospective, double blind, multicenter study to correlate the findings on esophageal capsule studies to those on standard endoscopy.

Balloon cytology has been reported as a cost-effective method for the diagnosis and surveillance of Barrett's esophagus patients. Falk *et al.* compared balloon cytology with biopsies and brush cytology in patients with Barrett's esophagus [44]. They were able to obtain adequate columnar epithelium in 83% patients with balloon cytology in comparison with 97% with brush cytology. The costs associated with

balloon cytology were six times less than that of endoscopy, in part due to lack of sedation. Other results have not been as promising. In a study of 10 unselected patients with known Barrett's esophagus, balloon cytology was unable to identify goblet cells in any of the patients. This area needs further study before balloon cytology can be recommended for the diagnosis of Barrett's esophagus [45].

In summary, more research is needed to validate current methods and identify other techniques, non-invasive methods and serologic markers to diagnose Barrett's esophagus reliably and in a cost-effective manner.

Conclusion

Approximately, 10–15% of people with chronic GERD are diagnosed with Barrett's esophagus, a premalignant condition for esophageal and gastroesophageal adenocarcinoma. The diagnosis of Barrett's esophagus is based on a combination of endoscopic and histologic criteria. The displacement of SCJ proximal to the GEJ should raise the suspicion for Barrett's esophagus and lead to biopsies to confirm intestinal metaplasia. Barrett's esophagus has been classified into long and short segment based on the endoscopic extent. A new system called the Prague C and M criteria for the endoscopic diagnosis of Barrett's esophagus, if validated, may simplify the description of endoscopic findings of Barrett's esophagus both for clinical and research studies. The single most important histologic finding is the presence of goblet cells that confirms the presence of intestinal metaplasia. Special stains like Alcian blue, if used judiciously in conjunction with H&E staining may avoid the overdiagnosis of intestinal metaplasia. Intestinal metaplasia is a patchy lesion that may be missed on a single endoscopy and, although the yield of intestinal metaplasia increases on repeat endoscopies, the number of endoscopies a patient with should undergo to avoid false negative results is unclear. This problem may be overcome by application of newer techniques like magnification, chromoendoscopy, narrow band imaging, and optical coherence tomography to help focused biopsies from areas suspected to represent intestinal metaplasia. Application of molecular techniques to identify cdx-2, muc-2, sucrase-isomaltase etc., in biopsy specimens may increase the sensitivity of the diagnosis of Barrett's esophagus. In the future, newer methods like capsule endoscopy and balloon cytology may help screen for Barrett's esophagus in a cost-effective manner.

Acknowledgement

Supported by the Veterans Affairs Medical Center, Kansas City, MO.

References

1. Reid BJ. Barrett's esophagus and esophageal adenocarcinoma. *Gastroenterol Clin North Am* 1991;**20**(4):817–34.
2. Haggitt RC. Barrett's esophagus, dysplasia, and adenocarcinoma. *Hum Pathol* 1994;**25**(10):982–93.
3. Brown LM, Devesa SS. Epidemiologic trends in esophageal and gastric cancer in the United States. *Surg Oncol Clin N Am* 2002;**11**(2):235–56.
4. Devesa SS, Blot WJ, Fraumeni JF, Jr. Changing patterns in the incidence of esophageal and gastric carcinoma in the United States. *Cancer* 1998;**83**(10):2049–53.
5. Pera M, Cameron AJ, Trastek VF, Carpenter HA, Zinsmeister AR. Increasing incidence of adenocarcinoma of the esophagus and esophagogastric junction. *Gastroenterology* 1993;**104**(2):510–3.
6. Pohl H, Welch HG. The role of overdiagnosis and reclassification in the marked increase of esophageal adenocarcinoma incidence. *J Natl Cancer Inst* 2005;**97**(2):142–6.
7. Blot WJ, Devesa SS, Fraumeni JF, Jr. Continuing climb in rates of esophageal adenocarcinoma: an update. *JAMA* 1993;**270**(11):1320.
8. Sharma P, McQuaid K, Dent J *et al*. A critical review of the diagnosis and management of Barrett's esophagus: the AGA Chicago Workshop. *Gastroenterology* 2004;**127**(1):310–30.
9. Barrett NR. Chronic peptic ulcer of the oesophagus and 'oesophagitis'. *Br J Surg* 1950;**38**(150):175–82.
10. Paull A, Trier JS, Dalton MD *et al*. The histologic spectrum of Barrett's esophagus. *N Engl J Med* 1976;**295**(9):476–80.
11. Haggitt RC, Tryzelaar J, Ellis FH, Colcher H. Adenocarcinoma complicating columnar epithelium-lined (Barrett's) esophagus. *Am J Clin Pathol* 1978;**70**(1):1–5.
12. Hamilton SR, Smith RR. The relationship between columnar epithelial dysplasia and invasive adenocarcinoma arising in Barrett's esophagus. *Am J Clin Pathol* 1987;**87**(3):301–12.
13. Lee RG. Dysplasia in Barrett's esophagus. A clinicopathologic study of six patients. *Am J Surg Pathol* 1985;**9**(12):845–52.
14. Thompson JJ, Zinsser KR, Enterline HT. Barrett's metaplasia and adenocarcinoma of the esophagus and gastroesophageal junction. *Hum Pathol* 1983;**14**(1):42–61.
15. Skinner DB, Walther BC, Riddell RH *et al*. Barrett's esophagus. Comparison of benign and malignant cases. *Ann Surg* 1983;**198**(4):554–65.
16. Sharma P, Morales TG, Sampliner RE. Short segment Barrett's esophagus—the need for standardization of the definition and of endoscopic criteria. *Am J Gastroenterol* 1998;**93**(7):1033–6.
17. Armstrong D. Review article: towards consistency in the endoscopic diagnosis of Barrett's oesophagus and columnar metaplasia. *Aliment Pharmacol Ther* 2004;**20**(suppl 5):40–7; discussion 61–2.
18. Eloubeidi MA, Provenzale D. Does this patient have Barrett's esophagus? The utility of predicting Barrett's esophagus at the index endoscopy. *Am J Gastroenterol* 1999;**94**(4):937–43.
19. Sharma P, Weston AP, Morales T *et al*. Relative risk of dysplasia for patients with intestinal metaplasia in the distal oesophagus and in the gastric cardia. *Gut* 2000;**46**(1):9–13.
20. Hayward J. The lower end of the oesophagus. *Thorax* 1961;**16**:36–41.
21. Hirota WK, Loughney TM, Lazas DJ *et al*. Specialized intestinal metaplasia, dysplasia, and cancer of the esophagus and esophagogastric junction: prevalence and clinical data. *Gastroenterology* 1999;**116**(2):277–85.
22. Schnell TG, Sontag SJ, Chejfec G. Adenocarcinomas arising in tongues or short segments of Barrett's esophagus. *Dig Dis Sci* 1992;**37**(1):137–43.
23. Rudolph RE, Vaughan TL, Storer BE *et al*. Effect of segment length on risk for neoplastic progression in patients with Barrett esophagus. *Ann Intern Med* 2000;**132**(8):612–20.
24. Cameron AJ, Souto EO, Smyrk TC. Small adenocarcinomas of the esophagogastric junction: association with intestinal metaplasia and dysplasia. *Am J Gastroenterol* 2002;**97**(6):1375–80.
25. Pera M. Trends in incidence and prevalence of specialized intestinal metaplasia, barrett's esophagus, and adenocarcinoma of the gastroesophageal junction. *World J Surg* 2003;**27**(9):999–1008; discussion 1006–8.
26. Wallner B, Sylvan A, Stenling R, Janunger KG. The esophageal Z-line appearance correlates to the preva-

lence of intestinal metaplasia. *Scand J Gastroenterol* 2000;**35**(1):17–22.

27. Peuchmaur M, Potet F, Goldfain D. Mucin histochemistry of the columnar epithelium of the oesophagus (Barrett's oesophagus): a prospective biopsy study. *J Clin Pathol* 1984;**37**(6):607–10.

28. Lee RG. Mucins in Barrett's esophagus: a histochemical study. *Am J Clin Pathol* 1984;**81**(4):500–3.

29. Jass JR. Mucin histochemistry of the columnar epithelium of the oesophagus: a retrospective study. *J Clin Pathol* 1981;**34**(8):866–70.

30. Weinstein WM, Ippoliti AF. The diagnosis of Barrett's esophagus: goblets, goblets, goblets. *Gastrointest Endosc* 1996;**44**(1):91–5.

31. Kim SL, Waring JP, Spechler SJ *et al*. Diagnostic inconsistencies in Barrett's esophagus. Department of Veterans Affairs Gastroesophageal Reflux Study Group. *Gastroenterology* 1994;**107**(4):945–9.

32. Spechler SJ, Zeroogian JM, Antonioli DA, Wang HH, Goyal RK. Prevalence of metaplasia at the gastro-oesophageal junction. *Lancet* 1994;**344**(8936):1533–6.

33. Iftikhar SY, James PD, Steele RJ, Hardcastle JD, Atkinson M. Length of Barrett's oesophagus: an important factor in the development of dysplasia and adenocarcinoma. *Gut* 1992;**33**(9):1155–8.

34. Jones TF, Sharma P, Daaboul B *et al*. Yield of intestinal metaplasia in patients with suspected short-segment Barrett's esophagus (SSBE) on repeat endoscopy. *Dig Dis Sci* 2002;**47**(9):2108–11.

35. Oberg S, Johansson J, Wenner J *et al*. Endoscopic surveillance of columnar-lined esophagus: frequency of intestinal metaplasia detection and impact of antireflux surgery. *Ann Surg* 2001;**234**(5):619–26.

36. Groisman GM, Amar M, Meir A. Expression of the intestinal marker Cdx2 in the columnar-lined esophagus with and without intestinal (Barrett's) metaplasia. *Mod Pathol* 2004;**17**(10):1282–8.

37. Lopes CV, Pereira-Lima JC, Hartmann AA. Correlation between Alcian blue-periodic acid-Schiff stain and immunohistochemical expression of mucin 2 in Barrett's oesophagus. *Histopathology* 2004;**45**(2):198–9.

38. Couvelard A, Cauvin JM, Goldfain D *et al*. Cytokeratin immunoreactivity of intestinal metaplasia at normal oesophagogastric junction indicates its aetiology. *Gut* 2001;**49**(6):761–6.

39. Ormsby AH, Vaezi MF, Richter JE *et al*. Cytokeratin immunoreactivity patterns in the diagnosis of short-segment Barrett's esophagus. *Gastroenterology* 2000;**119**(3):683–90.

40. El-Zimaity HM, Graham DY. Cytokeratin subsets for distinguishing Barrett's esophagus from intestinal metaplasia in the cardia using endoscopic biopsy specimens. *Am J Gastroenterol* 2001;**96**(5):1378–82.

41. Glickman JN, Wang H, Das KM *et al*. Phenotype of Barrett's esophagus and intestinal metaplasia of the distal esophagus and gastroesophageal junction: an immunohistochemical study of cytokeratins 7 and 20, Das-1 and 45 MI. *Am J Surg Pathol* 2001;**25**(1):87–94.

42. Mohammed IA, Streutker CJ, Riddell RH. Utilization of cytokeratins 7 and 20 does not differentiate between Barrett's esophagus and gastric cardiac intestinal metaplasia. *Mod Pathol* 2002;**15**(6):611–6.

43. Eliakim R, Yassin K, Shlomi I, Suissa A, Eisen GM. A novel diagnostic tool for detecting oesophageal pathology: the PillCam oesophageal video capsule. *Aliment Pharmacol Ther* 2004;**20**(10):1083–9.

44. Falk GW, Chittajallu R, Goldblum JR *et al*. Surveillance of patients with Barrett's esophagus for dysplasia and cancer with balloon cytology. *Gastroenterology* 1997;**112**(6):1787–97.

45. Fennerty MB, DiTomasso J, Morales TG *et al*. Screening for Barrett's esophagus by balloon cytology. *Am J Gastroenterol* 1995;**90**(8):1230–2.

CHAPTER 2

The Epidemiology and Prevalence of Barrett's Esophagus

Alan J. Cameron

Historical Background

Norman Barrett, a London thoracic surgeon, wrote a paper in 1950 entitled "Chronic peptic ulcer of the oesophagus and 'oesophagitis' [1]." He described cases of esophageal ulcers found at autopsy that were surrounded by columnar mucosa. Most had died from ulcer perforation. One case that Barrett reviewed had been reported by Alexander Lyall in 1937, possibly the first case recognized. Barrett suggested that the ulcers developed in the stomach which was displaced upward, due to a congenital short esophagus, and that this was a separate entity from reflux esophagitis. In 1953 Allison and Johnstone published a paper entitled "Oesophagus lined with gastric mucous membrane" [2]. They described in detail seven cases in whom the lower esophagus had a columnar lining. All seven had reflux esophagitis and a hiatal hernia. They suggested that "Barrett's ulcers" might be a consequence of chronic gastroesophageal reflux. Present opinion agrees with the views of Allison and Johnson that "Barrett's esophagus" is an acquired disorder caused by reflux.

Definition of Barrett's Esophagus

The changing definition of Barrett's esophagus over the years needs to be taken into account in a review of epidemiology. In 2002, the Practice Parameters Committee of the American College of Gastroenterology recommended that Barrett's esophagus be defined as "a change in the esophageal epithelium of any length that can be recognized at endoscopy and is confirmed to have intestinal metaplasia by biopsy of the tubular esophagus and excludes intestinal metaplasia of the cardia" [3]. This definition has evolved over some 30 years from columnar lining in the esophagus, to 3 cm or more of columnar lining, to 3 cm or more with esophageal intestinal metaplasia, to intestinal metaplasia in the esophagus without regard to length. The earlier requirement of 3 cm or more of columnar epithelium was often used because it was quite easily recognized as distinct from an irregular but normal squamocolumnar junction. At the present time, short segment Barrett's esophagus is diagnosed when there is visible red columnar epithelium in the esophagus less than 3 cm in length, with intestinal metaplasia. However, there is difficulty in the diagnosis of short segment Barrett's esophagus. One reason is overlap with intestinal metaplasia of the cardia. Biopsies taken below a normally located squamocolumnar junction show intestinal metaplasia in about 15% of patients having endoscopy [4,5]. On the other hand, an endoscopic suspicion of short segment Barrett's esophagus is confirmed by finding intestinal metaplasia on biopsy in only 36–50% of cases [6,7]. It is just not possible on routine endoscopy to distinguish reliably between a 1 or 2 cm length of Barrett's esophagus and a normal variation of the Z line. However, in the writer's experience, when a long segment of Barrett's esophagus is clearly identified at endoscopy, biopsy shows intestinal metaplasia in at least 95% of cases. In this epidemiologic review, therefore, Barrett's esophagus will generally refer to long segments of columnar epithelium in the lower esophagus.

Prevalence of Long Segment Barrett's Esophagus

Prevalence and incidence are sometimes confused in medical writing. Prevalence refers to the proportion of a given population having a particular condition at a specified time. Incidence refers to the proportion of a population developing a condition over a specified time interval, often 1 year.

Barrett's esophagus was rarely found before the widespread and increasing use of flexible endoscopy in the last few decades. In 1971 Burgess *et al.* reported 85 Mayo Clinic patients with this diagnosis between 1950 and 1969, about four cases per year [8]. In 1972, Naef and Savary reported the largest series up to that time, finding 62 cases of Barrett's esophagus in 4950 esophagoscopies they performed in Switzerland 1963–1971 [9]. In that era, most endoscopic examinations were done with rigid endoscopes.

Prevalence at Endoscopy

Many reports have used retrospective data from patients having routine clinical upper endoscopy. Table 2.1 shows the results for long segment Barrett's esophagus in nine large series from Western countries [9–17]. Note that many patients in these series did not have biopsy confirmation. In the studies summarized in Table 2.1, a mean of 1.5% of patients having endoscopy had Barrett's esophagus. This only approximates the true population prevalence of the condition. Endoscopy is performed for multiple

different indications, although most patients are investigated for symptoms other than reflux. Indications for endoscopy vary with time and geographic location. Patients having endoscopy are, on average, older than the general population. At endoscopy, under-diagnosis of Barrett's esophagus can occur due to lack of recognition of the disorder, and also over-diagnosis due to enthusiasm and lack of biopsy confirmation. Of note, the data in the above table does not suggest much change in the endoscopy prevalence of Barrett's esophagus over the past 30 years.

Prevalence in Persons with Reflux Symptoms

Most patients with Barrett's esophagus have symptoms of GERD, especially heartburn and acid regurgitation. In 1991, Philips and Wong reviewed reports of patients having routine clinical endoscopy for reflux disease [18]. Summarizing the findings in 14 papers, a total of 31 133 patients had endoscopy, of which 5385 (17%) had GERD. Barrett's esophagus was found in 1.7% of all patients having endoscopy and in 9.6% of patients with GERD. These older reports included large numbers but were retrospective. Later, prospective studies were performed.

Winters *et al.* investigated 97 patients with at least two of the three following symptoms; heartburn, regurgitation or dysphagia, occurring at least every week [19]. Those with previous endoscopy were excluded. Twelve of the 97 (12%) had Barrett's esophagus. However, only six (6%) had intestinal

Table 2.1 Prevalence of Barrett's esophagus (BE) in patients at routine clinical endoscopy.

Authors	Patients (*n*)	BE (*n*)	BE (%)
Naef & Savary 1972 [9]	6368	140	2.2
Burbidge & Radigan 1979 [10]	203	8	3.9
Cooper & Barbezat 1987 [11]	4448	52	1.2
Gruppo (Italian multicenter) 1991 [12]	14898	111	0.7
Cameron & Lomboy 1992 [13]	51311	57	0.9
Hirota *et al.* 1999 [14]	889	40	4.5
Caygill *et al.* 1999 [15]	44721	636	1.4
Todd *et al.* 2002 (1995 data) [16]	9620	139	1.4
Ford *et al.* 2004 (Whites) [17]	15063	690	4.6
Total	147521	2273	1.5

metaplasia on biopsy, and the diagnosis might be questioned without this histological finding. Also, the patients were at a naval hospital, so presumably most were male. The prevalence of Barrett's esophagus is higher in men.

Mann *et al.* examined 180 male patients with reflux symptoms [20]. Biopsies were taken 2 and 4 cm above the lower esophageal sphincter. Twelve patients (6.7%) had long segment Barrett's esophagus with intestinal metaplasia.

We investigated 200 male and female patients with reflux symptoms occurring at least every week, with no previous endoscopy [21]. A 3 cm or longer Barrett's esophagus, with intestinal metaplasia, was found in seven cases (3.5%). In a further prospective series from our group [22,23], we found a long segment Barrett's esophagus in 12 of 287 (4.2%) consecutive male and female patients with reflux symptoms.

The estimated prevalence of long segment Barrett's esophagus is therefore approximately 5% in patients with reflux symptoms, the number being higher in men and lower in women.

Age and Prevalence

Overall figures for the prevalence of Barrett's esophagus do not take into account the considerable variations with age and gender. A strong piece of evidence for Barrett's esophagus being an acquired disorder is the increasing incidence with age. In two endoscopic series, the prevalence of Barrett's esophagus at different ages was recorded [12,13]. The numerator was the number of patients with Barrett's esophagus in a particular age group, the denominator being the total number of patients in that age group having endoscopy for any indication. In the Italian multicenter study the prevalence of Barrett's esophagus rose progressively from age 30 to 70 years [12]. In our Mayo Clinic report, we had information on all ages from childhood to old age [13]. We found a very low prevalence in children, after which the prevalence rose fairly steadily with increasing age to reach about 1% after age 60 years (Fig. 2.1 [24]). In a more recent study, we again found the prevalence of Barrett's esophagus increasing with age from 20 to over 70 years [23]. We found that 50% of the maximum prevalence was reached about age 40 years, representing the median age of developing Barrett's esophagus [13]. However, the mean age of diagnosing Barrett's esophagus was 63 years [13]. We suggested that, on average, a newly diagnosed Barrett's esophagus had actually been present but undetected for over 20 years.

Barrett's Esophagus in Children

Although rare, Barrett's esophagus may occur in children. In our endoscopic series, we found Barrett's esophagus in none of 176 patients aged 0–9 years and in 1 of 679 patients aged 10–19 years [13]. El-Serag *et al.* reported 402 children, mean age 9.7

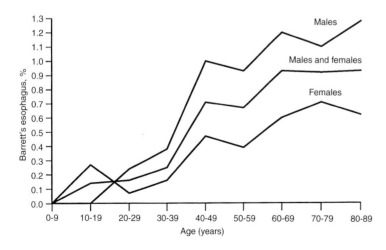

Fig. 2.1 The prevalence of Barrett's esophagus in patients having clinically indicated endoscopy. Prevalence increases with age. Half the maximum prevalence is reached about age 40 years. The male to female ratio was 2 : 1. Reproduced with permission from Cameron [24].

years, who had endoscopy for reflux disease [25]. Erosive esophagitis was found in 35%, but no case of biopsy proven Barrett's esophagus was found. In a literature review, Hassall found 36 reported cases of Barrett's esophagus in six series with biopsy proven intestinal metaplasia in children or young adults [26]. He concluded that Barrett's esophagus was much rarer in children than in adults. The youngest proven case was at age 7 years. The evidence reviewed by Hassall indicated that even in childhood the condition was acquired and associated with gastroesophageal reflux.

Gender

The prevalence of Barrett's esophagus is higher in men than in women. In the Italian multicenter study, Barrett's esophagus was found in 1.0 % of men versus 0.39% of women endoscoped, a ratio of 2.6 : 1.0 [12]. Likewise, at the Mayo Clinic, Barrett's esophagus was found in 0.97% of men and in 0.49% of women having endoscopy (see Fig. 2.1), a ratio of 2.0 : 1.0 [13]. A later report of 44 721 endoscopies showed 636 Barrett's esophagus, with a male to female ratio of 1.7 : 1.0 [15]. It is of interest to note that male predominance for adenocarcinoma of 3 : 1 in the UK [27] and 8 : 1 in US Whites [28] is even greater than the approximately 2 : 1 male predominance for Barrett's esophagus. The causes of the increased prevalence of Barrett's esophagus and adenocarcinoma in men are unknown.

Severity and Duration of Reflux Symptoms

Barrett's esophagus is found more often in patients with symptoms of esophageal reflux than in those without such symptoms. However, the severity of reflux symptoms has not proved helpful in distinguishing between patients with uncomplicated reflux esophagitis and those with Barrett's esophagus. The length of reflux symptoms may be more discriminating. Winters *et al.* found the mean duration of symptoms to be 15 years in Barrett's esophagus, not significantly different from 13.5 years in those found to have reflux esophagitis, both groups being longer than the mean 8.8 years in those with non-erosive reflux disease [19]. Lieberman *et al.* studied patients

having endoscopy for reflux symptoms [29]. Compared to patients with reflux symptoms for less than 1 year, the odds ratio for Barrett's esophagus in patients with symptoms for over 10 years was 6.4. In 1999 Hirota *et al.* found the mean duration of reflux symptoms to be 3.5 years in patients without long segment and 20 years in those with long segment Barrett's esophagus [14].

Barrett's Esophagus without Reflux Symptoms

If an estimated 5% of patients with reflux symptoms and 1.5% of all patients having endoscopy have Barrett's esophagus, then clearly the condition is found more often in symptomatic people. However, Barrett's esophagus may occur in patients with no history of heartburn or acid regurgitation. In a prospective Italian multicenter study of 14 98 patients having routine endoscopy, Barrett's esophagus was found in 8% of those with heartburn, 25 times the prevalence of 0.32% in those without heartburn [12]. In this report, 40% of subjects with Barrett's esophagus did not have reflux symptoms, being endoscoped for other indications. In patients with adenocarcinoma and Barrett's esophagus found simultaneously [30–32], only some 60% gave a reflux history preceding the onset of cancer-related symptoms. These results also showed that about 40% of subjects with Barrett's esophagus in the population do not have reflux symptoms. It follows that any proposal to screen people with reflux symptoms in the general population for cancer prevention by early detection of Barrett's esophagus would miss 40% of cases.

In two more recent studies, upper endoscopic screening for Barrett's esophagus was performed in subjects scheduled for lower gastrointestinal endoscopy. Gerson and Shetler reported long segment Barrett's esophagus in 7% and short segment Barrett's esophagus in 17% of 110 essentially asymptomatic subjects [33]. These frequency levels seem incongruent with other reports and clinical observations. In a similar study design, Rex *et al.* found long segment Barrett's esophagus in only 0.36% and short segment Barrett's esophagus in 5% of 556 subjects with no history of heartburn [34]. In 384 patients with a history of any heartburn, Rex *et al.*

found long segment Barrett's esophagus in 2.6% and short segment Barrett's esophagus in 6%. Thus, in this report, long segment Barrett's esophagus was seven times more prevalent in those with versus those without heartburn. In both these reports, short segment Barrett's esophagus was more prevalent than long segment Barrett's esophagus.

Race and Geographic Differences

The best available data regards the prevalence of Barrett's esophagus in patients having routine upper endoscopy for all indications. As noted previously (see Table 2.1), series from the USA, Western Europe, and Australasia showed long segment Barrett's esophagus in a mean of 1.5% of patients having endoscopy. Table 2.2 shows data for long segment Barrett's esophagus from non-Western countries [35–40]. Barrett's esophagus was found in comparable prevalence to the West in Iran and Turkey, but was rare in Oriental countries. Geographic variations in prevalence could be due to genetic differences between racial groups, or to environmental differences such as diet. It is therefore interesting to look at the prevalence of Barrett's esophagus in different racial groups living in the same country, who may share a more similar environment. For example, Mason and Bremner reported from South Africa that only 5% of their Barrett's esophagus patients were Black, in a city with an 80% Black population [41]. Table 2.3 shows data on the prevalence of long segment Barrett's esophagus in different racial groups examined in the same endoscopy units [14,17,37]. The data in Table 2.3 indicates that the low prevalence of Bar-

rett's esophagus in Blacks and Asians is maintained when they live in Western countries. The relative contribution of genes versus environment causing these racial differences is not known.

Barrett's esophagus is a consequence of gastroesophageal reflux. Although data are limited, a literature review showed that, as well as Barrett's esophagus, the community prevalence of reflux symptoms and the endoscopic prevalence of esophagitis were lower in Asian and Afro-Caribbean subjects than in Whites [42]. More prevalent reflux disease in Whites may account for their higher prevalence of Barrett's esophagus. One likely cause for increased reflux disease in Western countries is their greater dietary calorie and fat intake per capita [43], with associated obesity. For example, population energy intake per capita in 1998 was 2800 kcal/day in Japan, versus 3800 kcal/day in the USA. Another possible cause of increasing reflux disease and its complications is a declining prevalence of *Helicobacter pylori* infection.

Population Prevalence of Barrett's Esophagus

Gastroesophageal reflux symptoms are common in the general population. In the USA and Western Europe, about one in five adults have symptoms at least once weekly [44–47]. Assuming about one in 20 persons with weekly reflux have Barrett's esophagus, one can estimate that about one in 100 of the general population has Barrett's esophagus, an underestimate because some cases are asymptomatic. Allowing for 40% of cases being without reflux

Table 2.2 Prevalence of Barrett's esophagus (BE) at endoscopy in non-Western countries.

Authors	Country	Patients (*n*)	BE (*n*)	BE (%)
Nasseri-Moghaddam *et al.* 2003 [35]	Iran	269	10	3.70
Toruner *et al.* 2004 [36]	Turkey	395	7	1.50
Rajendra *et al.* 2004 [37]	Malaysia	985	32	1.60
Lee *et al.* 2003 [38]	Korea	1553	5	0.30
Azuma *et al.* 2000 [39]	Japan	650	4	0.60
Wong *et al.* 2002 [40]	China	16606	3	0.02

Table 2.3 Prevalence of Barrett's esophagus (BE) in patients of different racial groups examined in the same endoscopy units.

Authors	Country	Race	n	BE (n)	BE (%)
Hirota et al. 1999 [14]	USA	White	611	40	6.5
		Black	200	0	0.0
Rajendra et al. 2004 [37]	Malaysia	Malays	502	7	1.4
		Chinese	824	10	1.2
		Indians	659	15	2.3
Ford et al. 2004 [17]	UK	White	15 063	690	4.6
		Asian	5 297	45	0.8

symptoms, this estimate is similar to the 1.5% of all patients having endoscopy, for any indication, that have Barrett's esophagus.

We did an autopsy study to obtain a more direct measurement of the population prevalence of Barrett's esophagus [48]. Over 18 months, the esophagus at consecutive Mayo Clinic autopsies was examined by a gastroenterologist. In 733 autopsies, mean age 73 years, seven Barrett's esophagus cases were found, again approximately 1% of the total. There were four Barrett's esophagus cases in 226 cases in residents of Olmsted County. After adjusting for age and sex to correspond to the general population, the estimated prevalence of Barrett's esophagus in Olmsted was 376/100 000. In another study [49], no long segment Barrett's esophagus was found in 223 autopsies; two cases had short segment Barrett's esophagus. In summary, approximately 1.5% of older (over 60 years) persons in the general population has Barrett's esophagus.

Population Prevalence of Clinically Diagnosed Barrett's Esophagus

A distinction must be made between the true prevalence in the general population and the prevalence of clinically diagnosed cases, which is quite different.

Most esophageal adenocarcinomas can be shown to arise in Barrett's esophagus, if surgical resection specimens are carefully examined [50,51]. Following shrinkage of primary tumor with preoperative chemotherapy, Theisen et al. found Barrett mucosa in association with 97% of distal esophageal adenocarcinomas [52]. However, in most patients with

adenocarcinoma, the Barrett's esophagus is first recognized when the patient presents with tumor-related symptoms. Corley et al. found that only 5% of 333 esophageal adenocarcinomas had a Barrett's esophagus diagnosed more than 6 months before the cancer [53]. Dulai et al. reported that only 4.7% of 1503 patients undergoing resection for adenocarcinoma had a prior diagnosis of Barrett's esophagus [54]. It is probable that most of these cases had a Barrett's esophagus that would have remained undetected if cancer had not developed.

There is other evidence indicating that most cases of Barrett's esophagus in the population have not been diagnosed. We reported a population-based comparison of autopsy and clinically diagnosed prevalence of Barrett's esophagus in 1990 [48]. The Mayo Clinic is located in Olmsted County, Minnesota, and our medical record system allowed us to review records on essentially all residents of this county for research purposes. Clinically diagnosed cases were those with a previous endoscopy showing a 3 cm or longer Barrett's esophagus, and were still living in the county in January 1987. The age and sex adjusted prevalence was 22.6/100 000. The autopsy estimate, as discussed above, was 376/100 000, about 16 times greater. We concluded that most cases of Barrett's esophagus in the population had not been diagnosed. We repeated the clinically diagnosed Olmsted study [55]. In 1998, the prevalence of clinically diagnosed Barrett's esophagus was 82.6/100 000 in the county. We did not repeat the autopsy study, but if we assume that the true population prevalence is the same as 11 years earlier, we had now detected about one in five cases of Barrett's esophagus in our county. Clearly, most cases of Barrett's esophagus in the population remain undiagnosed, although more are being found with the increased use of endoscopy. The implication is that surveillance and treatment of early malignancy in presently known cases of Barrett's esophagus will have only a small impact on the population death rate from esophageal adenocarcinoma.

Is the True Prevalence of Barrett's Esophagus Changing?

The incidence of adenocarcinoma of the esophagus has increased greatly in the last few decades [27,56,57]. Barrett's esophagus is the principal precursor lesion, found in 60–90% of cases of adenocarcinoma [50–52]. More cases of Barrett's esophagus are now being diagnosed than 40–50 years ago.

Mayo population-based data from Olmsted County, Minnesota [55] showed a 28-fold increase in clinically diagnosed Barrett's esophagus (new cases) from 0.37/100000 in 1965–1969 to 10.5/100000 population in 1995–1997. Over the same time interval, the number of gastroscopic examinations per 100000 population increased 22-fold. We suggested that the increase in diagnosed cases was mostly due to increased use of endoscopy. Caygill et al. reviewed 44721 endoscopies at a single UK hospital; 636 had Barrett's esophagus [15]. The proportion of endoscopic examinations that showed a new case of Barrett's esophagus rose steadily from 0.2% of 6500 in 1977–1981 to 1.6% of 16500 in 1992–1996. The authors concluded that the increase might be due to an increasing real incidence, or to increased recognition of the disease by endoscopists, or to both. Todd et al., in Scotland, also used a large endoscopic database to determine the diagnosis rate of Barrett's esophagus (>3 cm) in patients having routine upper endoscopy [16]. New diagnosis of Barrett's esophagus rose from 0.08/100 endoscopies in 1980 to 1.45/100 in 1995, an 18-fold increase. The authors concluded that some of this increase, especially a rapid eightfold increase between 1987 and 1989, may have been due to increased awareness of the condition by endoscopists. A real increase in the incidence of Barrett's esophagus was also proposed.

Older reports show that Barrett's esophagus could be found if looked for. Allison and Johnstone reviewed the records of the Thoracic Surgical Department at Leeds, England, 1950–1953 [2]. Rigid endoscopy showed that 11 (9.6%) of 115 patients with esophageal stricture had Barrett's esophagus with a columnar lined segment of esophagus below the stricture but above the hiatal hernia. In another early paper, Naef and Savary in Switzerland reported on 4950 endoscopies 1963–1971; 62 patients (1.25%) had Barrett's esophagus [9]. This proportion is similar to series reported 25–30 years later, as seen in Table 2.1.

The author interprets the data to show that the real population prevalence of Barrett's esophagus may not have greatly increased past 40–50 years, and that greater recognition of the condition and more extensive use of endoscopy can explain most of the increased detection of new cases in recent years.

There is no epidemiologic data on Barrett's esophagus prior to the first description by Barrett in 1950 [1]. However, most esophageal adenocarcinomas arise in Barrett's esophagus, and the incidence of this cancer has greatly increased in the past 30–40 years, so it is very possible that the prevalence of Barrett's esophagus was lower earlier in the 20th century. It will be interesting to see in future, whether adoption of a more Western diet and lifestyle in non-Western countries is associated with an increasing prevalence of Barrett's esophagus.

Genetic and Familial Aspects

There are many reports of families with multiple relatives in successive generations having Barrett's esophagus, as illustrated in Fig. 2.2 [58–60]. Other members of these families had reflux disease without Barrett's esophagus, and an autosomal dominant liability to reflux, predisposing to Barrett's esophagus, was proposed.

Twin studies provide evidence for a genetic component in the causation of reflux disease. In two studies, concordance for reflux symptoms was greater for monozygotic than for dizygotic twins. Cameron et al. reported 8401 Swedish twin pairs age 55 years or older [61]. Heritability accounted for an estimated 31% of the liability to reflux. Mohammed et al. reported 1960 twin pairs in the UK,

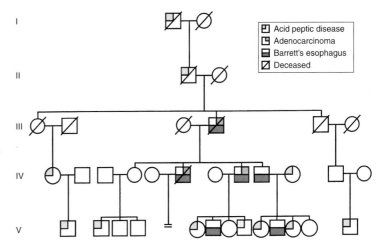

Fig. 2.2 Familial Barrett's esophagus. Six members of this family had Barrett's esophagus, three with esophageal adenocarcinoma. Other relatives had acid peptic (reflux) disease. An autosomal dominant inheritance of reflux in this family was proposed. Reproduced with permission from Jochem *et al.* [59].

mostly women [62]. It was estimated that additive genetic factors accounted for 43% of the liability to reflux. These twin studies did not address Barrett's esophagus.

We and Trudgill *et al.* used questionnaires to investigate symptoms in the first-degree relatives of consecutive patients with Barrett's esophagus [63,64]. Compared to matched controls, the Barrett's esophagus relatives had a 2.2 [63] to 4.8 [64] times increased risk for weekly or more frequent reflux symptoms. Our group then did endoscopy in symptomatic relatives of patients with Barrett's esophagus and in unrelated controls with similar reflux symptoms. [65,66]. We found long segment Barrett's esophagus in 8.4% of 191 symptomatic relatives, significantly more than in 4.2% of 287 symptomatic controls. Barrett's esophagus was rare in asymptomatic individuals.

These findings indicate that genetic factors contribute to the development of reflux disease, and also contribute to the progression from reflux disease to Barrett's esophagus. Studies to identify the genes involved are currently in progress.

Lifestyle Factors

As noted above, genes are partly responsible for the development of reflux disease and Barrett's esophagus, but cannot account for all; environmental factors are also important. Limited information on this is available. In a case-control study, Caygill *et al.* com-

pared 101 patients with Barrett's esophagus with an equal number with reflux esophagitis [67]. Obesity and smoking showed no difference between groups; alcohol use was about twice as common in the Barrett's esophagus group, but this did not reach statistical significance. Conio *et al.* used a questionnaire in 109 short segment Barrett's esophagus and 40 long segment Barrett's esophagus cases, and controls [68]. No significant difference was found for smoking, alcohol use, or coffee intake between the groups.

Short Segment Barrett's Esophagus

The above discussion relates to long segment Barrett' esophagus. In other cases red columnar epithelium extends into the lower esophagus in circumferential or tongue-like extensions less than 3 cm in length, with goblet cell metaplasia on biopsy. This is short segment Barrett's esophagus. It is a significant lesion, because adenocarcinomas may arise in short segment Barrett's esophagus [69]. In consecutive patients having endoscopy, the reported prevalence of short segment Barrett's esophagus varied, being 2.3% [70], 6.0% [14] and 8% [71] in three series. In our Mayo Olmsted County population-based study in progress, we found no cases until 1985. Before that time the diagnosis of short segment Barrett's esophagus was not recorded in our diagnostic index. By 1995–1997, the incidence of finding short segment Barrett's esophagus was 8.8/100 000, similar to the 10.5/100 000 person-years for new cases of long segment Barrett's esophagus. It is assumed that, as for long segments, most cases of short segment Barrett's esophagus in the population are not currently identified. The diagnosis of short segment Barrett's esophagus is often imprecise. Intestinal metaplasia of the cardia without short segment Barrett's esophagus is common [70,72] and it is often impossible at endoscopy to decide whether upward extensions of the Z line are normal variants or short segment Barrett's esophagus. In a prospective study, 112 patients were thought to have short segment Barrett's esophagus, mean length 2.1 cm, at endoscopy [6]. All had biopsies of the columnar appearing mucosa, but only 36% had histologic confirmation of intestinal metaplasia. These problems are further discussed in reviews [7,73].

Acknowledgements

The author acknowledges support from the Mayo General Clinical Research Center grant # RR-00585.

References

1. Barrett NR. Chronic peptic ulcer of the oesophagus and 'oesophagitis'. *Brit J Surg* 1950;**38**:175–82.
2. Allison PR, Johnstone AS. Oesophagus lined with gastric mucous membrane. *Thorax* 1953;**8**:87–101.
3. Sampliner RE and The Practice Parameters Committee of the American College of Gastroenterology. Updated guidelines for the diagnosis, surveillance, and therapy of Barrett's esophagus. *Amer J Gastroenterol* 2002;**97**:1888–95.
4. Spechler SJ, Zeroogian JM, Antonioli DA *et al.* Prevalence of metaplasia at the gastro-oesophageal junction. *Lancet* 1994;**344**:1533–6.
5. Morales TG, Sampliner RE, Bhattacharyya A. Intestinal metaplasia of the gastric cardia. *Amer J Gastroenterol* 1997;**92**:414–8.
6. Weinstein WM, Leh W, Lewin K *et al.* How often is short segment Barrett's esophagus proven histologically? A prospective study. *Gastroenterology* 2002;**122**(suppl 1):A293.
7. Sharma S, Morales TG, Sampliner S. Short segment Barrett's esophagus—the need for standardization of the definition and of endoscopic criteria. *Amer J Gastroenterol* 1998;**93**:1033–6.
8. Burgess JN, Payne WS, Andersen HA, Weiland LH, Carlson HC. Barrett esophagus. The columnar-epithelial lined esophagus. *Mayo Clin Proc* 1971;**46**: 728–34.
9. Naef AP, Savary M. Conservative operations for peptic esophagitis with stenosis in columnar-lined lower esophagus. *Ann Thoracic Surg* 1972;**13**:543–51.
10. Burbidge E, Radigan JJ. Characteristics of the columnar-lined (Barrett's) esophagus. *Gastroint Endosc* 1979;**25**:133–6.
11. Cooper BT, Barbezat GO. Barrett's esophagus: a clinical study of 52 patients. *Quart J Med* 1987;**62**:97–108.
12. Gruppo Operativo per lo studio delle precancerosi dell esophago (GOSPE). Barrett's esophagus: epidemiological and clinical results of a multicentric survey. *Int J Cancer* 1991;**48**:364–8.
13. Cameron AJ, Lomboy CT. Barrett's esophagus: age, prevalence and the extent of columnar epithelium. *Gastroenterology* 1992;**103**:1241–5.
14. Hirota WK, Loughney TM, Lazas DJ *et al.* Specialized intestinal metaplasia, dysplasia and cancer of the esophagus and esophagogastric junction: prevalence and clinical data. *Gastroenterology* 1999;**116**:277–85.
15. Caygill CPJ, Reed PI, Johnston BJ *et al.* A single center's 20-year experience of columnar-lined (Barrett's) oesophagus diagnosis. *Eur J Gastroenterol Hepatol* 1999;**11**:1355–8.
16. Todd JA, Johnston DA, Dillon JF. The changing spectrum of gastroesophageal reflux disease. *Eur J Cancer Prev* 2002;**11**:215–9.
17. Ford AC, Reynolds PD, Forman D, Cooper B, Moayyedi P. A retrospective case control study to determine the risk of Barrett's esophagus according to ethnic origin. *Gut* 2004;**53**(suppl 1):A26.
18. Philips RW, Wong RKH. Barrett's esophagus: natural history, incidence, etiology, and complications. *Gastroenterol Clin N Amer* 1991;**20**:791–816.
19. Winters C, Spurling TJ, Chobanian SJ *et al.* Barrett's esophagus. A prevalent, occult complication of gastroesophageal reflux disease. *Gastroenterology* 1987;**92**:118–24.
20. Mann NS, Tsai MF, Nair PK. Barrett's esophagus in patients with symptomatic reflux esophagitis. *Am J Gastroenterol* 1989;**84**:1494–6.
21. Cameron AJ, Kamath PS, Carpenter HA. Prevalence of Barrett's esophagus and intestinal metaplasia at the esophagogastric junction. *Gastroenterology* 1997; **112**:A82.
22. Romero Y, Cameron AJ, McDonnell SK *et al.* Family history doubles Barrett's esophagus risk. *Gastroenterology* 2002;**122**(suppl 1):A292.

23. Romero Y, Cameron AJ, Schaid DJ *et al*. Barrett's esophagus: prevalence in symptomatic relatives. *Am J Gastroenterol* 2002;**97**:1127–32.

24. Cameron AJ, Epidemiologic studies and the development of Barrett's esophagus. *Endoscopy* 1993;**25**(9):635–6.

25. El-Serag HB, Bailey NR, Gilger M, Rabeneck L. Endoscopic manifestations of gastroesophageal reflux disease in patients between 18 months and 25 years without neurological deficits. *Amer J Gastroenterol* 2002;**97**:1635–9.

26. Hassall E. Barrett's esophagus: congenital or acquired? *Amer J Gastroenterol* 1993;**88**:819–24.

27. Caygill CPJ, Watson A, Reed PI, Hill MJ. Characteristics and regional variations of patients with Barrett's esophagus in the UK. *Eur J Gastroent Hep* 2003;**15**:1217–22.

28. Blot WJ, Devesa SS, Kneller RW, Fraumeni JF, Jr. Rising incidence of adenocarcinoma of the esophagus and gastric cardia. *JAMA* 1991;**265**:1287–9.

29. Lieberman DA, Oehlke M, Helfand M, and the GORGE consortium. Risk factors for Barrett's esophagus in community-based practice. *Amer J Gastroenterol* 1997;**92**:1293–7.

30. Williamson WA, Ellis FH, Gibb SP *et al*. Barrett's esophagus. Prevalence and incidence of adenocarcinoma. *Arch Int Med* 1991;**151**:2212–6.

31. Van Sandick JW, Van Lanschot JJB, Kuiken BW *et al*. Impact of endoscopic biopsy surveillance of Barrett's oesophagus on pathololological stage and clinical outcome of Barrett's carcinoma. *Gut* 1998;**43**:216–22.

32. Menke-Pluymers MBE, Schoute NW, Mulder AH *et al*. Outcome of surgical treatment of adenocarcinoma in Barrett's oesophagus. *Gut* 1992;**33**:1454–8.

33. Gerson LB, Shetler K, Triadafilopoulos G. Prevalence of Barrett's esophagus in asymptomatic individuals. *Gastroenterology* 2002;**123**:461–7.

34. Rex DK, Cummings OW, Shaw S *et al*. Screening for Barrett's esophagus in colonoscopy patients with and without heartburn. *Gastroenterology* 2003;**125**:1670–7.

35. Nasseri-Moghaddam S, Malekzadeh R, Sotoudeh M *et al*. Lower esophagus in dyspeptic Iranian patients: a prospective study. *J Gastroentero Hepatol* 2003;**18**:315–21.

36. Toruner M, Soykan I, Enzari A *et al*. Barrett's esophagus: prevalence and its relationship with dyspeptic symptoms. *J Gastroentero Hepatol* 2004;**19**:535–40.

37. Rajendra S, Kutty K, Karim N. Ethnic differences in the prevalence of endoscopic esophagitis and Barrett's esophagus: the long and the short of it. *Dig Dis Sci* 2004;**39**:237–42.

38. Lee JI, Park H, Jung HW *et al*. Prevalence of Barrett's esophagus in an urban Korean population. *J Gastroenterol* 2003;**38**:23–7.

39. Azuma N, Endo T, Arimura Y *et al*. Prevalence of Barrett's esophagus and expression of mucin antigens detected by a panel of monoclonal antibodies in Barrett's esophagus and esophageal adenocarcinoma in Japan. *J Gastroenterol* 2000;**35**:583–92.

40. Wong WM, Lam SK, Hui WM *et al*. Long-term prospective follow-up of endoscopic oesophagitis in southern Chinese—prevalence and spectrum of the disease. *Aliment Pharmacol Ther* 2002;**16**:2037–42.

41. Mason RJ, Bremner CG. The columnar-lined (Barrett's) oesophagus in black patients. *S Afr J Surg* 1998;**36**:61–2.

42. Kang JY. Systematic review: geographical and ethnic differences in gastro-esophageal reflux disease. *Aliment Pharmacol Ther* 2004;**20**:705–17.

43. Hongo M, Shoji T. Epidemiology of reflux disease and CLE in East Asia. *J Gastroenterol* 2003;**38**(suppl XV):25–30

44. Nebel OT, Fornes MF, Castell DO. Symptomatic gastrosophageal reflux: incidence and precipitating factors. *Dig Dis Sci* 1976;**21**:953–6.

45. Locke GR, III, Talley NJ, Fett SR, Zinsmeister AR, Melton LJ, III. Prevalence and clinical spectrum of gastroesophageal reflux: a population based study in Olmsted County, Minnesota. *Gastroenterology* 1997;**112**:1448–56.

46. Thompson WG, Heaton KW. Heartburn and globus in apparently healthy people. *Canad Med Ass J* 1982;**126**:46–8.

47. Isolauri J, Laippala P. Prevalence of symptoms suggestive of gastroesophageal reflux in an adult population. *Ann Med* 1995;**27**:67–70.

48. Cameron AJ, Zinsmeister AR, Ballard DJ, Carney JA. Prevalence of columnar-lined (Barrett's) esophagus. Comparison of population-based clinical and autopsy findings. *Gastroenterology* 1990;**99**:918–22.

49. Ormsby AH, Kilgore SP, Goldblum JR *et al*. The location and frequency of intestinal metaplasia at the esophagogastric junction in 223 consecutive autopsies: implications for patient treatment and preventive strategies in Barrett's esophagus. *Mod Pathol* 2000;**13**:614–20.

50. Cameron AJ, Lomboy CT, Pera M, Carpenter HA. Adenocarcinoma of the esophagogastric junction and Barrett's esophagus. *Gastroenterology* 1995;**109**:1541–6.

51. Hamilton SR, Smith RRL, Cameron JL. Prevalence and characteristics of Barrett esophagus in patients with adenocarcinoma of the esophagus or esophagogastric junction. *Hum Pathol* 1988;**19**:942–8.

52. Theisen J, Stein HJ, Dittler HJ *et al.* Preoperative chemotherapy unmasks underlying Barrett's mucosa in patients with adenocarcinoma of the distal esophagus. *Surg Endosc* 2002;**16**:671–3.

53. Corley DA, Levin TR, Habel LA *et al.* Surveillance and survival in Barrett's adenocarcinomas: a population-based study. *Gastroenterology* 2002;**122**:633–40.

54. Dulai GS, Guha S, Kahn KL, Gornbein J, Weinstein WM. Preoperative prevalence of Barrett's esophagus in esophageal adenocarcinoma: a systematic review. *Gastroenterology* 2002;**122**:26–33.

55. Conio M, Cameron AJ, Romero Y *et al.* Secular trends in the epidemiology and outcome of Barrett's oesophagus in Olmsted County, Minnesota. *Gut* 2001;**48**:304–9.

56. Pera M, Cameron AJ, Trastek VF, Carpenter HA, Zinsmeister AR. Increasing incidence of adenocarcinoma of the esophagus and esophagogastric junction. *Gastroenterology* 1993;**104**:510–3.

57. Devesa SS, Blot WJ, Fraumeni JF. Changing patterns in the incidence of esophageal and gastric carcinoma in the United States. *Cancer* 1998;**83**:2049–53.

58. Crabb DW, Berk MA, Hall TR *et al.* Familial gastroesophageal reflux and development of Barrett's esophagus. *Ann Int Med* 1985;**103**:52–4.

59. Jochem VJ, Fuerst PA, Fromkes JJ. Familial Barrett's esophagus associated with adenocarcinoma. *Gastroenterology* 1992;**102**:1400–2.

60. Fahmy N, King JF. Barrett's esophagus: an acquired condition with genetic predisposition. *Am J Gastroenterol* 1993;**88**:1262–5.

61. Cameron AJ, Lagergren J, Henriksson C *et al.* Gastroesophageal reflux disease in monozygotic and dizygotic twins. *Gastroenterology* 2002;**122**:55–9.

62. Mohammed I, Cherkas LF, Riley SA, Spector TD, Trudgill NJ. Genetic influences in gastro-oesophageal reflux disease: a twin study. *Gut* 2003;**52**:1085–9.

63. Romero Y, Cameron AJ, Locke GR, III *et al.* Familial aggregation of gastroesophageal reflux in patients with Barrett's esophagus and esophageal adenocarcinoma. *Gastroenterology* 1997;**113**:1449–56.

64. Trudgill NJ, Kapur KC, Riley AS. Familial clustering of reflux symptoms. *Am J Gastroenterol* 1999;**94**:1172–8.

65. Romero Y, Cameron AJ, Schaid DJ *et al.* Barrett's esophagus: prevalence in symptomatic relatives. *Am J Gastroenterol* 2002;**97**:1127–32.

66. Romero Y, Cameron AJ, McDonnell S *et al.* Family history doubles Barrett's esophagus risk. *Gastroenterology* 2002;**122**(suppl 1):A292.

67. Caygill CPJ, Johnston DA, Lopez M *et al.* Lifestyle factors and Barrett's esophagus. *Amer J Gastroenterol* 2002;**97**:1328–31.

68. Conio M, Filiberti R, Blanchi S *et al.* Risk factors for Barrett's esophagus: a case-control study. *Int J Cancer* 2002;**97**:226–9.

69. Schnell TG, Sontag SJ, Chejfec G. Adenocarcinomas arising in tongues or short segments of Barrett's esophagus. *Dig Dis Sci* 1992;**37**:137–43.

70. Johnston MH, Hammond AS, Laskin W, Jones DM. The prevalence and clinical characteristics of short segments of specialized intestinal metaplasia in the distal esophagus on routine endoscopy. *Amer J Gastroenterol* 1996;**91**:1507–11.

71. Weston AP, Krmpotich P, Makdisi WF *et al.* Short segment Barrett's esophagus: clinical and histological features, associated endoscopic findings, and association with gastric intestinal metaplasia. *Amer J Gastroenterol* 1996;**91**:981–6.

72. Voutilanen M, Farkkila M, Juhola M *et al.* Specialized columnar epithelium of the esophagogastric junction: prevalence and associations. *Am J Gastroenterol* 1999;**94**:913–8.

73. Nandurkar S, Talley NJ. Barrett's esophagus: the long and short of it. *Amer J Gastroenterol* 1999;**94**:30–40.

CHAPTER 3

Esophageal Adenocarcinoma— Epidemiology and Association with Barrett's Esophagus

Jesper Lagergren

Incidence

The incidence esophageal adenocarcinoma (EAC) has been increasing steeply since the mid 1970s in most industrialized populations. This increase has been most pronounced in the UK, Australia, Netherlands, and USA, and less so in Eastern Europe and in Scandinavia [1–5]. The increase is generally greater among men and more so among Caucasians. In contrast, the incidence of esophageal squamous-cell carcinoma is more stable or has decreased slightly in these populations [1–5]. Due to these incidence changes, the occurrence of adenocarcinomas has surpassed that of squamous-cell carcinomas in several countries. Although the incidence of adenocarcinoma of the esophagus has increased, it has to be stressed that this is still an uncommon disease. In countries in which population-based incidence figures are available, the number of new cases per 100 000 White men during year 2000 varied between 1 and 5 [5].

Tumor Classification

It has been suggested that the increasing incidence of adenocarcinomas is explained by improvements in diagnostic methods, mainly the introduction of endoscopy, and an increased general awareness of these tumors among endoscopists and others. This is an unlikely explanation, however, since the trend differs distinctly between men and women and the incidence is still increasing during a period without major changes in diagnostic procedures. Nor can the increasing trend be explained by changes in tumor classification of, i.e., a proximal shift of the classification of tumors located near the gastroesophageal junction, since there is an increase in both adenocarcinoma of the esophagus and the gastric cardia, and again the increase is continuing. Therefore, the increasing incidence is not likely to be explained by misclassification.

Age, Sex, Race, and Socioeconomic Factors

The age distribution is in line with most other cancers, with an increased risk with increasing age. The median age at diagnosis is about 60 years. A striking and probably important, but yet unexplained feature of the incidence of EAC is the strong (7 : 1) male predominance, similar in all populations studied [1–5]. The incidence of EAC is higher among Caucasians as compared to non-Caucasians [1–5], which is possibly explained by differences in socioeconomic variables [1]. The knowledge of any influence of various socioeconomic factors is very limited and the available reports are contradictory [6]. There are indications that low socioeconomic status, based on measures of income and education, might increase the risk also of these tumors [7–10], but inconsistent results [9,11] and the use of different measures of socioeconomic status makes comparisons and interpretations difficult.

Heredity

Familial clustering of Barrett's esophagus as well as EAC has been reported [12,13]. However, in three large population-based studies of familial occurrence, no evidence of family history of gastrointestinal cancer among cases of EAC was found [14]. Therefore, the influence of genetic factors in the population-based setting seems to be limited. Moreover, a change of gene pool in 20–30 years that can explain the increase in incidence of this tumor is unlikely.

Barrett's Esophagus and Gastroesophageal Reflux

Patients with Barrett's esophagus have an excess risk of developing adenocarcinoma ranging between 30 and 400-fold [17–24]. In studies of large sample size, the excess risk has been estimated to be 30 to 60-fold relative to the risk of the general population [18,19,22,24], and a majority, if not all, cases with adenocarcinoma of the esophagus arise from a Barrett's mucosa [25]. The role of gastroesophageal reflux—or reflux symptoms—*per se* in the development of EAC has been investigated in four recent large epidemiological studies. In a medical record-based case-control study in the USA, a twofold increased risk of esophageal or cardia adenocarcinoma was found among persons with a recorded history of gastroesophageal reflux disease (GERD), hiatus hernia, esophagitis/esophageal ulcer, or difficulty in swallowing [26]. In a Swedish population-based, nationwide case-control study, information on the subject's history of gastroesophageal reflux was collected in personal interviews [27]. Among persons with recurrent symptoms of reflux occurring at least once per week, the risk of EAC was increased eightfold. The more frequent, more severe, and longer-lasting the symptoms of reflux, the greater the risk. Among persons with both long-standing and severe symptoms of reflux, the odds ratio was 43.5 for EAC. Since this relative risk was in the level of that observed for the relation between Barrett's esophagus and EAC, and due to the finding that the relation between reflux and this cancer seemed to be independent on the occurrence of Barrett's esophagus the critical role of Barrett's before in the etiology of EAC was challanged [27]. However, the accumulated data seem to support that Barrett's esophagus is truly a necessary intermediate step in the causal pathway between reflux and EAC [25]. In a case-control study of similar design in the USA, there was also a dose–response relation between reflux symptoms and EAC [28]. A more recent population-based cohort study of 65 000 male patients with a diagnosis of heartburn, hiatus hernia, or esophagitis revealed a ninefold increased risk of EAC among patients with an endoscopically verified esophagitis [29]. The risk estimates increased with increasing follow-up time (P for trend = 0.03). Based on available studies, it is possible to establish that reflux is a major risk factor for EAC.

Body Mass

A high body mass index (BMI) has been found to be a risk factor for adenocarcinoma of the esophagus in several epidemiological case-control studies [30–32]. Three recent large population-based studies all show similar results; i.e., a strong and dose-dependent association between increasing BMI and risk of EAC, seemingly independent of reflux symptoms [30–32]. Among persons with a historical BMI above 30, the relative risk of developing EAC has been found to be as high as 16 compared with the leanest (BMI < 22) [31]. Moreover, the first prospective study of this association reveals a clear association between obesity and this cancer [33]. However, the mechanism behind this association remains to be identified [34]. Although obesity is common in Western societies and the prevalence is increasing [35], the sex distribution and the steepness of the increase in prevalence do not match that of the incidence of EAC well; therefore, the increasing incidence of EAC is not entirely explained by this association.

Tobacco Smoking

Several studies have reported a moderately increased risk of adenocarcinoma of the esophagus among tobacco smokers [9,32], while a few studies did not [36]. A recent study with prospective exposure collection revealed a moderate association [33].

Taken together, there seems to be an association between smoking and EAC, but the strength is considerably weaker than that with squamous cell carcinoma [9,32,33,36].

Alcohol Drinking

There seems to be no positive relation between alcohol consumption and the risk of adenocarcinoma of the esophagus. The results from four large population-based case-control studies [9,32,33,36], including one study with prospective data collection [33], are all in agreement that no such association exists, independent of the type of alcoholic beverage consumed.

Helicobacter pylori

In a case-control study by Chow *et al.* it was found that infection with *Helicobacter pylori* as measured by positive results for both immunoglobulin G (IgG)-serology and CagA-positivity decreased the risk of esophageal or cardia adenocarcinoma by 60% [37]. However, a study of similar design by Wu *et al.* revealed no association between *H. pylori*-infection and EAC [38]. A recent Swedish population-based case-control study revealed that regardless of whether IgG enzyme linked immunosorbent assay (ELISA), CagA, or both were used as indicator of infection, there was a significantly 50–80% reduced risk for EAC [39]. Hence, an inverse relation between *H. pylori* infection and risk of adenocarcinoma of the esophagus is likely, but not yet clearly proven [37–39]. The postulated mechanism for the protective effect of *H. pylori* is through its ability to cause atrophic gastritis, and possibly also by increasing intragastric ammonia production [40]. This mechanism was recently challanged in the Swedish case-control study, however, since the inverse association between *H. pylori* and EAC remained unaffected after adjustment for gastric atrophy [39].

Diet

The knowledge of the influence of dietary factors is sparse and the available studies are susceptible to bias [41]. Confounding by dietary variables is a source of error that is difficult to reliably adjust for. However, low intake of fruit and vegetables is an established dietary risk factor [42,43]. The antioxidants in these dietary items might have a particular protective effect [42,44]. Furthermore, low intake of dietary fiber seems to increase the risk according to two large population-based case-control studies [42,45]. Other potential dietary risk factors include high intake of dietary fat, dietary cholesterol, and animal protein [42].

Lower Esophageal Sphincter Relaxing Drugs

Some data suppport that a continuous and long-standing use of medications that can relax the lower esophageal sphincter (LES), and thereby cause gastroesophageal reflux, may increase the risk of developing adenocarcinoma of the esophagus [46]. Groups of medications that were introduced before the increase in incidence of EAC started included nitroglycerins, aminophylline, β-receptor agonists, anticholinergics, and benzodiazepines. A use of any of the medications in these five groups for more than 5 years increased the risk of EAC significantly and more than twofold. After adjustment for reflux symptoms, this association disappeared, indicating that the mechanism behind the association might be reflux as hypothesized [46]. In a study from the USA, there was no clear sign of an association between drugs that can relax the LES and the risk of EAC [47]. Hence, the relation needs to be further studied.

Non-Steroidal Anti-Inflammatory Drugs

Numerous studies have indicated an antitumoral effect on gastrointestinal tumors by the use of non-steroidal anti-inflammatory drugs (NSAIDs), especially by using selective cyclooxygenase-2 (COX-2) inhibitors [48,49]. Overexpression of COX-2 has been identified in EAC [50–52]. Tumor growth in esophageal cancer is reduced by the treatment with COX-2 inhibitors [53]. Epidemiological studies have shown a reduced risk of developing esophageal cancer among individuals using NSAIDs [54–56].

However, a large, prospective nested case-control study has suggested that the occurrence of upper gastrointestinal disorders could distort the association between NSAIDs and esophageal cancer risk [57]. The inverse association in previous research might be explained by lack of appropriate adjustment for such disorders. Therefore, the relation between NSAIDs and EAC remains uncertain.

Explanations for the Increasing Incidence

Gastroesophageal reflux is the strongest risk factor for EAC, but it is uncertain whether this factor can explain the increasing incidence of this tumor. If reflux is the main reason for the increasing incidence of EAC, the incidence of reflux disease should have risen during recent decades. There is, unfortunately, no data available on the incidence of GERD, only prevalence figures. In a study of hospitalization for reflux disease, the prevalence of diagnoses representing GERD had increased [58], but the recording of reflux disease in the medical records might not mirror the true incidence of the disease. In that sense, it might be more appropriate to evaluate the prevalence of reflux symptoms in population-based studies. According to such studies, there are no clear signs of an increasing prevalence in earlier studies as compared to more recent ones [59–61]. However, differences in design and populations in these studies makes comparisons difficult. Hence, there are as yet no data that establishes any increasing incidence of reflux disease. Moreover, the strong male predominance among patients with EAC is not compatible with the even sex distribution of reflux in the population [62].

If the incidence of reflux is rising, this increase in turn could be caused by some environmental factor. One such potential factor is the use of medications that relax the LES and thereby facilitate reflux. As discussed above, a positive association between previous use of such medications and the risk of EAC has been identified [46]. However, another study of similar design in the USA showed conflicting results [47]. The increasing use of these drugs in the 1960s and 1970s may still have contributed to the increase in incidence of EAC.

It would be tempting to attribute the increase in the incidence of EAC to the increase in average body mass observed in Western populations [35]. However, the apparently sudden deflection of the incidence curve for EAC, [1–5], the rapidity of the increase, [1–5], and the marked, six to eightfold, male predominance, [1–5] are observations not consistent with this interpretation.

Tobacco smoking has been proposed to be a risk factor contributing to the rising incidence of adenocarcinoma of the esophagus [9]. The association between smoking and squamous cell carcinoma of the esophagus is much stronger than that with adenocarcinoma [9,32,33,36]. Furthermore, smoking has declined markedly among men, as reflected by a decreasing incidence of lung cancer [63], while the increasing incidence of EAC is strongest among men [1–5]. Taken together, tobacco smoking does not seem to be the main reason for the increasing incidence of these tumors.

It has been suggested that this increase is linked to falling rates of *H. pylori* infection in Western societies [37], and the majority of available studies point to an inverse relation between infection with *H. pylori* and risk of EAC [37–39]. There are a limited number of studies, and the sex distribution of the infection does not fit with the distribution of patients with EAC.

In conclusion, gastroesophageal reflux, use of medications that might cause such reflux, obesity, and decreasing occurrence of infection with *H. pylori* might all be factors that contribute to the increasing incidence of adenocarcinoma of the esophagus. A general problem is that the sex distribution of these factors does not match the strong male predominance of EAC. It is probably a key task to thoroughly address the reasons behind this sex distribution before we can confidently establish the reasons for the increasing incidence of this tumor.

Prognosis

Although the survival rates among patients with EAC have improved during recent years [64,65], the 5-year survival of 10% is still a dismal figure [66]. The poor survival rates indicate that all attempts to improve the therapy have only to a limited degree contributed to an improved overall survival. Surgery alone remains the only potentially curative treatment [67]. Some authors have reported a better survival rate among patients with cancer emerging from a Barrett's mucosa [68,69] compared with esophageal malignancies without this metaplasia. This might be explained by more prevalent symptoms of gastroesophageal reflux in the Barrett's group, leading to earlier endoscopy and confirmation of the diagnosis at an earlier tumor stage. Furthermore, the recent introduction of endoscopic surveillance programs among patients with Barrett's mucosa in many endoscopy units might improve the long-term survival in this defined group of patients. To reduce the mortality in EAC, it is important not only to optimize the therapy but, probably even more importantly, to identify risk factors that might make primary prevention possible.

Endoscopic Screening or Surveillance

The poor survival rates for adenocarcinoma of the esophagus are improved mainly by early tumor detection [70]. Therefore, it is important to identify absolute high-risk persons in whom endoscopic screening or surveillance might be warranted. Since reflux symptoms are common [62] and EAC is still an uncommon disease, endoscopic screening in reflux patients would rapidly overtax available health care resources [27]. The possible benefits of endoscopic screening should not exceed the costs and inconveniences for patients and health care systems. In a re-analysis of Swedish nation-wide case-control data, the number of endoscopies needed to identify one esophageal or cardia adenocarcinoma in persons with various combinations of both obesity and reflux was determined [71]. The risks were combined in a multiplicative manner, and among obese persons with recurrent reflux symptoms the odds ratio was 184 for EAC compared with lean persons without reflux. We then estimated the number needed to survey to detect one esophageal or cardia adenocarcinoma among men aged 50–79 years. Six percent had the combination of BMI ≥ 25 kg/m^2 and reflux symptoms, but only 0.3% of men aged 50–79 years had reflux and BMI > 30 kg/m^2. The number of persons needed to screen to detect one adenocarci-

noma varied from 2189 in the former stratum, to 594 in the latter. Thus, if 60 obese men aged 50–79 years with reflux symptoms are followed for 10 years, one esophageal or cardia adenocarcinoma will be observed. In some other countries, the incidence figures of EAC are higher compared to those in Sweden. According to a recent analysis based on data accrued in the literature, screening endoscopy, but not surveillance, might play a role among men over 50 years with severe reflux symptoms [72]. In conclusion, it is possible to identify a limited group with a relative risk that greatly exceeds that of the general population, but the absolute risk for the individual person is closely linked with the incidence of the cancer. Given the poor results of treatment of the cancer when it occurs and if the incidence of these tumors continues to increase, future studies might find that surveillance may be worthwhile.

References

1. Devesa SS, Blot WJ, Fraumeni JF, Jr. Changing patterns in the incidence of esophageal and gastric carcinoma in the United States. *Cancer* 1998;**83**:2049–53.
2. Powell J, McConkey CC. The rising trend in oesophageal adenocarcinoma and gastric cardia. *Eur J Cancer Prev* 1992;**1**:265–9.
3. Armstrong RW, Borman B. Trends in incidence rates of adenocarcinoma of the oesophagus and gastric cardia in New Zealand, 1978–1992. *Int J Epidemiol* 1996;**25**:941–7.
4. Hansson LE, Sparén P, Nyrén O. Increasing incidence in both histological types of esophageal carcinomas among men in Sweden. *Int J Cancer* 1993;**54**:402–7.
5. Bollschweiler E, Wolfgarten E, Gutschow C, Holscher AH. Demographic variations in the rising incidence of esophageal adenocarcinoma in white males. *Cancer* 2001;**92**:549–55.
6. Wong A, Fitzgerald RC. Epidemiologic risk factors for Barrett's esophagus and associated adenocarcinoma. *Clin Gastroenterol Hepatol* 2005;**3**:1–10.
7. Brown LM, Silverman DT, Pottern LM *et al*. Adenocarcinoma of the esophagus and esophagogastric junction in white men in the United States: alcohol, tobacco, and socioeconomic factors. *Cancer Causes Control* 1994;**5**:333–40.
8. Zhang ZF, Kurtz RC, Sun M *et al*. Adenocarcinomas of the esophagus and gastric cardia: medical conditions,

tobacco, alcohol, and socioeconomic factors. *Cancer Epidemiol Biomarkers Prev* 1996;**5**:761–8.

9. Gammon MD, Schoenberg JB, Ahsan H *et al*. Tobacco, alcohol, and socioeconomic status and adenocarcinomas of the esophagus and gastric cardia. *J Natl Cancer Inst* 1997;**89**:1277–84.

10. van Loon AJ, Goldbohm RA, van den Brandt PA. Socioeconomic status and stomach cancer incidence in men: results from The Netherlands Cohort Study. *J Epidemiol Community Health* 1998;**52**:166–71.

11. Brewster DH, Fraser LA, McKinney PA, Black RJ. Socioeconomic status and risk of adenocarcinoma of the oesophagus and cancer of the gastric cardia in Scotland. *Br J Cancer* 2000;**83**:387–90.

12. Romero Y, Cameron AJ, Locke GR, III *et al*. Familial aggregation of gastroesophageal reflux in patients with Barrett's esophagus and esophageal adenocarcinoma. *Gastroenterology* 1997;**113**:1449–56.

13. Chak A, Lee T, Kinnard MF *et al*. Familial aggregation of Barrett's oesophagus, oesophageal adenocarcinoma, and oesophagogastric junctional adenocarcinoma in Caucasian adults. *Gut* 2002;**51**:323–28.

14. Zhang ZF, Kurtz RC, Sun M *et al*. Adenocarcinomas of the esophagus and gastric cardia: medical conditions, tobacco, alcohol, and socioeconomic factors. *Cancer Epidemiol Biomark Prev* 1996;**5**:761–8.

15. Lagergren J, Ye W, Lindgren A, Nyrén O. Heredity and risk of cancer of the esophagus and gastric cardia. *Cancer Epidemiol Biomarkers Prev* 2000;**9**:757–60.

16. Dhillon PK, Farrow DC, Vaughan TL *et al*. Family history of cancer and risk of esophageal and gastric cancers in the United States. *Int J Cancer* 2001;**93**:148–52.

17. Spechler SJ, Goyal RK. Barrett's esophagus. *N Engl J Med* 1986;**315**:362–71.

18. Spechler SJ, Robbins AH, Rubins HB *et al*. Adenocarcinoma and Barrett's esophagus. An overrated risk. *Gastroenterology* 1984;**87**:927–33.

19. Cameron AJ, Ott BJ, Payne WS. The incidence of adenocarcinoma in columnar-lined (Barrett's) esophagus. *N Engl J Med* 1985;**313**:857–8.

20. Robertson CS, Mayberry JF, Nicholson DA, James PD, Atkinson M. Value of endoscopic surveillance in the detection of neoplastic change in Barrett's oesophagus. *Br J Surg* 1988;**72**:760–3.

21. Hameeteman W, Tytgat GNJ, Houthoff HJ, Van der Tweel JG. Barrett's esophagus: development of dysplasia and adenocarcinoma. *Gastroenterology* 1989;**96**:1249–56.

22. Van Der Veen AH, Dees J, Blankenstein JD, Blankenstein M. Adenocarcinoma in Barrett's esophagus: an overrated risk. *Gut* 1989;**10**:14–8.

23. Ovaska J, Miettinen M, Kivilaksko E. Adenocarcinoma arising in Barrett's esophagus. *Dig Dis Ci* 1989;**34**:1336–9.

24. Drewitz DJ, Sampliner RE, Garewal HS. The incidence of adenocarcinoma in Barrett's esophagus: a prospective study of 170 patients followed 4.8 years. *Am J Gastroenterol* 1997;**92**:212–5.

25. Enzinger PC, Mayer RJ. Esophageal cancer. *N Engl J Med* 2003;**349**:2241–52.

26. Chow WH, Finkle WD, McLaughlin JK *et al*. The relation of gastroesophageal reflux disease and its treatment to adenocarcinomas of the esophagus and gastric cardia. *JAMA* 1995;**274**:474–7.

27. Lagergren J, Bergström R, Lindgren A, Nyrén O. Symptomatic gastroesophageal reflux is a strong risk factor for esophageal adenocarcinoma. *N Engl J Med* 1999;**340**:825–31.

28. Farrow DC, Vaughan TL, Sweeney C *et al*. Gastroesophageal reflux disease, use of H2 receptor antagonists, and risk of esophageal and gastric cancer. *Cancer Causes Control* 2000;**11**:231–8.

29. Ye W, Chow WH, Lagergren J, Yin L, Nyrén O. Risk of adenocarcinomas of the oesophagus and gastric cardia in patients with gastroesophageal reflux diseases and after antireflux surgery. *Gastroenterology* 2001;**121**:1286–93.

30. Chow WH, Blot WJ, Vaughan TL *et al*. Body mass index and risk of adenocarcinoma of the esophagus and gastric cardia. *J Natl Cancer Inst* 1998;**90**:150–5.

31. Lagergren J, Bergström R, Nyrén O. Association between body mass and adenocarcinoma of the esophagus and gastric cardia. *Ann Intern Med* 1999;**130**:883–90.

32. Wu AH, Wan P, Bernstein L. A multiethnic population-based study of smoking, alcohol and body size and risk of adenocarcinomas of the stomach and esophagus (United States). *Cancer Causes Control* 2001;**12**:721–32.

33. Lindblad M, Rodríguez LG, Lagergren J. Body mass, tobacco and alcohol and risk of esophageal, cardia, and gastric adenocarcinoma among men and women in a nested case-control study. *Cancer Causes Control* 2005;**16**:285–94.

34. Buttar NS, Wang KK. Mechanisms of disease: carcinogenesis in Barrett's esophagus. *Nature Clin Practice* 2004;**1**:106–12.

35. Seidell JC, Flegal KM. Assessing obesity: classification and epidemiology. *Br Med Bull* 1997;**53**:238–52.

36. Lagergren J, Bergström R, Lindgren A, Nyrén O. The role of tobacco, snuff and alcohol use in the aetiology of cancer of the oesophagus and gastric cardia. *Int J Cancer* 2000;**85**:340–6.

37. Chow WH, Blaser MJ, Blot WJ *et al*. An inverse relation between CagA⁺ strains of *Helicobacter pylori* infection and risk of esophageal and gastric cardia adenocarcinoma. *Cancer Res* 1998;**58**:588–90.

38. Wu AH, Crabtree JE, Bernstein L *et al*. Role of *Helicobacter pylori* CagA⁺ strains and risk of adenocarcinoma of the stomach and esophagus. *Int J Cancer* 2003;**103**:815–21.

39. Ye W, Held M, Lagergren J *et al*. *Helicobacter pylori* infection and gastric atrophy: risk of adenocarcinoma and squamous-cell carcinoma of the esophagus and gastric cardia adenocarcinoma. *J Natl Cancer Inst* 2004;**96**:388–96.

40. Richter JE, Falk GW, Vaezi MF. *Helicobacter pylori* and gastroesophageal reflux disease: the bug may not be all bad. *Am J Gastroenterol* 1998;**93**:1800–2.

41. Mayne ST, Navarro SA. Diet, obesity and reflux in the etiology of adenocarcinomas of the esophagus and gastric cardia in humans. *J Nutr* 2002;**132**:3467S–70S.

42. Mayne ST, Risch HA, Dubrow R *et al*. Nutrient intake and risk of subtypes of esophageal and gastric cancer. *Cancer Epidemiol Biomark Prev* 2001;**10**:1055–62.

43. Terry P, Lagergren J, Hansen H, Wolk A, Nyrén O. Fruit and vegetable consumption in the prevention of esophageal and cardia cancers. *Eur J Cancer Prev* 2001;**10**:365–9.

44. Terry P, Lagergren J, Ye W, Nyrén O, Wolk A. Antioxidants and cancers of the esophagus and gastric cardia. *Int J Cancer* 2000;**87**:750–4.

45. Terry P, Lagergren J, Ye W, Wolk A, Nyrén O. Inverse association between intake of cereal fiber and risk of gastric cardia cancer. *Gastroenterology* 2001;**120**:387–91.

46. Lagergren J, Bergström R, Adami HO, Nyrén O. Association between medications that relax the lower esophageal sphincter and risk for esophageal adenocarcinoma. *Ann Intern Med* 2000;**133**:165–75.

47. Vaughan TL, Farrow DC, Hansten PD *et al*. Risk of esophageal and gastric adenocarcinomas in relation to use of calcium channel blockers, asthma drugs, and other medications that promote gastroesophageal reflux. *Cancer Epidemiol Biomarkers Prev* 1998;**7**:749–56.

48. Taketo MM. Cyclooxygenase-2 inhibitors in tumorigenesis (Part I). *J Natl Cancer Inst* 1998;**90**:1529–36.

49. Taketo MM. Cyclooxygenase-2 inhibitors in tumorigenesis (Part II). *J Natl Cancer Inst* 1998;**90**:1609–20.

50. Wilson KT, Fu S, Ramanujam KS, Meltzer SJ. Increased expression of inducible nitric oxide synthase and cyclooxygenase-2 in Barrett's esophagus and associated adenocarcinomas. *Cancer Res* 1998;**58**:2929–34.

51. Zimmermann KC, Sarbia M, Weber AA *et al*. Cyclooxygenase-2 expression in human esophageal carcinoma. *Cancer Res* 1999;**59**:198–204.

52. Shirvani VN, Ouatu-Lascar R, Kaur BS, Omary MB, Triadafilopoulos G. Cyclooxygenase 2 expression in Barrett's esophagus and adenocarcinoma: *ex vivo* induction by bile salts and acid exposure. *Gastroenterology* 2000;**118**:487–96.

53. Souza RF, Shewmake K, Beer DG, Cryer B, Spechler SJ. Selective inhibition of cyclooxygenase-2 suppresses growth and induces apoptosis in human esophageal adenocarcinoma cells. *Cancer Res* 2000;**60**:5767–72.

54. Funkhouser EM, Sharp GB. Aspirin and reduced risk of esophageal carcinoma. *Cancer* 1995;**76**:1116–9.

55. Thun MJ, Namboodiri MM, Calle EE, Flanders WD, Heath CW. Aspirin and risk of fatal cancer. *Cancer Res* 1993;**53**:1322–7.

56. Farrow DC, Vaughan TL, Hansten PD *et al*. Use of aspirin and other nonsteroidal anti-inflammatory drugs and risk of esophageal and gastric cancer. *Cancer Epidemiol Biomarkers Prev* 1998;**7**:97–102.

57. Lindblad M, Lagergren J, Rodríguez LG. Nonsteroidal anti-inflammatory drugs and risk of esophageal and gastric cancer. *Cancer Epidemiol Biomarkers Prev* 2005;**14**:444–50.

58. el-Serag HB, Sonnenberg A. Opposing time trends of peptic ulcer and reflux disease. *Gut* 1998;**43**:327–33.

59. Locke GR, Talley NJ, Fett SL, Zinsmeister AR, Melton LJ. Prevalence and clinical spectrum of gastroesophageal reflux: a population-based study in Olmsted County, Minnesota. *Gastroenterology* 1997;**112**:1448–56.

60. Nebel OT, Fornes MF, Castell DO. Symptomatic gastroesophageal reflux: incidence and precipitating factors. *Am J Dig Dis* 1976;**21**:953–6.

61. Thompson WG, Heaton KW. Heartburn and globus in apparently healthy people. *Can Med Assoc J* 1982;**126**:46–8.

62. Nilsson M, Johnsen R, Ye W, Hveem K, Lagergren J. The prevalence of gastroesophageal reflux among adults. *Scand J Gastroenterology* 2004;**39**:1040–5.

63. Cancer Registry. *Cancer Incidence in Sweden 1993, 1994 and 1995*. Stockholm: National Board of Health and Welfare, 1998.

64. Sundelöf M, Ye W, Dickman P, Lagergren J. Improved survival in both histological types of oesophageal cancer in Sweden. *Int J Cancer* 2002;**99**:751–4.

65. Farrow DC, Vaughan TL. Determinants of survival following the diagnosis of esophageal adenocarcinoma (United States). *Cancer Causes Control* 1996;**7**:322–7.

66. Berrino F. *Survival of Cancer Patients in Europe: The EUROCARE II Study*. Lyon: International Agency for Research on Cancer, 1999.

67. Wu PC, Posner MC. The role of surgery in the management of oesophageal cancer. *Lancet Oncol* 2003;**4**:481–8.

68. Johansson J, Johnsson F, Walther B *et al.* Adenocarcinoma in the distal esophagus with and without Barrett esophagus. Differences in symptoms and survival rates. *Arch Surg* 1996;**131**:708–13.

69. Thomas P, Doddoli C, Lienne P *et al.* Changing patterns and surgical results in adenocarcinoma of the oesophagus. *Br J Surg* 1997;**84**:119–25.

70. Altorki NK, Skinner DB. Adenocarcinoma in Barrett's esophagus. *Semin Surg Oncol* 1990;**6**:274–8.

71. Lagergren J, Ye W, Bergström R, Nyrén O. Utility of endoscopic screening for upper gastrointestinal adenocarcinoma. *JAMA* 2000;**284**:961–2.

72. Inadomi JM, Sampliner R, Lagergren J *et al.* Screening and surveillance for Barrett's esophagus in high-risk patients: a cost-utility analysis. *Ann Intern Med* 2003;**138**:176–86.

CHAPTER 4
Pathogenesis of Barrett's Esophagus

Nicholas J. Clemons, Rebecca. C. Fitzgerald, and Michael J. G. Farthing

Introduction

The link between Barrett's esophagus and esophageal adenocarcinoma is widely accepted; however, the etiopathogenesis of Barrett's esophagus is currently unclear. Although reflux of gastric contents into the esophagus certainly plays an important role, it is likely that inflammatory, environmental, and genetic factors are also involved. Understanding the pathogenesis of Barrett's esophagus will be important to define those at highest risk of developing esophageal adenocarcinoma in order to develop preventative and therapeutic strategies.

Cell of Origin

Following the first referral to the columnar-lined distal esophagus as Barrett's esophagus [1], several theories have evolved as to the origin of the metaplastic cells. It was not until 1970 that an experimental animal model conclusively demonstrated that Barrett's esophagus is in fact an acquired rather than a congenital condition [2]. However, the conversion of squamous to columnar epithelium is a poorly understood process, particularly in comparison to epithelial metaplasias at other sites such as the cervix [3]. Furthermore, the cell of origin for Barrett's esophagus has not yet been definitively described although there are three major hypotheses: (i) proximal migration of gastric or junctional columnar epithelium to replace the damaged epithelium ("transitional zone metaplasia"); (ii) transdifferation of damaged stem cells in the exposed papillae of inflamed squamous mucosa ("*de novo* metaplasia"); and (iii) migration of stem cells in the glandular neck region of esophageal ducts following squamous mucosal damage ("duct cell metaplasia") (Fig. 4.1). Interestingly, theories for the mechanism of squamous re-epithelialization of Barrett's esophagus following acid suppression combined with either potassium titanyl phosphate (KTP) laser photoablation or photodynamic therapy are essentially the same as those listed above [4]. Thus, it is possible the same stem cell may be responsible for the production of squamous epithelium under normal conditions and columnar epithelium of Barrett's esophagus following chronic reflux. Once metaplasia is initiated in the esophagus, it is thought that columnar cells colonize the mucosa rapidly within 3 years, with only 5–10% of metaplasias increasing in surface area thereafter [5]. Others have reported that Barrett's esophagus develops in a matter of weeks [6].

Animal models have provided some information regarding the metaplastic cell origin. Early experiments in dogs by Bremner *et al.* suggested that, following denuding of the squamous epithelium, the columnar epithelium originates by proximal migration of gastric or junctional columnar epithelium [2]. Importantly, this study also showed that maximal columnarization of the esophagus requires mucosal damage, an impaired lower esophageal sphincter (LES), chronic reflux and low gastric clearance. In addition, at least in the dog, a minimum of 8 weeks is required for maximal changes following mucosal damage. However, other studies have challenged the theory of proximal migration and provided evidence that the metaplastic epithelium originates from cells in the native esophagus [7]. In another canine study, a modification of that performed by Bremner *et al.*, a ring of squamous epithelium was left intact distal to the denuded area, which demonstrated that the resultant columnar epithelium regeneration could not have originated from the stomach. Instead, the metaplastic cells appeared to have arisen from

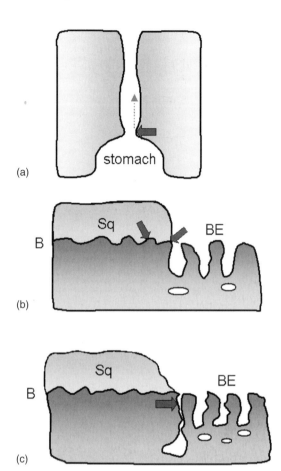

(a)

(b)

(c)

Fig. 4.1 Three theories for the cell of origin in Barrett's esophagus. (a) Transitional zone metaplasia—gastric or junctional columnar epithelium (wide arrow) migrates proximally to replace the damaged squamous of the lower esophagus. (b) *De novo* metaplasia—stem cells located in the papillae of the basal layer (B) of the squamous epithelium (Sq) transdifferentiate to form Barrett's epithelium (BE). (c) Duct cell metaplasia—stem cells in the glandular neck region of esophageal ducts (arrow) migrate to form the columnar-type epithelium following squamous mucosal damage.

undifferentiated cells in the glands or ducts within the esophagus (*de novo* or duct cell metaplasia) [7]. In addition, the presence of cytokeratin 13 in Barrett's epithelium, which is characteristic of squamous epithelia but is not present in the columnar epithelium of the cardia, further suggested that Barrett's esophagus may originate from cells in the native epithelium [8].

It has been proposed that the stem cells of the squamous epithelium or adjacent esophageal glandular tissue are induced to undergo an altered program of differentiation following chronic damage [9]. Furthermore, the cell of origin is likely to be a pluripotential stem cell since cells, such as goblet and parietal cells, not normally found in the esophagus may be present in the regenerated epithelium. Meyer *et al.* hypothesized that basal cells of the esophagus exposed by erosive reflux damage, are induced to transdifferentiate into columnar epithelium (*de novo* metaplasia) [10]. In keeping with this theory, it has been proposed that Barrett's esophagus develops directly from erosions in reflux esophagitis. However, reflux esophagitis typically induces scattered erosions in the distal squamous epithelium, while Barrett's esophagus usually involves the whole circumference of the esophagus distally with tongues of columnar cells extending proximally [11]. Thus, it is unlikely that Barrett's esophagus originates and spreads from small erosions created by reflux esophagitis.

Definitive studies on the cell of origin for Barrett's esophagus have been hampered by the lack of good animal models, but also because it is rare to observe the metaplastic change as it occurs *in vivo*. Recently, a multilayered epithelium with morphological and ultrastructural characteristics of both squamous and columnar epithelium, was described at the squamocolumnar junction and within the columnar mucosa of patients with Barrett's esophagus [12–14]. Using scanning electron microscopy, Shields *et al.* identified a unique surface cell at the squamocolumnar junction that was only found in patients with Barrett's esophagus. These surface cells displayed the concomitant presence of microvilli, intercellular ridges, and surface microridges [12]. This is interesting because microvilli are distinctive features of glandular epithelium, whereas intercellular ridges and surface microridges are distinctive of squamous epithelium. In a second study, the same group detected this unique cell in 37.5% of Barrett's esophagus patients but not in control patients without Barrett's esophagus and this cell was found to overlie normal squamous epithelium [14]. A study of cytokeratin expression in this multilayered epithelium detected cytokeratin 8 and 19 expression (columnar cell markers) and focal groups of cells with cytokeratin 4 and 13 expression (squamous markers) [15]. Confirmation of a unique, mixed cellular phenotype of multilayered epithelium has been provided by similar studies from another group [16]. Together, these results have led to the proposal that this multilayered epithelium may represent an intermediate stage in the metaplastic process secondary to the transformation of pluripopptent basal cells originating from squamous epithelium or submucosal gland ducts.

Extrinsic factors providing appropriate signals are required for stem cells to alter their differentiation program. Two such microenvironmental factors that might mediate esophageal metaplasia are the refluxate and inflammatory signals.

The Role of the Refluxate

It is well established that Barrett's esophagus develops as a consequence of chronic reflux, and indeed the theories for the cell of origin discussed above depend upon reflux-induced damage to initiate the metaplastic process. The prevalence of Barrett's esophagus is less than 1% in people without gastroesophageal reflux disease (GERD), but is approximately 10% in those with GERD [17,18]. In a case-control study, reflux symptoms were associated with a sixfold increased risk of developing Barrett's esophagus and were strongest in individuals with chronic symptoms [19]. Under normal circumstances damage to the mucosa of the esophagus is repaired by regeneration with squamous epithelium from squamous stem cells located in the basal compartment (reviewed in [20]). It has been proposed that when reflux exposure is repetitive and chronic, denuded areas of the esophagus may be replaced with metaplastic columnar epithelium as a protective mechanism. This new epithelium is more acid resistant and pluripotent, thus it continues to regenerate in the presence of a toxic luminal environment. In a rat reflux model, damage to the esophagus was more readily regenerated with columnar epithelium than with squamous epithelium, particularly under low pH conditions, suggesting that columnar cells are inherently more resistant to acid [21]. However, the exact role of reflux components

in the development of Barrett's esophagus is presently unclear.

The key physiological determinants of whether a patient with GERD develops Barrett's esophagus or not, appear to be low LES pressure, hiatal hernia, the presence of acid and bile salts in the refluxate, and longer episodes of reflux [22]. These will be discussed in turn.

LES Pressure Patients with Barrett's esophagus have been reported to have lower LES pressure than patients with uncomplicated GERD [23,24], which may result in inappropriate LES relaxations producing more frequent reflux episodes. In addition, peristalsis in Barrett's esophagus patients may be impaired, leading to poor clearance of refluxate and thus longer episodes of reflux exposure [25].

Hiatal Hernia Hiatal hernia may also contribute to an increased exposure to reflux. The combined statistics from several early studies reported that more than 90% of patients had hiatal hernia [1,26,27]. A recent study reported that hernia length and hiatal openings are greater in patients with Barrett's esophagus than in control subjects with or without esophagitis [28]. In this study, 96% of patients with Barrett's esophagus and 71% of patients with esophagitis also had hiatal hernia. Hiatal hernia may increase reflux and impair esophageal clearance by a number of mechanisms including lowering LES pressure, trapping refluxate in the sac and reducing the protective pressure of the crural diaphragm [29–32]. Thus, given the strong association of Barrett's esophagus with the presence of hiatal hernia and the increased exposure to reflux in patients with hiatal hernia, it is likely that hiatal hernia plays a significant role in the development of Barrett's esophagus.

Gastric Refluxate Contents This is highly heterogeneous and its components can include saliva, food, acid, mucous, and pepsin. In many patients with Barrett's esophagus, duodenal components including bile salts, trypsin, lipase, and cholesterol are also present [33]. Of these components, most attention has been given to acid and bile in the development of Barrett's esophagus and their role is discussed in further detail in Chapter 5.

Reflux components other than acid and bile have also been implicated in the pathogenesis of Barrett's esophagus. In a rabbit model, the addition of pepsin to acid has been shown to be more damaging to the mucosa than acid alone [34]. Gastrin has been shown to induce proliferation and activate antiapoptotic pathways in Barrett's metaplasia, suggesting that it may aid in the development and progression of Barrett's esophagus [35,36]. In another recent study, expression of gastrin was shown to be increased in non-dysplastic Barrett's esophagus biopsies compared to biopsies from normal, dysplastic and esophageal adenocarcinoma tissue [37]. Expression of gastrin is associated with induction of cyclooxygenase-2 (COX-2) in Barrett's esophagus before development of dysplasia. Together with the finding that gastrin induced proliferation in a COX-2-dependent manner, these studies suggest that autocrine production of gastrin may be involved in the pathogenesis of Barrett's esophagus, at least partly through induction of COX-2 [37]. These studies give credence to the proposal to use proton pump inhibitors in combination with COX-2 inhibitors as a chemopreventive strategy.

Despite a wealth of evidence linking reflux and the development of Barrett's esophagus summarized above, the molecular pathways involved are still largely unknown. It is hoped that mouse models, such as the combined surgical and carcinogen mouse model of Barrett's esophagus and esophageal adenocarcinoma developed by Xu *et al.* [38], may help to understand the interplay between luminal factors and the molecular mechanisms involved in the pathogenesis of Barrett's esophagus. For example, use of this model on a *p27* null background nearly doubled the incidence of Barrett's esophagus from 14% in wild-type animals to 26% in *p27* null animals [39]. In a further study, chronic administration of a pan-inhibitor of cyclin-dependent kinases, flavopiridol, markedly reduced the incidence of Barrett's esophagus on the *p27* null background [40]. The molecular mechanisms of Barrett's carcinogenesis will be discussed in more detail in a later chapter.

As only 5–10% of people with GERD have intestinal metaplasia [41], it is evident that factors other than reflux are involved in the pathogenesis of Barrett's esophagus. For example, a manometric and pH study to determine the role of GERD in Barrett's esophagus showed that patients with Barrett's esophagus had similar quantities of acid reflux than people with severe esophagitis without Barrett's esophagus [42]. Furthermore, use of proton pump inhibitors to normalize esophageal pH improves heartburn symptoms but does not lead to significant regression of Barrett's esophagus, suggesting that suppression of acid is insufficient for reversing Barrett's esophagus [43]. Other studies also indicate that surgical or pharmaceutical therapy to reduce or ablate reflux of acid and bile only result in partial regression of the metaplastic mucosa [4,44–46]. This may be due to the fact that a mild chronic inflammatory infiltrate can remain despite correction of reflux disease by acid suppressing drugs [4]. Thus, it is possible that inflammation plays a large role in the development and maintenance of Barrett's esophagus.

Inflammation in Barrett's Esophagus

Inflammation produced as a result of chronic reflux may play an important role in creating the microenvironment around the cell of origin from which the Barrett's esophagus arises. Native esophageal mucosa that has been damaged by acid and bile is commonly infiltrated by inflammatory cells of mixed lineages [47,48]. Infiltration by acute inflammatory cells is followed by T lymphocytes particularly at the site of metaplastic foci [48]. T-cell infiltrates are present in persistent areas of Barrett's esophagus following endoscopic ablation therapy, but are absent in the new squamous epithelium, suggesting that lymphocytes may be important in the maintenance of the metaplastic tissue [4,49]. One of the consequences of the inflammatory cell infiltrate is the localized production of reactive oxygen species (ROS). Indeed, increased production of ROS has been detected in the mucosa of patients with Barrett's esophagus and/or esophagitis compared to normal mucosa; however, there was no significant difference between Barrett's esophagus and esophagitis [50]. ROS can have a plethora of biological effects on cells including roles in cell cycle progression, signal transduction, protein degradation, and DNA damage (reviewed in [51]). Increased levels of DNA strand breaks, pro-mutagenic 8-hydroxydeoxyguanosine DNA lesions and lipid membrane damage have been reported in Barrett's esophagus compared to the normal mucosa [52,53]. Upregulation of genes involved in the production of ROS, such as COX-2 and nitric oxide synthase (NOS), has also been reported in Barrett's esophagus [54–56]. To compound the problem, the levels of glutathione and vitamin C, two mediators of antioxidant defence, are reduced in Barrett's epithelium [52,57]. Thus, ROS-induced DNA damage may be important not only in the development of Barrett's esophagus but may also contribute to the development of dysplasia and ultimately esophageal adenocarcinoma since DNA strand breaks may increase the neoplastic potential of a cell.

ROS can also induce the production of cytokines that can stimulate epithelial proliferation, survival, and migration. For example, inflammatory infiltrates have been shown to induce expression of Fas ligand on metaplastic cells, which may support survival of metaplastic tissue by protecting from immune surveillance [58]. Cytokines produced by the inflammatory cells and by the Barrett's epithelium in response to inflammation may include transforming growth factor-β (TGF-β), interleukin-1β (IL-1β), IL-10, IL-4, interferon-γ (IFN-γ), and tumor necrosis factor-α (TNF-α) [49,59]. It is possible that the specific cytokine profile may influence the esophageal mucosal response to reflux. Individuals who develop esophagitis display an acute inflammatory response characterized by a Th1-type pro-inflammatory cytokine profile with increased levels of IL-1β, IL-8 and IFN-γ [59]. This type of response is associated with a cellular immune response against infection and malignancy. In contrast, a Th2-type cytokine profile characterized by a small increase in IL-10 and an increase in IL-4 is associated with Barrett's esophagus [59]. Interestingly, IL-4 has been demonstrated to induce goblet cell metaplasia and mucin gene expression in airway epithelial cells [60]. A Th2-type

response is indicative of a predominantly anti-inflammatory response. In addition, this particular cytokine profile in Barrett's metaplasia does not seem to be simply a result of the development of an intestinal phenotype as this profile differed from that of gastric antrum and duodenum, which displayed a similar profile to each other [59].

The unique cytokine environment in Barrett's esophagus may be genetically predetermined. An analogous example is observed in the development of duodenal ulcer disease versus intestinal metaplasia and gastric cancer in patients with *Helicobacter pylori* infection [61]. El-Omar *et al.* demonstrated that the outcome of infection is determined by specific IL-1β polymorphisms, which influence IL-1β expression in the gastric mucosa [61]. Similarly, specific cytokine profiles may determine whether patients develop Crohn's disease or ulcerative colitis [62]. However, it is yet to be determined whether the cytokine profile is a causative factor in the development of Barrett's esophagus.

Role of Inherited Factors

There is some evidence from small case studies that genetic factors may play a role in a proportion of Barrett's esophagus cases due to strong familial clustering [63–68]. The more extensive of these studies reported a high prevalence of reflux symptoms, esophagitis, Barrett's esophagus (in some cases with associated esophageal adenocarcinoma), and other associated esophageal disorders within the families of affected individuals over several generations [64,66–68]. The pattern of affected individuals in these studies suggest that there may be autosomal dominant inheritable factors involved [64,66].

Indirect evidence for a role of inherited factors comes from a much larger study comparing the prevalence of reflux in families of patients with esophageal adenocarcinoma, Barrett's esophagus, or esophagitis to that in the families of their spouses [69]. Reflux symptoms were more common in relatives of patients with esophageal adenocarcinoma and Barrett's esophagus than in spouse-control relatives. However, recently it was reported that a higher incidence of reflux symptoms in relatives of Barrett's esophagus patients did not correlate with an increased risk of Barrett's esophagus when compared to control cases with reflux symptoms but with no family history of Barrett's esophagus [70]. A study of GERD in monozygotic and dizygotic twins also showed a genetic effect involved in the development of the disease, with an increased concordance for reflux in monozygotic twins compared with dizygotic twins [71]. However, the incidence of Barrett's esophagus was not examined.

Drovdlic *et al.* and Chak *et al.* have produced several large studies on familial predisposition to Barrett's esophagus [72–74]. One study compared 58 subjects with Barrett's esophagus, esophageal adenocarcinoma, or gastroesophageal junction adenocarcinoma and 106 control subjects with symptomatic GERD without Barrett's esophagus [74]. The prevalence of Barrett's esophagus, esophageal adenocarcinoma, or gastroesophageal junction adenocarcinoma was approximately fivefold greater (24% vs. 5%) in first- or second-degree relatives of case subjects compared with control subjects. An endoscopic study to identify new cases of Barrett's esophagus in relatives of probands known to have familial Barrett's esophagus versus relatives of probands with "isolated" Barrett's esophagus found significantly more new cases in the former group than the later, consistent with an autosomally dominant inherited trait [73].

However, despite these studies, the actual genetic mechanisms responsible for the proposed predisposition to Barrett's esophagus or esophageal adenocarcinoma are largely unknown. One candidate gene may be *GSTP1*, which encodes for glutathione *S*-transferase (GST), an enzyme involved in detoxification. A higher occurrence of a polymorphic variant of this gene, *GSTP1b*, which results in a significantly lower GST enzyme activity and thus impaired detoxification, has been reported in patients with Barrett's esophagus compared to normal controls [75]. Large-scale association studies are required to investigate the role of such candidate genes in the pathogenesis of Barrett's esophagus.

While the studies described above indicate that a subset of all Barrett's esophagus cases may be accounted for by an autosomal dominant transmission of a high penetrance germline genetic predisposition, this is unlikely to be true for the majority of

Barrett's esophagus cases. However, the majority of "isolated" Barrett's esophagus cases are likely to be influenced by the effects of multiple low penetrance genes, which may modify the response to environmental and lifestyle factors.

Host, Dietary, and Lifestyle Factors

The short time frame for the observed increase in esophageal adenocarcinoma suggests environmental factors as etiological agents, possibly interacting with genetically determined characteristics that define personal susceptibility. There are a number of studies examining the association between diet and the development of esophageal adenocarcinoma, but there are little data available with regards to Barrett's esophagus. A recent study reported that the plasma concentration of antioxidants, particularly vitamin C, was significantly lower in Barrett's esophagus patients than in matched controls [57]. In addition, lower levels of vitamin C were also found in Barrett's mucosa compared to the normal squamous mucosa from the same patients. Hence, there may be a defect in the antioxidant status of the esophageal mucosa, which makes these individuals more susceptible to the actions of ROS. However, it is not clear whether the lower vitamin C levels are due to a dietary insufficiency or a defect in absorption [57]. These data may explain the epidemiological evidence linking low consumption of fruit and vegetables with an increased risk of esophageal adenocarcinoma [76]. In addition, the tendency for lower plasma vitamin C to occur more frequently in male compared with female Barrett's esophagus patients is interesting in view of the higher frequency of Barrett's esophagus and esophageal adenocarcinoma in men [57].

Dietary nitrates have also been implicated in the development of Barrett's esophagus. Nitrates are absorbed from the small intestine into the bloodstream and approximately 25% of this is secreted into the mouth by the salivary glands, where it is rapidly converted to nitrite by bacteria (reviewed in [77]). Nitrite in swallowed saliva is converted to nitrous acid and nitrosating species upon contact with acidic gastric juice [78]. These nitrosating species have the potential to form carcinogenic *N*-nitroso compounds and can also induce oxidative stress through depletion of antioxidant species. Ascorbic acid in the gastric juice can convert the nitrosating species into nitric oxide (NO) [79,80], thus protecting against the effects of nitrosating species. However, NO reacts with oxygen to form N_2O_3, which can damage DNA directly or indirectly via reformation of *N*-nitroso compounds (reviewed in [77]). In addition, NO itself can interfere with DNA repair mechanisms, thus contributing to mutagenesis [81]. A recent study using an *in vitro* model demonstrated that NO can diffuse from the lumen into the epithelial cells [82]. In normal subjects, the highest production of NO occurs at the gastroesophageal junction where saliva and gastric acid meet [83]. Therefore, in patients with GERD the location where NO production is highest is likely to be more proximal in the esophagus.

Nitrite chemistry might be an attractive explanation for the epidemiologic characteristics of esophageal adenocarcinoma. The rising incidence of esophageal adenocarcinoma over the past few decades coincides with a 20-fold increase in the use of chemical nitrogenous fertilizers following World War II [84]. In addition, esophageal adenocarcinoma is more common in the middle socioeconomic classes [85], who might be expected to be higher consumers of green leafy vegetables, which are a common dietary source of nitrates. In contrast, *H. pylori* infection is known to lower gastric juice ascorbic acid concentrations [86] and is also negatively associated with esophageal adenocarcinoma in one study [87]. Presently it is unknown whether nitrite chemistry in the esophagus is a direct contributing factor to the pathogenesis of Barrett's esophagus, however the possibility requires further investigation.

There is no association between the existence of Barrett's esophagus and coffee intake [19]; this is despite a positive association between coffee intake and

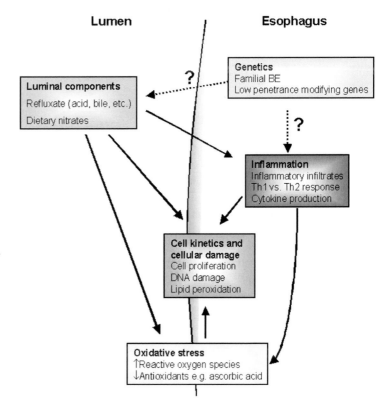

Fig. 4.2 Pathogenesis of Barrett's esophagus is multifactorial. The combination of luminal components and inflammation of the esophagus mucosa create a potent microenvironment, involving oxidative stress, cytokine production, and altered cellular kinetics, which together induce metaplastic change. This process is likely to be influenced by underlying genetic differences that define individual susceptibility.

reflux episodes in healthy subjects [88]. Alcohol and tobacco smoking are unlikely to play a major role in the development of esophageal adenocarcinoma from existing Barrett's esophagus [89], however there is some suggestion that they may influence the development of Barrett's esophagus. A history of tobacco [90] and alcohol use [19,91] has been more frequently reported in patients with Barrett's esophagus than healthy subjects. More studies with larger numbers are required to fully ascertain the role of alcohol and tobacco in Barrett's esophagus.

While a case-control study has demonstrated a strong correlation between obesity and esophageal adenocarcinoma [92], to our knowledge there are no published reports specifically examining the relationship between body mass index and Barrett's esophagus. It could be hypothesized that obesity may have a role in the pathogenesis of Barrett's esophagus indirectly through effects on gastric reflux. Increased abdominal pressure could lead to more severe reflux and may explain the predominance of Barrett's esophagus in men since fat is deposited around the abdomen more readily in men than in women. Obesity also increases risk of hiatal hernia, which as stated above is capable of promoting GERD by several mechanisms. However, further work is required in view of the contradictory evidence that currently exists on this subject.

Summary

In summary, while the pathogenesis of Barrett's esophagus is presently unclear, it is likely to be multifactorial (Fig. 4.2). Because of the strong links between esophageal adenocarcinoma and Barrett's esophagus and between Barrett's esophagus and GERD, factors involved in the development of GERD have been the focus of attention in attempts to explain the rise in incidence of esophageal adenocarcinoma. While reflux certainly plays a major role in the development of Barrett's esophagus, there is increasing evidence that associated inflammatory and other environmental factors, perhaps interacting with genetically determined characteristics, also play important roles. We propose that the microenvironment created by the combination of these factors around the cell of origin produces the selective pressure required for the generation and development of clones of cells that give rise to the metaplastic tissue.

References

1. Allison PR, Johnstone AS. The oesophagus lined with gastric mucous membrane. *Thorax* 1953;**8**(2): 87–101.
2. Bremner CG, Lynch VP, Ellis FH, Jr. Barrett's esophagus: congenital or acquired? An experimental study of esophageal mucosal regeneration in the dog. *Surgery* 1970;**68**(1):209–16.
3. Smedts F, Ramaekers FC, Vooijs PG. The dynamics of keratin expression in malignant transformation of cervical epithelium: a review. *Obstet Gynecol* 1993;**82**(3): 465.
4. Biddlestone LR, Barham CP, Wilkinson SP, Barr H, Shepherd NA. The histopathology of treated Barrett's esophagus: squamous reepithelialization after acid suppression and laser and photodynamic therapy. *Am J Surg Pathol* 1998;**22**(2):239–45.
5. Barrett MT, Sanchez CA, Prevo LJ *et al.* Evolution of neoplastic cell lineages in Barrett oesophagus. *Nat Genet* 1999;**22**(1):106–9.
6. Cameron AJ, Lomboy CT. Barrett's esophagus: age, prevalence, and extent of columnar epithelium. *Gastroenterology* 1992;**103**(4):1241–5.
7. Gillen P, Keeling P, Byrne PJ, West AB, Hennessy TP. Experimental columnar metaplasia in the canine oesophagus. *Br J Surg* 1988;**75**(2):113–5.
8. Salo JA, Kivilaakso EO, Kiviluoto TA, Virtanen IO. Cytokeratin profile suggests metaplastic epithelial transformation in Barrett's oesophagus. *Ann Med* 1996;**28**(4):305–9.
9. Jankowski JA, Wright NA, Meltzer SJ *et al.* Molecular evolution of the metaplasia–dysplasia–adenocarcinoma sequence in the esophagus. *Am J Pathol* 1999; **154**(4):965–73.
10. Meyer W, Vollmar F, Bar W. Barrett-esophagus following total gastrectomy. A contribution to its pathogenesis. *Endoscopy* 1979;**11**(2):121–6.
11. Cameron AJ, Arora AS. Barrett's esophagus and reflux esophagitis: is there a missing link? *Am J Gastroenterol* 2002;**97**(2):273–8.
12. Shields HM, Zwas F, Antonioli DA *et al.* Detection by scanning electron microscopy of a distinctive

esophageal surface cell at the junction of squamous and Barrett's epithelium. *Dig Dis Sci* 1993;**38**(1):97–108.

13. Shields HM, Sawhney RA, Zwas F *et al.* Scanning electron microscopy of the human esophagus: application to Barrett's esophagus, a precancerous lesion. *Microsc Res Tech* 1995;**31**(3):248–56.

14. Sawhney RA, Shields HM, Allan CH *et al.* Morphological characterization of the squamocolumnar junction of the esophagus in patients with and without Barrett's epithelium. *Dig Dis Sci* 1996;**41**(6):1088–98.

15. Boch JA, Shields HM, Antonioli DA *et al.* Distribution of cytokeratin markers in Barrett's specialized columnar epithelium. *Gastroenterology* 1997;**112**(3):760–5.

16. Glickman JN, Chen YY, Wang HH, Antonioli DA, Odze RD. Phenotypic characteristics of a distinctive multilayered epithelium suggests that it is a precursor in the development of Barrett's esophagus. *Am J Surg Pathol* 2001;**25**(5):569–78.

17. Winters C, Jr., Spurling TJ, Chobanian SJ *et al.* Barrett's esophagus. A prevalent, occult complication of gastroesophageal reflux disease. *Gastroenterology* 1987;**92**(1):118–24.

18. Mann NS, Tsai MF, Nair PK. Barrett's esophagus in patients with symptomatic reflux esophagitis. *Am J Gastroenterol* 1989;**84**(12):1494–6.

19. Conio M, Filiberti R, Blanchi S *et al.* Risk factors for Barrett's esophagus: a case-control study. *Int J Cancer* 2002;**97**(2):225–9.

20. Jankowski JA, Harrison RF, Perry I, Balkwill F, Tselepis C. Barrett's metaplasia. *Lancet* 2000;**356**(9247):2079–85.

21. Seto Y, Kobori O. Role of reflux oesophagitis and acid in the development of columnar epithelium in the rat oesophagus. *Br J Surg* 1993;**80**(4):467–70.

22. Campos GM, DeMeester SR, Peters JH *et al.* Predictive factors of Barrett esophagus: multivariate analysis of 502 patients with gastroesophageal reflux disease. *Arch Surg* 2001;**136**(11):1267–73.

23. Singh P, Taylor RH, Colin-Jones DG. Esophageal motor dysfunction and acid exposure in reflux esophagitis are more severe if Barrett's metaplasia is present. *Am J Gastroenterol* 1994;**89**(3):349–56.

24. Coenraad M, Masclee AA, Straathof JW *et al.* Is Barrett's esophagus characterized by more pronounced acid reflux than severe esophagitis? *Am J Gastroenterol* 1998;**93**(7):1068–72.

25. Lidums I, Holloway R. Motility abnormalities in the columnar-lined esophagus. *Gastroenterol Clin North Am* 1997;**26**(3):519–31.

26. Burgess JN, Payne WS, Andersen HA, Weiland LH, Carlson HC. Barrett esophagus: the columnar-epithelial-lined lower esophagus. *Mayo Clin Proc* 1971;**46**(11):728–34.

27. Borrie J, Goldwater L. Columnar cell-lined esophagus: assessment of etiology and treatment. A 22 year experience. *J Thorac Cardiovasc Surg* 1976;**71**(6):825–34.

28. Cameron AJ. Barrett's esophagus: prevalence and size of hiatal hernia. *Am J Gastroenterol* 1999;**94**(8):2054–9.

29. Mittal RK, Lange RC, McCallum RW. Identification and mechanism of delayed esophageal acid clearance in subjects with hiatus hernia. *Gastroenterology* 1987;**92**(1):130–5.

30. Sloan S, Kahrilas PJ. Impairment of esophageal emptying with hiatal hernia. *Gastroenterology* 1991;**100**(3):596–605.

31. Sloan S, Rademaker AW, Kahrilas PJ. Determinants of gastroesophageal junction incompetence: hiatal hernia, lower esophageal sphincter, or both? *Ann Intern Med* 1992;**117**(12):977–82.

32. Mittal RK, Balaban DH. The esophagogastric junction. *N Engl J Med* 1997;**336**(13):924–32.

33. Wild CP, Hardie LJ. Reflux, Barrett's oesophagus and adenocarcinoma: burning questions. *Nat Rev Cancer* 2003;**3**(9):676–84.

34. Tobey NA, Hosseini SS, Caymaz-Bor C *et al.* The role of pepsin in acid injury to esophageal epithelium. *Am J Gastroenterol* 2001;**96**(11):3062–70.

35. Haigh CR, Attwood SE, Thompson DG *et al.* Gastrin induces proliferation in Barrett's metaplasia through activation of the CCK2 receptor. *Gastroenterology* 2003;**124**(3):615–25.

36. Harris JC, Clarke PA, Awan A, Jankowski J, Watson SA. An antiapoptotic role for gastrin and the gastrin/CCK-2 receptor in Barrett's esophagus. *Cancer Res* 2004;**64**(6):1915–9.

37. Abdalla SI, Lao-Sirieix P, Novelli MR *et al.* Gastrin-induced cyclooxygenase-2 expression in Barrett's carcinogenesis. *Clin Cancer Res* 2004;**10**(14):4784–92.

38. Xu X, LoCicero J, III, Macri E, Loda M, Ellis FH, Jr. Barrett's esophagus and associated adenocarcinoma in a mouse surgical model. *J Surg Res* 2000;**88**(2):120–4.

39. Ellis FH, Jr., Xu X, Kulke MH, LoCicero J, III, Loda M. Malignant transformation of the esophageal mucosa is enhanced in *p27* knockout mice. *J Thorac Cardiovasc Surg* 2001;**122**(4):809–14.

40. Lechpammer M, Xu X, Ellis FH *et al.* Flavopiridol reduces malignant transformation of the esophageal

mucosa in *p27* knockout mice. *Oncogene* 2005; **24**(10): 1683–8.

41. Cameron AJ. Epidemiology of columnar-lined esophagus and adenocarcinoma. *Gastroenterol Clin North Am* 1997;**26**(3):487–94.

42. Parrilla P, Ortiz A, Martinez de Haro LF, Aguayo JL, Ramirez P. Evaluation of the magnitude of gastro-oesophageal reflux in Barrett's oesophagus. *Gut* 1990;**31**(9):964–7.

43. Sharma P, Sampliner RE, Camargo E. Normalization of esophageal pH with high-dose proton pump inhibitor therapy does not result in regression of Barrett's esophagus. *Am J Gastroenterol* 1997;**92**(4):582–5.

44. Ouatu-Lascar R, Fitzgerald RC, Triadafilopoulos G. Differentiation and proliferation in Barrett's esophagus and the effects of acid suppression. *Gastroenterology* 1999;**117**(2):327–35.

45. Li H, Walsh TN, O'Dowd G *et al*. Mechanisms of columnar metaplasia and squamous regeneration in experimental Barrett's esophagus. *Surgery* 1994; **115**(2):176–81.

46. Gore S, Healey CJ, Sutton R *et al*. Regression of columnar lined (Barrett's) oesophagus with continuous omeprazole therapy. *Aliment Pharmacol Ther* 1993;**7**(6):623–8.

47. Weston AP, Cherian R, Horvat RT *et al*. Mucosa-associated lymphoid tissue (MALT) in Barrett's esophagus: prospective evaluation and association with gastric MALT, MALT lymphoma, and *Helicobacter pylori*. *Am J Gastroenterol* 1997;**92**(5):800–4.

48. Goldblum JR, Vicari JJ, Falk GW *et al*. Inflammation and intestinal metaplasia of the gastric cardia: the role of gastroesophageal reflux and *H. pylori* infection. *Gastroenterology* 1998;**114**(4):633–9.

49. Harrison RF, Perry I, Jankowski JA. Barrett's mucosa: remodelling by the microenvironment. *J Pathol* 2000;**192**(1):1–3.

50. Olyaee M, Sontag S, Salman W *et al*. Mucosal reactive oxygen species production in oesophagitis and Barrett's oesophagus. *Gut* 1995;**37**(2):168–73.

51. Boonstra J, Post JA. Molecular events associated with reactive oxygen species and cell cycle progression in mammalian cells. *Gene* 2004;**337**:1–13.

52. Wetscher GJ, Hinder RA, Klingler P *et al*. Reflux esophagitis in humans is a free radical event. *Dis Esophagus* 1997;**10**(1):29–32; discussion 33.

53. Olliver JR, Hardie LJ, Dexter S, Chalmers D, Wild CP. DNA damage levels are raised in Barrett's oesophageal mucosa relative to the squamous epithelium of the oesophagus. *Biomarkers* 2003;**8**(6):509–21.

54. Sihvo EI, Salminen JT, Rantanen TK *et al*. Oxidative stress has a role in malignant transformation in Barrett's oesophagus. *Int J Cancer* 2002;**102**(6):551–5.

55. Morris CD, Armstrong GR, Bigley G, Green H, Attwood SE. Cyclooxygenase-2 expression in the Barrett's metaplasia–dysplasia–adenocarcinoma sequence. *Am J Gastroenterol* 2001;**96**(4):990–6.

56. Wilson KT, Fu S, Ramanujam KS, Meltzer SJ. Increased expression of inducible nitric oxide synthase and cyclooxygenase-2 in Barrett's esophagus and associated adenocarcinomas. *Cancer Res* 1998;**58**(14):2929–34.

57. Fountoulakis A, Martin IG, White KL *et al*. Plasma and esophageal mucosal levels of vitamin C: role in the pathogenesis and neoplastic progression of Barrett's esophagus. *Dig Dis Sci* 2004;**49**(6):914–9.

58. Younes M, Schwartz MR, Finnie D, Younes A. Overexpression of Fas ligand (FasL) during malignant transformation in the large bowel and in Barrett's metaplasia of the esophagus. *Hum Pathol* 1999;**30**(11): 1309–13.

59. Fitzgerald RC, Onwuegbusi BA, Bajaj-Elliott M *et al*. Diversity in the oesophageal phenotypic response to gastro-oesophageal reflux: immunological determinants. *Gut* 2002;**50**(4):451–9.

60. Dabbagh K, Takeyama K, Lee HM *et al*. IL-4 induces mucin gene expression and goblet cell metaplasia *in vitro* and *in vivo*. *J Immunol* 1999;**162**(10):6233–7.

61. El-Omar EM, Carrington M, Chow WH *et al*. Interleukin-1 polymorphisms associated with increased risk of gastric cancer. *Nature* 2000;**404**(6776):398–402.

62. Inoue S, Matsumoto T, Iida M *et al*. Characterization of cytokine expression in the rectal mucosa of ulcerative colitis: correlation with disease activity. *Am J Gastroenterol* 1999;**94**(9):2441–6.

63. Gelfand MD. Barrett esophagus in sexagenarian identical twins. *J Clin Gastroenterol* 1983;**5**(3):251–3.

64. Crabb DW, Berk MA, Hall TR *et al*. Familial gastroesophageal reflux and development of Barrett's esophagus. *Ann Intern Med* 1985;**103**(1):52–4.

65. Prior A, Whorwell PJ. Familial Barrett's oesophagus? *Hepatogastroenterology* 1986;**33**(2):86–7.

66. Jochem VJ, Fuerst PA, Fromkes JJ. Familial Barrett's esophagus associated with adenocarcinoma. *Gastroenterology* 1992;**102**(4 Pt 1):1400–2.

67. Fahmy N, King JF. Barrett's esophagus: an acquired condition with genetic predisposition. *Am J Gastroenterol* 1993;**88**(8):1262–5.

68. Eng C, Spechler SJ, Ruben R, Li FP. Familial Barrett esophagus and adenocarcinoma of the gastroesophageal junction. *Cancer Epidemiol Biomarkers Prev* 1993;**2**(4):397–9.

69. Romero Y, Cameron AJ, Locke GR, III *et al.* Familial aggregation of gastroesophageal reflux in patients with Barrett's esophagus and esophageal adenocarcinoma. *Gastroenterology* 1997;**113**(5):1449–56.

70. Romero Y, Cameron AJ, Schaid DJ *et al.* Barrett's esophagus: prevalence in symptomatic relatives. *Am J Gastroenterol* 2002;**97**(5):1127–32.

71. Cameron AJ, Lagergren J, Henriksson C *et al.* Gastroesophageal reflux disease in monozygotic and dizygotic twins. *Gastroenterology* 2002;**122**(1):55–9.

72. Drovdlic CM, Goddard KA, Chak A *et al.* Demographic and phenotypic features of 70 families segregating Barrett's oesophagus and oesophageal adenocarcinoma. *J Med Genet* 2003;**40**(9):651–6.

73. Chak A, Faulx A, Kinnard M *et al.* Identification of Barrett's esophagus in relatives by endoscopic screening. *Am J Gastroenterol* 2004;**99**(11):2107–14.

74. Chak A, Lee T, Kinnard MF *et al.* Familial aggregation of Barrett's oesophagus, oesophageal adenocarcinoma, and oesophagogastric junctional adenocarcinoma in Caucasian adults. *Gut* 2002;**51**(3):323–8.

75. van Lieshout EM, Roelofs HM, Dekker S *et al.* Polymorphic expression of the glutathione *S*-transferase P1 gene and its susceptibility to Barrett's esophagus and esophageal carcinoma. *Cancer Res* 1999;**59**(3): 586–9.

76. Zhang ZF, Kurtz RC, Yu GP *et al.* Adenocarcinomas of the esophagus and gastric cardia: the role of diet. *Nutr Cancer* 1997;**27**(3):298–309.

77. McColl KEL. When saliva meets acid: chemical warfare at the oesophagogastric junction. *Gut* 2005;**54**(1):1–3.

78. Mirvish SS. Role of *N*-nitroso compounds (NOC) and *N*-nitrosation in etiology of gastric, esophageal, nasopharyngeal and bladder cancer and contribution to cancer of known exposures to NOC. *Cancer Lett* 1995;**93**(1):17–48.

79. Suzuki H, Iijima K, Moriya A *et al.* Conditions for acid catalysed luminal nitrosation are maximal at the gastric cardia. *Gut* 2003;**52**(8):1095–101.

80. Iijima K, Fyfe V, McColl KE. Studies of nitric oxide generation from salivary nitrite in human gastric juice. *Scand J Gastroenterol* 2003;**38**(3):246–52.

81. Liu L, Xu-Welliver M, Kanugula S, Pegg AE. Inactivation and degradation of O_6-alkylguanine-DNA alkyl-transferase after reaction with nitric oxide. *Cancer Res* 2002;**62**(11):3037–43.

82. Iijima K, Grant J, McElroy K *et al.* Novel mechanism of nitrosative stress from dietary nitrate with relevance to gastro-oesophageal junction cancers. *Carcinogenesis* 2003;**24**(12):1951–60.

83. Iijima K, Henry E, Moriya A *et al.* Dietary nitrate generates potentially mutagenic concentrations of nitric oxide at the gastroesophageal junction. *Gastroenterology* 2002;**122**(5):1248–57.

84. Spechler SJ. Carcinogenesis at the gastroesophageal junction: free radicals at the frontier. *Gastroenterology* 2002;**122**(5):1518–20.

85. Brewster DH, Fraser LA, McKinney PA, Black RJ. Socioeconomic status and risk of adenocarcinoma of the oesophagus and cancer of the gastric cardia in Scotland. *Br J Cancer* 2000;**83**(3):387–90.

86. Banerjee S, Hawksby C, Miller S *et al.* Effect of *Helicobacter pylori* and its eradication on gastric juice ascorbic acid. *Gut* 1994;**35**(3):317–22.

87. Chow WH, Blaser MJ, Blot WJ *et al.* An inverse relation between *cag*A⁺ strains of *Helicobacter pylori* infection and risk of esophageal and gastric cardia adenocarcinoma. *Cancer Res* 1998;**58**(4):588–90.

88. Van Deventer G, Kamemoto E, Kuznicki JT, Heckert DC, Schulte MC. Lower esophageal sphincter pressure, acid secretion, and blood gastrin after coffee consumption. *Dig Dis Sci* 1992;**37**(4):558–69.

89. Levi F, Ollyo JB, La Vecchia C *et al.* The consumption of tobacco, alcohol and the risk of adenocarcinoma in Barrett's oesophagus. *Int J Cancer* 1990;**45**(5):852–4.

90. Hirota WK, Loughney TM, Lazas DJ *et al.* Specialized intestinal metaplasia, dysplasia, and cancer of the esophagus and esophagogastric junction: prevalence and clinical data. *Gastroenterology* 1999;**116**(2):277–85.

91. Pehl C, Pfeiffer A, Wendl B, Kaess H. Different effects of white and red wine on lower esophageal sphincter pressure and gastroesophageal reflux. *Scand J Gastroenterol* 1998;**33**(2):118–22.

92. Lagergren J, Bergstrom R, Nyren O. Association between body mass and adenocarcinoma of the esophagus and gastric cardia. *Ann Intern Med* 1999;**130**(11):883–90.

CHAPTER 5

Role of Acid and Bile in Barrett's Esophagus

Joel E. Richter

Barrett's esophagus represents a metaplastic process in which the normal squamous epithelium of the lower esophagus is replaced by specialized columnar epithelium. This condition develops in approximately 10% of patients with gastroesophageal reflux disease (GERD) [1], and represents the most severe form of GERD. Patients with Barrett's esophagus may present with serious complications in the form of strictures, ulcerations, or adenocarcinoma. The role of acid and bile reflux in the development of Barrett's esophagus and its complications is controversial and has been the subject of many animal and human studies.

Barrett's Esophagus is an Acquired Condition

Columnar epithelium lining the distal esophagus was first described in 1950 by Norman Rupert Barrett [2]. He believed that this condition was a congenital abnormality secondary to arrested regression of the esophageal glandular epithelium that normally lines the fetal esophagus. However, in 1953, Allison and Johnstone suggested an acquired nature for Barrett's esophagus based on the presence of reflux symptoms, esophagitis, and hiatal hernia in association with esophageal columnar epithelium [3]. The controversy persisted until 1970, when the landmark study by Bremner *et al.* using an experimental model of esophageal mucosal regeneration in dogs, showed columnar rather than squamous cell regeneration after severe mucosal injury from chronic gastroesophageal reflux [4]. Bremner suggested that the columnar cells in the esophagus resulted from the proximal migration of cardiac

columnar epithelium. However, later studies [5] demonstrated that columnar cells were not a direct extension of the surface lining of the adjacent stomach, but rather the metaplasia of a submucosal pleuripotential stem cell in the esophagus. The current hypothesis is that Barrett's mucosa develops from multipotent cells present in the basal layer of the esophageal mucosa, which become transformed into glandular cells after injury from the gastric contents.

Barrett's Esophagus: Acid, Bile or Both?

There is now overwhelming evidence supporting the association of GERD and Barrett's esophagus. However, the role of individual constituents of the gastric refluxate in the development of Barrett's esophagus and its associated complications still remains uncertain. Gastric acid and pepsin have received the most attention; however, the development of Barrett's esophagus in a few achlorhydric and postgastrectomy patients suggests a possible role for duodenal contents. The duodenal contents suspected of causing esophageal mucosal injury include bile acids and lysolecithin present in the bile secretions as well as the pancreatic enzyme trypsin (Fig. 5.1). We will review the role of gastric and duodenal contents in the formation of Barrett's esophagus.

Importance of Acid and Pepsin

Substantial experimental and clinical evidence strongly supports the importance of acid and pepsin in causing esophageal mucosal injury. In fact, the

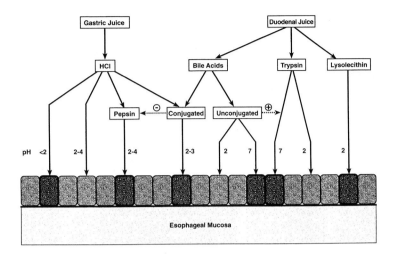

Fig 5.1 Proposed agents responsible for esophageal mucosal injury. Darkly shaded mucosal cells represent injury from the gastric refluxate.

original studies by Bremner *et al.* implicate acid reflux in formation of columnar epithelium and Barrett's esophagus [4]. In this study, high acid output produced by repeated histamine injections resulted in epithelial metaplasia and Barrett's formation. Other animal studies [6] suggested that esophageal exposure to acid alone at high concentrations, or a lower concentration in combination with pepsin, results in macroscopic and microscopic esophageal mucosa injury, predisposing the patient to columnar metaplasia and Barrett's formation (see Fig. 5.1).

Clinical studies have confirmed the presence of severe gastroesophageal reflux in patients with Barrett's esophagus. In general, these patients are characterized by decreased lower esophageal sphincter (LES) pressure, increased frequency and duration of esophageal acid exposure, and delayed esophageal acid clearance [7].

Iascone *et al.* reported a direct relationship between the severity of esophageal mucosal injury and the degree and frequency of mucosal exposure to acid reflux [8]. Subsequently, multiple studies have found that patients with Barrett's esophagus have a greater amount and more frequent acid exposure than patients with erosive esophagitis and non-erosive disease [9,10] (Fig. 5.2). Overall, these studies observe that greater than 90% of Barrett's esophagus patients, 75% with erosive esophagitis, and 50% of patients with non-erosive reflux disease have abnormal pH tests.

Other studies have attempted to define the relationship between the degree, extent, and constituents of the acid contents and the presence of Barrett's esophagus. Stein *et al.* reported that patients with Barrett's esophagus had greater exposure times to more caustic gastric acid concentrations (pH < 3.0 or 2.0), compared to those with erosive or non-erosive GERD [11]. Fass *et al.* studied 27 patients with Barrett's esophagus of various lengths, finding a significant correlation between percent total time pH < 4 and the length of Barrett's mucosa ($r = 0.6234$, $P = 0.005$) [12] (Fig. 5.3). In addition, there was a significant correlation between percent upright and supine time pH < 4 and the length of Barrett's mucosa. Patients with short segment Barrett's esophagus had significantly less esophageal acid exposure than patients with long segment Barrett's esophagus, in terms of both total acid exposure and supine time pH < 4. On the other hand, Avidan *et al.* studying 256 patients with Barrett's esophagus compared to a similar large control group, found no relationship between total acid, upright, or supine acid exposure times in the development of Barrett's esophagus [13]. Rather, their study noted that hiatal hernia and the number of reflux episodes per 24 h were critical to the development of Barrett's esophagus. They observed that the rate of hiatal hernia was 76% in Barrett's patients versus 36% in subjects without Barrett's esophagus and the reflux episodes per 24 h averaged 106 episodes in Barrett's patients versus 53 episodes in patients without Barrett's esophagus.

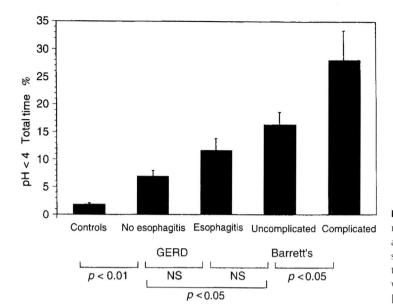

Fig. 5.2 Esophageal acid exposure, measured as percent total time pH < 4 across the spectrum of gastroesophageal reflux disease (GERD) patients. NS, not significant. Reproduced with permission from Vaezi and Richter [10].

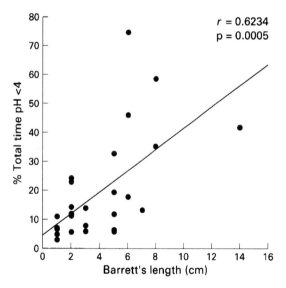

Fig. 5.3 Correlation between length of Barrett's mucosa and percent total time pH < 4, suggesting that degree of acid reflux partially contributes to the length of Barrett's esophagus. Reproduced with permission from Fass *et al.* [12].

Finally, studies show a positive correlation between the degree of abnormal acid and pepsin exposure and the severity of esophagitis in Barrett's esopha-gus. Gotley *et al.* found that esophageal aspirates from patients with esophagitis had significantly higher concentrations of acid and pepsin than the aspirates from healthy controls [14].

However, it is important to note that the frequency and duration of esophageal acid exposure is not always predictive of the degree of esophageal mucosal injury. This suggests the importance of other factors including the inherent resistance of esophageal mucosa to acid injury, the role of saliva and bicarbonate producing submucosal glands in the distal esophagus to neutralize refluxed acid, or the possibility of duodenal contents (bile or pancreatic enzymes) contributing to esophageal injury.

Importance of Bile

Although commonly referred to as "bile reflux," it is important to remember that reflux of duodenal contents contains more than just bile. Furthermore, the term "alkaline reflux" is often used interchangeably, suggesting that pH 7.0 represents the reflux of duodenal contents into the lower esophagus. However, recent studies have confirmed the inaccuracy of pH monitoring under these circumstances, suggesting that alkaline reflux is a misnomer. Therefore, duodenogastroesophageal reflux (DGER) is a more appropriate term representing the retrograde reflux of duodenal contents (bile and pancreatic enzymes) into the stomach with subsequent reflux into the esophagus. DGER is a normal phenomenon that occurs usually at night, and when extensive, it may produce symptoms or mucosal injury.

Conjugated bile acids are the predominant constituent of DGER in normal individuals and may produce esophageal mucosal injury at an acidic pH (see Fig. 5.1). Meanwhile, animal studies suggest that unconjugated bile acids and the pancreatic enzyme trypsin may cause mucosal injury at a more neutral pH value [15] (see Fig. 5.1). Some surgical groups have interpreted the latter findings to mean that aggressive acid suppression, although protective against the injurious effects of acid and possibly conjugated bile acids, may in fact perpetuate DGER, potentially causing complications in patients with Barrett's esophagus. However, the clinical importance of DGER in the absence of acid reflux in patients with esophageal mucosal injury and Barrett's esophagus remains controversial.

Methods for Measuring DGER

Prior methods used for measuring DGER have included endoscopy, aspiration studies (both gastric and esophageal), scintigraphy, and ambulatory pH monitoring; all of these have technical difficulties and do not accurately measure DGER (Table 5.1). Currently, the most commonly used methods of assessing DGER are ambulatory esophageal bilirubin monitoring and impedance monitoring of non-acidic reflux.

A few comments should be made about ambulatory 24-h pH monitoring, as it was this method of testing that raised suspicion of alkaline reflux as an important factor in Barrett's esophagus. By defining "alkaline reflux" as pH > 7.0 as an indirect marker for DGER, Attwood *et al.* reported that this phenomenon was greater in patients with Barrett's esophagus when compared to patients with esophagitis or normal controls [16]. Furthermore, they found that a pH > 7.0 was significantly higher in complicated Barrett's patients (stricture, ulcer, dysplasia) than in Barrett's patients without complications, whereas a pH < 4 did not distinguish the two groups.

Table 5.1 Current available methods for detecting duodenogastroesophageal reflux (DGER).

Method	Advantages	Disadvantages
Endoscopy	Easy to visualize bile	Poor sensitivity, specificity Requires sedation High cost
Aspiration studies	Less invasive than endoscopy No sedation, less cost	Short duration of study Requires familiarity with enzyme assay of bile acids
Scintigraphy	Non-invasive	Semi-quantitative at best Radiation exposure, high cost
pH monitoring	Ambulatory, testing up to 24 h Easy to perform Relatively non-invasive	pH > 7.0 not a marker for DGER
Bilirubin (Bilitec) monitoring	Same as above Good correlation with gastric bile acid concentrations	Underestimates DGER by about 30% in acid pH (< 3.5) Requires modified liquid diet
Multichannel intraluminal impedance	Most accurate ambulatory technique to measure non-acid reflux	Must be combined with Bilitec to measure duodenal reflux

Unfortunately, the measurement of esophageal pH > 7.0 as a marker for DGER is confounded by several problems. Precautions must be taken to use only glass electrodes; patients must observe a dietary restriction of foods with pH > 7.0; and patients must be inspected for periodontal disease and have dilation of strictures to avoid pooling of saliva. Furthermore, several investigators found that the most common reason for an increased pH in the esophagus was the increased production of saliva, probably generated by the irritation from the pH catheter [17,18]. Finally, using an ambulatory bilirubin monitoring device combined with pH monitoring, my group found no difference in the degree of the percent total time pH > 7.0 between controls, patients with GERD, and those with Barrett's esophagus [19]. With these compelling observations, the era of "alkaline reflux" as a surrogate marker for DGER ended.

The pivotal instrumentation for helping us understand DGER was the development in the early 1980s of the Bilitec 2000 system. This is an ambulatory, fiber optic probe that uses the optical property of bilirubin, the most common bile pigment, to detect DGER spectrophotometrically, independent of pH [20]. Bilirubin has a characteristic spectrophotometric absorption band at 450 nm. The basic working principal of the system is that any absorption near this wavelength implies the presence of bilirubin and, therefore, represents DGER. Several reports have indicated good correlation between Bilitec readings and bile acid concentration measured by duodenal aspiration studies ($r = 0.71$, $P \leq 0.1$ [20] and $r = 0.82$, $P \leq 0.001$) [21].

Unfortunately, this technology is only a semi-quantitative measure for detecting DGER. Validation studies from our group [21] found that this instrument underestimates bile reflux by at least 30% in an acidic medium (pH < 3.5). In solutions with pH < 3.5, bilirubin undergoes a monomer to dimer isomerization which is reflected by the shift in the absorption wavelength from 453 nm to 400 nm. Because Bilitec readings are based on the detection of absorption at 470 nm, this shift underestimates the degree of DGER. Therefore, Bilitec measurements of DGER must always be accompanied by the simultaneous measurements of acid exposure using prolonged pH monitoring. Furthermore, a variety of substances can cause false positive readings by the Bilitec, because it indiscrimately records any substance absorbing around 470 nm. This necessitates use of a modified diet to avoid interference and false readings [22]. Finally, it is important to remember that Bilitec measures reflux of bilirubin, and not bile acids or pancreatic enzymes; this, therefore, presumes that the presence of bilirubin in the refluxate is accompanied by other duodenal contents. Although this is true in most cases, a few medical conditions (Gilbert's and Dubin–Johnson syndromes) may result in a disproportionate secretion of bilirubin as compared to other duodenal contents, especially bile acids.

Multi-channel intraluminal impedance is a new technique that measures the electrical impedance of the esophagus, the opposite of conductivity, using a catheter system similar to standard manometry [23]. Based on the principal that the non-distended esophagus and esophageal mucosa have a baseline impedance (approximately 1000–2000 ohmns), material passing down or refluxing up into the esophagus generally cause a decrease in resting impedance. The only exception is air, which causes an increase in baseline impedance. When combined with a pH probe measuring acid, this technology allows measurements of both acid and non-acidic reflux as well as its migration into the proximal esophagus. However, unlike the Bilitec device, it does not identify the origin of the non-acidic reflux (i.e. duodenal contents versus neutralized gastric contents after a meal). Impedance reflux monitoring has been especially useful in defining non-acidic reflux in patients with troubling regurgitation symptoms or atypical complaints despite taking BID proton pump inhibitors (PPIs). Unfortunately, impedance is not useful in studying most patients with Barrett's esophagus because the columnar lined mucosa has a much lower baseline impedance than squamous mucosa, making it difficult to identify reflux episodes [24].

Human Studies Assessing Role of Simultaneous Acid and DGER

Despite its limitations, Bilitec is an important advancement in the assessment of DGER in the clinical

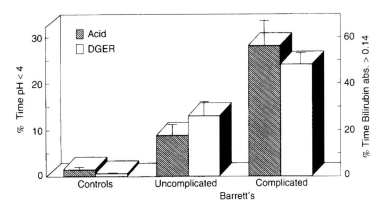

Fig. 5.4 Esophageal acid (percent of time pH < 4) and duodenogastroesophageal reflux (DGER) (percent time at bilirubin absorbance > 0.14) in controls and in patients with uncomplicated and complicated Barrett's esophagus. This study finds that acid reflux parallels DGER and both factors are highest in patients with complicated Barrett's esophagus. abs, absorbance. Reproduced with permission from Vaezi and Richter [10].

arena. Several studies using this new device have provided important insights into the role of DGER in causing esophageal mucosal injury in humans. These studies show a significant but graded increase in both acid and DGER from controls to esophagitis patients, with the highest values in patients with Barrett's esophagus. Furthermore, it appears that DGER occurs more commonly in association with acid reflux.

Recent studies of patients with and without complications of Barrett's esophagus found increased reflux of bile and acid into the lower esophagus of both groups as compared to controls [10,19]. More importantly, reflux of acid paralleled DGER, and both were significantly higher in patients with complicated Barrett's than in the uncomplicated group (Fig. 5.4). The results of these studies were recently confirmed by other investigators [25,26]. Marshall *et al.* studied 55 patients with GERD and found a good correlation between the degree of acid and DGER (*r* = 0.55) [25]. Furthermore, expanded studies by Vaezi and Richter found that simultaneous esophageal exposure to both acid and DGER was the most prevalent reflux pattern, occurring in 95% of patients with Barrett's esophagus and 79% of GERD patients [10] (Fig. 5.5). In fact, they found a strong correlation (*r* = 0.73) between acid and DGER in controls, reflux patients, and those with Barrett's esophagus. Thus, these studies support the earlier findings in animals suggesting a possible synergy between acid and DGER in the development of esophagitis and Barrett's esophagus.

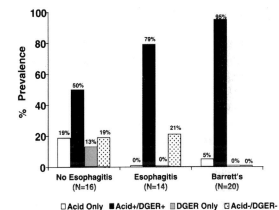

Fig. 5.5 Prevalence of esophageal acid and duodenogastroesophageal reflux (DGER) in gastroesophageal reflux disease (GERD) subgroups. Combined exposure to acid and DGER occurred in 50% of patients with non-erosive GERD, 79% of esophagitis patients and 95% of patients with Barrett's esophagus. Reproduced with permission from Vaezi and Richter [10].

Human Studies Assessing Role of DGER Alone

The role of DGER in producing esophageal mucosal injury in the absence of acid reflux has not been completely clarified. Using prolonged pH and bilirubin monitoring, studies by Marshall *et al.* of 55 patients with GERD found that DGER in the absence of acid reflux was a rare event (6%) in patients without prior gastric surgery [25]. This confirmed our earlier observations finding DGER without acid reflux in only 7% of 30 GERD patients and none of 20 patients with Barrett's esophagus [10] (see Fig. 5.5). Additionally, in our study of 32 partial gastrectomy patients who exhibited reflux symptoms, we found increased DGER either alone or combined with acid reflux in 78% of patients [26]. This patient population represents an excellent human model for increased DGER because of the incompetent pylorus and free regurgitation of duodenal contents into the stomach, resulting in gastric bile acid concentrations (0.5–3.0 mol/L) known to cause esophageal mucosal injury in the animal model (>1 mol/L). Endoscopic esophagitis, however, was present only in those who had concomitant acid reflux.

On the other hand, several recent studies suggest that DGER alone may cause esophageal mucosal injury. European studies report that DGER with acid reflux may be responsible for esophageal injury in three out of five patients with reflux esophagitis [27] or in mechanically ventilated intensive care patients [28]. However, the latter group was treated with only ranitidine, which is not the most optimal acid suppressive agent; this raises the possibilities that the origin of the esophageal mucosal injury in these ventilated patients was secondary to combined acid and DGER. A more convincing study came from Japan, where 30 patients having undergone total gastrectomy were studied with concurrent 24-h esophageal pH and Bilitec monitoring, and divided into two groups based on the endoscopic presence with ($n = 6$) and without ($n = 24$) reflux esophagitis [29]. The percent total time of esophageal bilirubin reflux was over 50% in all subjects with reflux esophagitis, whereas all but one patient without esophagitis had bile reflux values of less then 40%. The follow-up of these patients ranged from 3–48 months (median 8 months) and no patient developed Barrett's esophagus. However, isolated cases of Barrett's esophagus in human subjects after total gastrectomy have been reported [30]. This last study is convincing evidence that large amounts of bile reflux may cause reflux esophagitis and possibly Barrett's esophagus; however, the implication in most patients with an intact stomach cannot be defined by these human case series.

Two human studies have attempted to address the relationship between bile reflux and Barrett's esophagus, one by statistical modeling and the other by a clinical case series. Campo *et al.* performed a multivariate analysis of 502 patients with GERD [31]. All had undergone complete demographic, endoscopic, and physiologic evaluation including 24-h esophageal pH and Bilitec monitoring. The group was divided into 328 patients without Barrett's esophagus and 174 patients with Barrett's esophagus (67 short segment and 107 long segment Barrett's esophagus). Seven factors were identified as predictors of Barrett's esophagus. They included abnormal bile reflux, hiatal hernia larger than 4 cm, a defective LES, male gender, defective esophageal peristalsis, abnormal number of reflux episodes lasting longer than 5 min, and GERD symptoms lasting for more than 5 years. Only abnormal bile reflux (OR 4.8; 95% CI 1.7–13.2) was identified as a predictor of short segment Barrett's esophagus. Three factors were identified as predictors of long segment Barrett's esophagus—hiatal hernia, defective LES, and abnormal longest acid reflux episode. These authors argued for the primary importance of bile reflux in the development of Barrett's esophagus and the subsequent need for antireflux surgery.

Another method of addressing the importance of bile reflux alone in developing Barrett's esophagus would be to study patients after partial gastrectomy, where bile reflux is common. This was recently done by Avidan *et al.* who evaluated 650 patients with short segment and 366 patients with long segment Barrett's esophagus, comparing them to a control population of 3047 patients with GERD but without Barrett's esophagus [32]. In the case population, 25 (4%) patients with short segment and 15 (4%) patients with long segment Barrett's esophagus presented with a history of gastric surgery compared with 162 (5%) patients in the control population. Similar results were obtained in separate analyses of patients with Billroth 1 gastrectomy, Billroth 2 gastrectomy or vagotomy and pyloroplasty. Therefore, gastric surgery for benign peptic ulcer disease, with its associated reflux of bile without acid, is not sufficient to cause Barrett's esophagus.

Thus, current studies in patients with intact stomachs show that duodenal contents mix with gastric contents and both, usually in an acid milieu, reflux into the esophagus. The degree and extent of this reflux parallels the severity of GERD, increasing from healthy controls to patients with esophagitis to those with Barrett's esophagus. These findings by several groups strongly suggest the possibility that synergism between acid, pepsin, and conjugated bile acids may contribute to Barrett's metaplasia and possibly adenocarcinoma. On the other hand, evidence that bile reflux alone is injurious to the esophagus is still unresolved. After total gastrectomy, massive bile reflux may cause reflux esophagitis and possibly Barrett's esophagus. On the other hand, patients with intact stomach or only partial surgical resections show minimal evidence of bile alone causing esophageal mucosal damage.

Clinical Implications

Recent studies in patients with severe GERD found that aggressive acid suppression with PPIs dramatically decreased both acid and DGER [19,33,34]. Champion *et al.* were the first to show this phenomenon in nine patients with severe GERD (three with esophagitis, six with Barrett's esophagus) who were aggressively treated with acid suppression (omeprazole, 20 mg, twice daily) [19] (Fig. 5.6). Their findings were later reproduced by two other independent groups of investigators. Marshall *et al.*

studied esophageal and gastric bile reflux in 23 patients with Barrett's esophagus; they found a significant ($P \leq 0.005$) reduction of both esophageal and gastric acid (pH monitoring) and bile (Bilitec) reflux after 6–10 weeks of treatment with omeprazole (20 mg, twice daily) [33]. Similarly, Menges *et al.* found that esophageal acid and DGER were both significantly ($P = 0.001$) reduced after 2 weeks of treatment with 20–40 mg of omeprazole or pantoprazole [34]. Median percent time pH was <4 and bilirubin absorbance was >0.2 before and during therapy was 18.2% versus 2.3% and 29.8% versus 0.7% respectively in patients with Barrett's esophagus. These studies suggest that the decrease in DGER measured after treatment with PPIs may be due to the inhibition of both gastric acidity and volume, making less gastric contents available to reflux into the esophagus, despite a low LES pressure. Therefore, medical therapy with aggressive acid suppression may not only protect the esophageal mucosa from the damaging effects of acid, and eliminate the synergy between acid, pepsin, and bile, but also may decrease the volume of both acid and bile reflux into the esophagus.

Based on recent data, protection against the damaging effects of acid and bile reflux may only be achieved if the suppression of gastric reflux is nearly complete. Recent *ex vivo* studies from Fitzgerald *et al.* and Ouatu-Lascar *et al.* suggest that intermittent

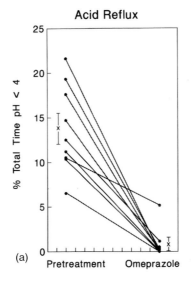
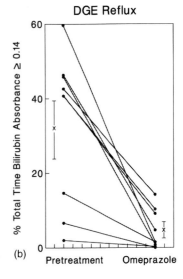

Fig. 5.6 Omeprazole 20 mg, twice daily, markedly decreases both acid reflux (a) and duodenogastroesophageal (DGE) reflux (b) in nine patients with severe gastroesophageal reflux disease (GERD). Reproduced with permission from Champion *et al.* [19]

"pulses" of acid result in enhanced Barrett's epithelial cell proliferation, possibly increasing the risk of dysplasia or adenocarcinoma [35,36]. In clinical practice, intermittent pulses of gastric acid reflux into the esophagus may occur naturally or may be due to inadequate acid suppression, despite being on PPIs. Recently, Gerson *et al.* studied 110 patients with GERD (48 with Barrett's esophagus) who were asymptomatic on PPI therapy [37]. Forty-four patients with GERD (71%) and 27 patients with Barrett's esophagus (56%) required PPIs twice daily to achieve adequate symptom control. Thirty-six patients (58%) with GERD and 24 patients (50%) with Barrett's esophagus ($P = 0.4$) normalized their intraesophageal pH profiles on PPI. Compared with GERD, patients with Barrett's esophagus were more likely to have a higher degree of pathologic acid reflux despite PPI therapy, and exhibited less intragastric acid suppression, particularly at night. In combination, these data suggest that despite symptom control, only about 50% of patients with Barrett's esophagus have their esophageal acid reflux eliminated, which may increase their chance of developing esophageal dysplasia or adenocarcinoma.

As the result of the above studies, possibly all patients with Barrett's esophagus, regardless of symptoms, should undergo serial pH testing in order to titrate the adequacy of PPI therapy. However, this approach would be time consuming, expensive, and it might interfere in the more important need for routine endoscopic surveillance. Another alternative would be to reserve serial pH testing for acid control in those patients with persistent low-grade or high-grade dysplasia, both groups more likely to develop adenocarcinoma. Nevertheless, this is a much-debated subject in the treatment of Barrett's esophagus and future studies are needed to resolve this issue before we can recommend routine esophagus pH testing to all our patients with Barrett's esophagus.

Patients with Barrett's esophagus who have a prior partial gastrectomy for peptic ulcer disease may have mild upper gastrointestinal symptoms due to nonacidic DGER. Administration of aluminum hydroxide containing antacids (30 mL, four times a day), cholestyramine (1 g, four times a day), or ursodeoxycholic acid may improve symptoms [38]. Addition-

ally, in a recent randomized double blind crossover study, cisapride (20 mg, four times a day) was found to significantly reduce both DGER measured by the Bilitec and associated upper gastrointestinal symptoms (i.e. abdominal pain, bloating, belching, regurgitation, nausea, and vomiting) in patients after vagotomy and antrectomy or pyloromyotomy for chronic ulcer disease [39]. Thus, medical therapy with promotility drugs is an alternative to surgical Roux-en-Y diversion, although cisapride's limited availability due to safety issues reduces its utility.

These observations have important implications for treating patients with both acid and bile reflux. Medical therapy may decrease both acid and DGER to a similar degree as antireflux surgery. Medical therapy has the advantage of avoiding a surgical procedure and its associated complications, which is an important consideration for older Barrett's patients and those with contraindications to surgery. However, in younger patients in whom long term medical therapy is anticipated, antireflux surgery may be a more suitable and cost-effective alternative.

References

1. Spechler SJ, Goyal RK. Barrett's esophagus. *N Engl J Med* 1986;**315**:362–71.
2. Barrett NR. Chronic peptic ulcer of the esophagus and "esophagitis." *Br J Surg* 1950;**38**:175–82.
3. Allison PR, Johnstone AS. The esophagus lined with gastric mucous membrane. *Thorax* 1953;**8**:87–101.
4. Bremner CG, Lynch VP, Ellis FH. Barrett's esophagus: congenital or acquired? An experimental study of esophageal mucosal regeneration in the dog. *Surgery* 1970;**68**:209–16.
5. Gillen P, Keeling P, Byrne PJ *et al.* Experimental columnar metaplasia in the canine esophagus. *Br J Surg* 1988;**75**:113–5.
6. Goldberg HI, Dodds, WJ, Gee S *et al.* Role of acid and pepsin in acute experimental esophagitis. *Gastroenterology* 1969;**56**:223–30.
7. Stein HJ, Hoeft S, DeMeester TR. Reflux and motility pattern in Barrett's esophagus. *Dis Esop* 1992;**5**:21–8.
8. Iascone C, DeMeester TR, Little AG, Skinner DB. Barrett's esophagus: functional assessment, proposed pathogenesis and surgical therapy. *Arch Surg* 1983;**118**:543–9.

9. Falk GW. Barrett's esophagus. *Gastroenterology* 2002;**122**:1569–91.

10. Vaezi MF, Richter JE. Role of acid and duodenogastroesophageal reflux in gastroesophageal disease. *Gastroenterology* 1996;**111**:1192–9.

11. Stein HJ, Hoeft S, DeMeester TR. Functional foregut abnormalities in Barrett's esophagus. *J Thorac Cardiovasc Surg* 1993;**105**:107–11.

12. Fass R, Hell RW, Garewal HS *et al.* Correlation of oesophageal acid exposure with Barrett's oesphagus length. *Gut* 2001;**48**:310–3.

13. Avidan B, Sonnenberg A, Schnell TG, Sontag SJ. Hiatal hernia and acid reflux frequency predict presence and length of Barrett's esophagus. *Dig Dis Sci* 2002;**47**:256–64.

14. Gotley DC, Morgan AP, Ball D *et al.* Composition of gasto-oesophageal refluxate. *Gut* 1991;**32**:1093–9.

15. Kivilaakso E, Fromn D, Silen W. Effect of bile salts and related compounds on isolated esophageal mucosa. *Surgery* 1980;**87**:280–5.

16. Attwood SEA, DeMeester TR, Bremner CG, Barlow AP, Hinder RA. Alkaline gastroesophageal reflux implications in the development of complications in Barrett's columnar-lined lower esophagus. *Surgery* 1989;**106**:764–76.

17. Singh S, Bradley LA, Richter JE. Determinants of oesophageal alkaline pH environment in controls and patients with gastro-oesophageal reflux disease. *Gut* 1993;**34**:309–16.

18. DeVault KR, Georgeson S, Castell DO. Salivary stimulation mimics esophageal exposure to refluxed duodenal contents. *Am J Gastroenterol* 1993;**88**:1040–3.

19. Champion G, Richter JE, Vaezi MF *et al.* Duodenogastroesophageal reflux: relationship to pH and importance in Barrett's esophagus. *Gastroenterology* 1994;**107**:747–54.

20. Bechi P, Paucciani F, Baldini F *et al.* Long-term ambulatory enterogastric reflux monitoring. Validation of a new fiber optic technique. *Dig Dis Sci* 1993;**38**:1297–306.

21. Vaezi MF, LaCamera RG, Richter JE. Validation studies of Bilitec 2000: an ambulatory duodenogastric reflux monitoring system. *Am J Physiol* 1994;**30**:G1050–7.

22. Tack J, Bisschops R, Koele G *et al.* Dietary restrictions during ambulatory monitoring of duodenogastroesophageal reflux. *Dig Dis Sci* 2003;**48**:1213–20.

23. Tutuian R, Vela MF, Shay SS, Castell DO. Multichannel intraluminal impedance in esophageal function testing and gastroesophageal reflux monitoring. *J Clinical Gastroenterol* 2003;**37**:206–15.

24. Orlando RC. Esophageal potential difference measurements in esophageal disease. *Gastroenterology* 1982;**83**:1026–31.

25. Marshall REK, Anggiansah A, Owen WA, Owen WJ. The relationship between acid and bile reflux and symptoms in gastroesophageal reflux disease. *Gut* 1997;**40**:182–7.

26. Vaezi MF, Richter JE. Contribution of acid and DGER to esophageal mucosal injury and symptoms in partial gastrectomy patients. *Gut* 1997;**41**:297–302.

27. Marshall REK, Anggiansah A, Owen WA, Owen WJ. Investigation of oesophageal reflux symptoms after gastric surgery with combined pH and bilirubin monitoring. *Br J Surg* 1999;**86**:271–5.

28. Wilmer A, Tack J, Frinas E *et al.* Duodenogastroesophageal reflux and esophageal mucosal injury in mechanically ventilated patients. *Gastroenterology* 1999;**116**:1293–9.

29. Yumiba T, Kawahara H, Nishikawa K *et al.* Impact of esophageal bile exposure on the genesis of reflux esophagitis in the absence of gastric acid after total gastrectomy. *Am J Gastroenterol* 2002;**97**:1647–52.

30. Westhoff BC, Weston A, Cherian R, Sharma P. Development of Barrett's esophagus 6 months after total gastrectomy. *Am J Gastroenterol* 2004;**99**:2271–7.

31. Campo GM, DeMeester SR, Peters JH *et al.* Predictive factors for Barrett's esophagus. Multivariate analysis of 502 patients with gastroesophageal reflux disease. *Arch Surg* 2001;**136**:1267–73.

32. Avidan B, Sonnenberg A, Schnell TG, Sontag SJ. Gastric surgery is not a risk for Barrett's esophagus or esophageal adenocarcinoma. *Gastroenterology* 2001;**121**:1288–5.

33. Marshall REK, Anggiansah A, Manifold DK *et al.* Reduction of gastroesophageal bile reflux by omeprazole in Barrett's esophagus: an initial experience. *Gut* 1998;**43**:603–6.

34. Menges M, Muller M, Zeitz M. Increased acid and bile reflux in Barrett's esophagus compared to reflux esophagitis, and effect of proton pump inhibitor therapy. *Am J Gastroenterol* 2001;**96**:331–7.

35. Fitzgerald RC, Omary MB, Triadafilopoulos G. Dynamic effect of acid on Barrett's esophagus. *J Clin Invest* 1996;**98**:2120–8.

36. Ouatu-Lascar R, Fitzgerald RC, Triadafilopoulos G. Differentiation and proliferation in Barrett's esophagus and the effect of acid suppression. *Gastroenterology* 1999;**117**:327–35.

37. Gerson LB, Bopara V, Ullah N, Triadafilopoulos G. Oesophageal and gastric pH profiles in patients with gastro-oesophageal reflux disease and Barrett's

oesophagus treated with proton pump inhibitors. *Aliment Pharmacol Ther* 2004;**20**:637–43.

38. Richter JE. Duodenogastric reflux-induced (alkaline) esophagitis. *Curr Treat Options in Gastroenterol* 2004;**7**:53–8.

39. Vaezi MF, Sears R, Richter JE. Double-blind placebo-controlled cross-over trial of cisapride in postgastrectomy patients with duodenogastric reflux. *Dig Dis Sci* 1996;**41**:754–63.

CHAPTER 6

Esophageal Motility Abnormalities in Barrett's Esophagus

John E. Pandolfino and Peter J. Kahrilas

Introduction

Although the etiology of Barrett's metaplasia is uncertain, it is clearly associated with gastroesophageal reflux disease (GERD) [1]. Early studies quantifying gastroesophageal reflux in Barrett's esophagus and GERD patients concluded that Barrett's esophagus patients represented an extreme end of the spectrum [2–4]. When studies were controlled for the grade of esophagitis it became evident that acid exposure was increased in Barrett's esophagus compared to patients with non-erosive GERD and mild to moderate esophagitis, but that the difference in acid exposure between patients with severe esophagitis and Barrett's esophagus were insignificant [5]. However, despite the general agreement that esophageal acid exposure is increased with Barrett's esophagus, there is less certainty as to whether or not there are unique motor abnormalities in Barrett's esophagus distinct from the GERD population in general.

Greater acid exposure in Barrett's esophagus is a consequence of both an increased frequency of reflux events and impaired esophageal acid clearance. Given the similarities between the acid exposure profile of severe esophagitis it is not surprising that the motility abnormalities are also comparable. Unfortunately, there is a paucity of data focused specifically on motor abnormalities in Barrett's esophagus and consequently, motility abnormalities in Barrett's esophagus will be discussed within the context of those associated with severe esophagitis. Owing to their importance in the pathogenesis of acid induced mucosal damage, abnormalities of the antireflux barrier, esophageal clearance, and gastric function will each be reviewed. Particular emphasis will be given to the discussion of the motility abnormalities associated with hiatal hernia because of the strong association of this condition with Barrett's esophagus.

Antireflux Barrier

A prerequisite for the development of GERD is the reflux of gastric contents into the esophagus, an event indicative of dysfunction of the esophagogastric junction (EGJ). The EGJ is a complex anatomic zone whose functional integrity is attributable to both the intrinsic lower esophageal sphincter (LES) pressure and extrinsic compression of the LES by the crural diaphragm. Loss of EGJ integrity occurs by three dominant mechanisms: (i) transient LES relaxations (tLESRs); (ii) LES hypotension; or (iii) anatomic disruption of the EGJ inclusive of but not limited to hiatal hernia [6,7]. Transient LES relaxations are the dominant mechanism of reflux in patients with mild to moderate GERD [6]. Patients with severe GERD differ from those with mild to moderate reflux in that a greater proportion of their reflux occurs in the context of decreased LES pressure and a co-existent hiatal hernia [8,9]. Given the fact that patients with Barrett's esophagus have comparable acid exposure to patients with severe GERD it should not be surprising that Barrett's esophagus is usually associated with decreased LES pressure [10–12] and hiatal hernia [13–16].

Lower Esophageal Sphincter

The LES is a 3–4 cm segment of tonically contracted smooth muscle at the EGJ. Resting LES tone varies among normal individuals from 10–30 cm Hg relative to intragastric pressure and continuous pressure monitoring reveals considerable temporal variation. Large fluctuations of LES pressure occur with the migrating motor complex; during phase III, LES pressure may exceed 80 mmHg. Lesser fluctuations occur throughout the day with pressure decreasing in the postcibal state and increasing during sleep [17]. The genesis of LES tone is a property of both the smooth muscle itself and of its extrinsic innervation [18]. At any given moment, LES pressure is affected by myogenic factors, intra-abdominal pressure, gastric distention, peptides, hormones, various foods, and many medications.

Early reports indicated that patients with Barrett's esophagus had lower LES pressures compared to either control subjects or patients with reflux disease [3,19]. However, in 1987 Gillen *et al.* reported no difference in LES pressure between patients with Barrett's esophagus and those with esophagitis [2]. This study, however, included a high proportion of patients with severe esophagitis (16 of 25 patients with grade 3–4 esophagitis). Given these conflicting results, subsequent investigations measured the LES pressure in patients with stratified grades of esophagitis and Barrett's esophagus [5,20]. These studies supported the observation that the LES pressure in patients with Barrett's esophagus were decreased to the same degree as seen with severe esophagitis. Furthermore analogous to the situation with esophageal acid exposure, patients with Barrett's esophagus and esophagitis had lower LES pressure than Barrett's esophagus patients without esophagitis [20].

Gastroesophageal reflux can occur in the context of low LES pressure either by strain-induced or free reflux. Manometric studies suggest that strain-induced reflux or free reflux is unlikely unless the LES pressure is below 10 and 4 cmHg respectively [21]. It is also a rare occurrence in patients without hiatus hernia [22]. Free reflux is characterized by a fall in intraesophageal pH without an identifiable change in either intragastric pressure or LES pressure. Episodes of free reflux are observed only when the LES pressure is within 0–4 cmHg of intragastric pressure. A wide-open or patulous hiatus will predispose to this free reflux as both the intrinsic and the extrinsic sphincter are compromised. From the above discussion it is apparent that many patients with Barrett's esophagus are at risk for strain induced or free reflux.

Compelling evidence exists that tLESRs are the most frequent mechanism for reflux during periods of normal LES pressure (>10 mmHg). Transient LES relaxations occur independently of swallowing, are not accompanied by peristalsis, are accompanied by crural diaphragm inhibition, and persist for longer periods than do swallow-induced LES relaxations (>10 s) [23,24]. Of note, prolonged manometric recordings have not consistently demonstrated an increased frequency of tLESRs in GERD patients compared to normal controls [25]. However, the frequency of acid reflux (as opposed to gas reflux) during tLESRs has been consistently reported to be greater in GERD patients [25,26]. Similar to patients with severe esophagitis and large hiatus hernias, Barrett's esophagus patients are also subject to tLESRs. Patel *et al.* studied seven patients with Barrett's esophagus using concurrent manometry and pH monitoring and reported that tLESRs accounted for 64% of reflux events [27]. This is similar to the frequency of tLESRs found in patients with severe esophagitis and hiatus hernia and further supports the hypothesis that both groups have a similar compromise of EGJ function [22,24,28].

Diaphragmatic Sphincter and Hiatal Hernia

Most patients with severe esophagitis have a hiatal hernia, and consequently there is a high prevalence of hiatal hernia in Barrett's esophagus. Cameron reported finding a ≥2 cm hernia in 96% of patients with Barrett's esophagus and 72% of patients with short segment Barrett's esophagus [13] (Fig. 6.1). The role that hiatal hernia plays in compromising the antireflux barrier is multifactorial. From an anatomical perspective, hiatal hernia may be associated with widening of the diaphragmatic hiatus, thus limiting the ability of the right crus to function as a sphincter (Fig. 6.2). In addition to this anatomical consideration, the physiologic function of the crural diaphragm may be compromised by its dissociation from the LES.

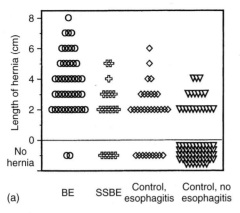

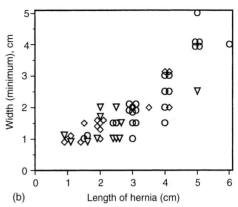

Fig 6.1 (a) Axial length of hiatal hernia in Barrett's esophagus. The prevalence of hiatal hernia and extent of axial herniation in four patient populations: (i) long segment Barrett's esophagus (intestinal metaplasia involving >3 cm of the esophagus); (ii) short segment Barrett's esophagus (intestinal metaplasia involving <3 cm of the esophagus); (iii) controls with esophagitis; and (iv) controls without esophagitis. The prevalence and size of hiatal hernia is increased in Barrett's esophagus. BE, Barrett's esophagus; SSBE, short segment Barrett's esophagus; circle, Barrett's esophagus; cross, short segment Barrett's esophagus; diamond, controls with esophagitis; triangle, controls without esophagitis. (b) Width of diaphragmatic hiatus in two dimensions measured endoscopically. Patients with Barrett's epithelium had wider openings than controls with and without esophagitis. Circle, Barrett's esophagus; diamond, controls with esophagitis; triangle, controls without esophagitis. Reproduced with permission from Cameron [13].

Fig 6.2 Anatomy of the diaphragmatic hiatus: normal and hiatus hernia. The right crus makes up the muscular component of the crural diaphragm. Arising from the anterior longitudinal ligament overlying the lumbar vertebrae. A single muscle band splits into an anterior and posterior muscular band that cross each other to form the walls of the hiatal canal and then fuse anteriorly. With hiatus hernia the muscle becomes thin and atrophic limiting its ability to function as a sphincter.

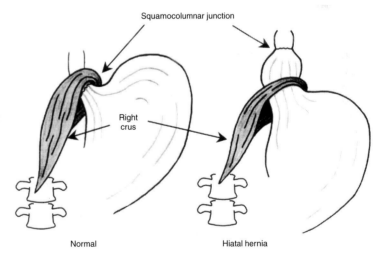

Evidence of a specialized role of the crural diaphragm in preventing reflux begins with the observation that the costal and crural diaphragm can function independently. During the LES relaxation associated with vomiting electrical activity is absent in the crural diaphragm but active in the costal diaphragmatic dome [29]. A similar pattern is evident during tLESR and belching [24]. Additional evidence of the sphincteric role of the hiatus are manometric data from patients after oncologically prompted removal of the distal esophagus [30]. These patients still exhibit a high-pressure zone within the hiatal canal. In addition to contributing to basal pressure, the crural diaphragm augments the EGJ during activities associated with increased intra-abdominal pressure. The importance of this function was evident in studies in which gastroesophageal reflux was elicited by straining maneuvers in individuals with graded severity of hiatus hernia [8]. Of several physiologic and anatomical variables tested, the size of the hiatal hernia was shown to have the highest correlation with the susceptibility to strain-induced reflux. The implication of this observation is that patients with hiatus hernia exhibit progressive impairment of the EGJ proportional to the length of axial herniation.

The patulous hiatal canal associated with large hiatal hernias also affects the antireflux barrier during swallowing. One of the differences between a swallow induced LES relaxation and a tLESR is the crural inhibition, which occurs only with the latter [24]. In the presence of a large hiatal hernia, as is often the case in Barrett's esophagus patients, the hiatal canal is distorted to the point where it becomes a patulous orifice incapable of achieving luminal closure during inspiration (see Fig. 6.2). Under these circumstances, deglutitive LES relaxation, which usually is accompanied by continued respiratory contraction, becomes indistinguishable from a tLESR. As a result, the EGJ opens at the onset of any LES relaxation, including deglutitive relaxation, thereby broadening the set of circumstances associated with reflux.

Yet another effect hiatal hernia exerts on the antireflux barrier pertains to diminishing both the length and intrinsic pressure of the LES. Relevant animal experiments revealed that simulating the effect of hiatal hernia by severing the phrenoesophageal ligament reduced the LES pressure and that the subsequent repair of the ligament restored the LES pressure to levels similar to baseline [31]. Similarly, manometric studies in humans using a topographic representation of the EGJ high pressure zone of hiatal hernia patients revealed a distinct intrinsic sphincter and hiatal canal pressure components, each of which was of lower magnitude than the EGJ pressure of a comparator group of normal controls [32]. However, simulating reduction of the hernia by arithmetically repositioning the intrinsic

sphincter back within the hiatal canal resulted in calculated EGJ pressures that were practically indistinguishable from those of the control subjects. These and previous studies also demonstrated that hiatus hernia may also affect the overall length of the LES high pressure zone [33]. Combined manometric and fluoroscopic studies found that both peak EGJ pressure and length negatively correlated with hiatal hernia size. This is likely due to disruption of the EGJ segment distal to the squamocolumnar junction attributable to the gastroesophageal flap valve [34].

Mechanical Properties of the Relaxed EGJ

For reflux to occur in the setting of a relaxed or hypotensive sphincter it is necessary for the relaxed sphincter to open. Recent physiologic studies exploring the role of compliance in GERD reported that GERD patients without and particularly with hiatus hernia had increased compliance at the EGJ compared to normal subjects [35] and patients with fundoplication [36]. These experiments utilized a combination of barostat-controlled distention, manometry, and fluoroscopy to directly measure the compliance of the EGJ. Several parameters of EGJ compliance were shown to be increased in hiatus hernia patients with GERD: (i) the EGJ opened at lower distention pressure; (ii) the relaxed EGJ opened at distention pressures that were at or near resting intragastric pressure; and (iii) for a given distention pressure the EGJ opened about 0.5 cm wider. Still significant, but lesser compliance related changes were demonstrated in the non-hernia GERD patients (Fig. 6.3). These alterations of EGJ mechanics are likely secondary to a disrupted, distensible crural aperture and may be the root causes of the physiological aberrations associated with GERD.

Increased EGJ compliance may help explain why patients with hiatus hernia have a distinct mechanistic reflux profile compared to patients without hiatus hernia [22]. Anatomical alterations, such as hiatal hernia, dilatation of the diaphragmatic hiatus, and disruption of the gastroesophageal flap valve may alter the elastic characteristics of the hiatus such that

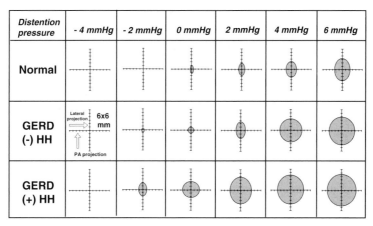

Distention pressure	- 4 mmHg	- 2 mmHg	0 mmHg	2 mmHg	4 mmHg	6 mmHg
Normal						
GERD (-) HH	*Lateral projection* 6x6 mm *PA projection*					
GERD (+) HH						

Fig 6.3 Dimensions and radial symmetry of the esophagogastric junction (EGJ). Measurements of EGJ opening diameters were made from posterior–anterior and lateral fluoroscopic projections and are plotted for each intrabag pressures relative to intragastric pressure distention pressure. Some degree of radial asymmetry of the hiatus was seen in all three groups; the lateral diameters were similar among the three groups but the hiatal hernia and non-hiatal hernia gastroesophageal reflux disease (GERD) patients had increased PA diameters compared to normal subjects. Reproduced with permission from Pandolfino *et al.* [35].

this factor is no longer protective in preventing gastroesophageal reflux. In that setting, reflux no longer requires "two hits" to the EGJ because the extrinsic sphincteric mechanism is chronically disrupted. Thus, the only prerequisite for reflux becomes LES relaxation, be that in the setting of swallow-induced relaxation, tLESR, or a period of prolonged LES hypotension. Patients with Barrett's esophagus will likely have abnormal compliance at the EGJ secondary to the high prevalence of hiatus hernia. Whether EGJ compliance is altered to a greater extent in Barrett's esophagus patients versus GERD patients with severe esophagitis with and without hiatus hernia is unclear.

Esophageal Clearance

Following reflux, the period that the esophageal mucosa remains at a pH < 4 is defined as the acid clearance time. Acid clearance begins with emptying of the refluxed fluid from the esophagus by peristalsis and is completed by the titration of residual acid by the buffering effect of swallowed saliva [37]. Prolongation of esophageal clearance among patients with esophagitis was demonstrated along with the initial description of an acid clearance test. Subsequent studies suggest that about 50% of patients with GERD exhibit prolonged esophageal acid clearance [1]. Clinical data from patients with Barrett's esophagus also suggest prolonged acid clearance. Scintigraphic studies demonstrated impaired esophageal emptying in 50–80% of Barrett's esophagus patients [38,39]. Ambulatory pH studies subsequently confirmed prolonged acid clearance in Barrett's esophagus patients and added further insight by stratifying the esophagitis patients by severity. Gillen *et al.* reported that after separating out patients with severe esophagitis and comparing them to patients with Barrett's esophagus there was no significant difference in acid clearance [2]. Several other reports have subsequently confirmed this observation and it is now generally accepted that patients with severe esophagitis and Barrett's esophagus have similar defects in esophageal clearance [5,20]. Investigations also confirm the additive effect of esophagitis and Barrett's esophagus on impairment of acid clearance with the combination being worse than either entity alone [5]. Ambulatory pH monitoring studies suggest that the heterogeneity within the GERD population, with respect to acid clearance, is at least partially attributed to hiatus hernia, as these individuals tended to have the most prolonged supine acid clearance [40].

Hiatal Hernia and Esophageal Clearance

Although, hiatal hernia is probably not an independent risk factor for developing Barrett's esophagus, it is an important contributor to the underlying pathogenesis of increased acid exposure both by compromising the antireflux barrier as discussed above and by impairing the process of acid clearance. Concurrent pH recording and scintigraphic scanning over the EGJ showed that impaired clearance was caused by reflux of fluid from the hernia sac during swallowing [41]. This observation was subsequently confirmed radiographically when Sloan and Kahrilas analyzed esophageal emptying in patients with reducing and non-reducing hiatal hernias [42]. The efficacy of emptying was significantly diminished in both hernia groups when compared to normal controls. Emptying was particularly impaired in the non-reducing hiatal hernia patients who exhibited complete emptying with only one third of test swallows. These patients with non-reducing hernias were the only group that exhibited retrograde flow of fluid from the hernia during deglutitive relaxation, consistent with the scintigraphic studies.

The mechanism of impaired esophageal emptying is evident from an analysis of esophageal emptying in the normal patient [43]. Typically, LES relaxation occurs within 3 s of the swallow but LES opening does not occur until the bolus reaches the distal esophagus. In order for the LES to open, pressure acting on the lumen of the sphincter must overcome the pressure acting extrinsic to the lumen. Since the normal position of the distal esophagus is intra-abdominal, the intragastric pressure acting to open the distal esophagus is negated by external pressure of equal magnitude. However, once the distal esophagus is positioned above the diaphragm the extrinsic pressure at the LES is reduced, more reflective of intrathoracic pressure. This leads to LES opening at the time of relaxation and early retrograde flow of gastric contents from the stomach into the low-pressure esophagus. Hiatal hernia also impairs the function of the crural diaphragm as a one-way valve during distal esophageal emptying owing to the persistence of a gastric pouch above the diaphragm. Both of these effects are particularly evident while in a recumbent posture.

Peristaltic Dysfunction

Peristaltic dysfunction in esophagitis has been described by a number of investigators. Failed peristalsis and hypotensive contractions (<30 mmHg) which result in incomplete emptying are of particular significance [44]. As esophagitis increases in severity, so does the incidence of failed peristalsis and hypotensive contractions [45] (Fig. 6.4). More recent investigations of peristaltic function has labeled this "ineffective esophageal motility," defined by the occurrence of >30% of hypotensive or failed contractions. Applying this definition, a significant increase in recumbent esophageal acid exposure time compared to patients with normal motility, esophageal spasm, nutcracker esophagus and hypertensive LES was reported [46]. With respect to the reversibility of

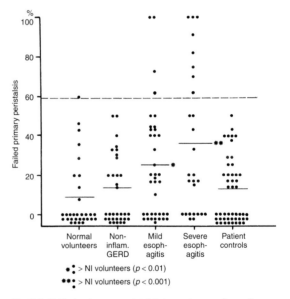

Fig 6.4 Failed primary peristalsis in gastroesophageal reflux disease (GERD). Primary peristalsis was classified as failed if either no peristaltic contraction followed deglutition or if peristalsis did not traverse the entire length of the esophagus. Compared with controls the mean failure rate of primary peristalsis was significantly greater in patients with esophagitis (P < 0.001). Non-parametric analysis of data from the control groups yielded a value of 51% as the upper limit of the 95% confidence interval (indicated by the horizontal dashed line). Each dot indicates the value for an individual subject. NI, non-inflammatory. Reproduced with permission from Kahrilas *et al.* [45].

peristaltic dysfunction, recent studies show no improvement after healing of esophagitis by acid inhibition [47], or by antireflux surgery [48].

Although early investigations reported normal peristaltic function in Barrett's esophagus [49,50], these studies can be criticized on methodological grounds and more recent data reveal that peristaltic dysfunction is prevalent in Barrett's esophagus patients. Similar to the case of esophagitis patients, patients with Barrett's esophagus exhibit both failed and ineffective contractions when compared to controls. Parrilla *et al.* reported that Barrett's esophagus patients had a higher incidence of failed peristalsis than both controls and patients with mild esophagitis [20]; there was no difference when he compared Barrett's esophagus patients to patients with severe esophagitis. However, when he separated the Barrett's esophagus population into those with esophagitis and without esophagitis there was a significant difference such that patients with concomitant esophagitis and Barrett's esophagus had failed peristalsis 23% of the time compared to 1.7% in patients without esophagitis. This suggests that the increased peristaltic dysfunction is more dependent on chronic inflammation than on metaplasia.

Esophageal contractility is impaired in a qualitatively similar way in patients with Barrett's esophagus and patients with severe esophagitis. Mean peristaltic amplitude is lower than in either controls [4] or patients with mild esophagitis [5]. Furthermore, patients with severe esophagitis and Barrett's esophagus both exhibit ineffective esophageal motility as previously defined [51]. Two studies evaluating peristaltic amplitude in Barrett's esophagus patients with and without esophagitis found no difference between the two groups [5,20]. However, Mason compared the esophageal contractility of patients with extensive Barrett's esophagus (>5 cm) to patients with more limited Barrett's esophagus (3–5 cm) and found that patients with extensive disease exhibited a significant decrease in peristaltic amplitude [52]. Adding to the controversy, Loughney *et al.* compared patients with long (>3 cm) and short segment (<3 cm) Barrett's esophagus and showed no difference in peristaltic contraction between the two groups [53]. However, the patients with long segment Barrett's esophagus did have significantly reduced peristaltic amplitude compared to normal subjects raising the issue of a type II error in this investigation.

Gastric Emptying and Duodenogastroesophageal Reflux

Gastric emptying may be impaired in 41–57% of patients with GERD [54]. Defects in gastric emptying may exacerbate reflux by increasing the gastroesophageal pressure gradient thereby promoting reflux or by increasing tLESR frequency as a result of increased gastric distention. However, contrary to what one would expect, patients with Barrett's esophagus have been shown to have relatively normal gastric emptying and two published series revealed no difference in either solid or liquid phase gastric emptying [55,56]. Probably of more interest, given the recent description of an unbuffered acid pocket after meals, are potential abnormalities in proximal stomach acid pooling [57]. Whether Barrett's esophagus patients, or GERD patients for that matter, have abnormalities in proximal stomach acid pooling has yet to be determined.

Normal gastric emptying in Barrett's esophagus is also surprising given the recent interest in duodenogastroesophageal reflux as a possible pathogenic mechanism in the development and progression of Barrett's esophagus. Studies suggest that duodenal contents may act synergistically with acid to damage the esophageal epithelium [58]. The motility abnormalities that promote duodenogastroesophageal reflux have not been determined; given the reported data, however, impaired gastric emptying does not appear to be a major mechanism. Studies of transpyloric flow and antroduodenal motility in patients with GERD similarly have revealed no functional abnormalities [59].

Therapy of Motor Abnormalities in Barrett's Esophagus

Medical Management

Most investigations of the effect of antireflux therapy on motor function suggest that no improvement is demonstrable after healing esophagitis [39,47]. Given the likely irreversibility of reflux related motor dysfunction, treatment with motility modifying agents may seem appropriate. Unfortunately the therapeutic efficacy of available agents is disappointing. The two most widely used motility agents in reflux are metoclopramide and cisapride. Metoclopramide has been shown to increase LES pressure via increased release of acetylcholine in the enteric nervous system; this has not been shown to have a beneficial impact on reflux [60]. Whether or not metoclopramide improves esophageal peristalsis is controversial. An early study suggested a 39% increase in peristaltic amplitude after intravenous metoclopramide [61] but two more recent randomized, controlled, double blinded studies in GERD patients failed to show any improvement [62,63]. Similar to the data with metoclopramide, cisapride has proven ineffective at augmenting LES pressure or esophageal peristalsis. Cisapride is a mixed serotonergic agent with 5HT-3 antagonist and 5HT-4 agonist properties that also enhances the release of acetylcholine from postganglionic fibers in the myenteric plexus. Several studies have reported minor increases in LES pressure and peristaltic amplitude with cisapride therapy, but as with metoclopramide, these effects were not clinically relevant [60]. Thus, the best available clinical evidence suggests that promotility drugs do not significantly improve esophageal motor function. The minimal increases in LES pressure observed are insignificant in patients with severely compromised LESs. Similarly, the mild increase in peristaltic amplitude is unlikely to improve esophageal clearance. Other than hiatus hernia, failed peristalsis is the more important mechanism of impaired esophageal emptying and unfortunately, neither metoclopramide nor cisapride impact that feature of peristaltic dysfunction. In summary, poor efficacy and a poor side effect profile make these agents unsuitable for treatment of motility abnormalities in Barrett's esophagus.

Surgical Treatment

Antireflux surgery improves the antireflux barrier in patients with GERD with several studies demonstrating a significant increase in EGJ pressure after fundoplication [3,64,65]. Along with improved EGJ pressure, the anatomic defect of hiatal hernia is also repaired. A more controversial and debated question is whether or not fundoplication improves esophageal peristalsis in patients with esophagitis and Barrett's esophagus. A number of studies suggest that antireflux surgery increases peristaltic amplitude [65,66]. However, even if real and not a methodological artifact attributable to the operation, these changes would be unlikely to improve impaired clearance which is largely attributable to failed peristalsis. No study has shown a reduction in the frequency of failed peristalsis or restoration of peristalsis in an aperistaltic patient as a result of antireflux surgery.

Conclusion

Barrett's epithelium is a result of increased esophageal acid exposure similar to that seen with severe esophagitis. Thus, it is not surprising that these two groups of reflux patients have similar motility abnormalities with both patient populations exhibiting a compromised antireflux barrier and prolonged esophageal acid clearance. Central to the mechanism of these defects is the association of both Barrett's esophagus and severe esophagitis with hiatal hernia. Why some patients with severe esophagitis develop Barrett's esophagus, and some do not, remains to be determined, but the epidemiological literature suggests that this is at least partially a function of genetic predisposition. Other factors, such as the role of duodenogastroesophageal reflux, are being explored. Neither medical nor surgical therapy corrects the peristaltic defect associated with Barrett's esophagus, although antireflux therapy clearly creates an effective antireflux barrier.

Acknowledgements

This work was supported by grant RO1 DC00646 (PJK) from the Public Health Service and K23 DK062170-01 (JEP) from the Public Health Service.

References

1. Lidums I, Holloway R. Motility abnormalities in the columnar-lined esophagus. *Gastroenterol Clin North Am* 1997;**26**(3):519–31.
2. Gillen P, Keeling P, Byrne PJ, Hennessy TP. Barrett's oesophagus: pH profile. *Br J Surg* 1987;**74**(9):774–6.

3. Iascone C, DeMeester TR, Little AG, Skinner DB. Barrett's esophagus. Functional assessment, proposed pathogenesis, and surgical therapy. *Arch Surg* 1983; **118**(5):543–9.

4. Singh P, Taylor RH, Colin-Jones DG. Esophageal motor dysfunction and acid exposure in reflux esophagitis are more severe if Barrett's metaplasia is present. *Am J Gastroenterol* 1994;**89**(3):349–56.

5. Coenraad M, Masclee AA, Straathof JW *et al*. Is Barrett's esophagus characterized by more pronounced acid reflux than severe esophagitis? *Am J Gastroenterol* 1998;**93**(7):1068–72.

6. Dodds WJ, Dent J, Hogan WJ *et al*. Mechanisms of gastroesophageal reflux in patients with reflux esophagitis. *N Engl J Med* 1982;**307**(25):1547–52.

7. Kahrilas PJ. GERD revisited: advances in pathogenesis. *Hepatogastroenterology* 1998;**45**(23):1301–7.

8. Sloan S, Rademaker AW, Kahrilas PJ. Determinants of gastroesophageal junction incompetence: hiatal hernia, lower esophageal sphincter, or both? *Ann Intern Med* 1992;**117**(12):977–82.

9. Barham CP, Gotley DC, Mills A, Alderson D. Precipitating causes of acid reflux episodes in ambulant patients with gastro-oesophageal reflux disease. *Gut* 1995; **36**(4):505–10.

10. Brandt MG, Darling GE, Miller L. Symptoms, acid exposure and motility in patients with Barrett's esophagus. *Can J Surg* 2004;**47**(1):47–51.

11. Zentilin P, Reglioni S, Savarino V. Pathophysiological characteristics of long- and short-segment Barrett's oesophagus. *Scand J Gastroenterol Suppl* 2003;**239**: 40–3.

12. Oberg S, DeMeester TR, Peters JH *et al*. The extent of Barrett's esophagus depends on the status of the lower esophageal sphincter and the degree of esophageal acid exposure. *J Thorac Cardiovasc Surg* 1999;**117**(3): 572–80.

13. Cameron AJ. Barrett's esophagus: prevalence and size of hiatal hernia. *Am J Gastroenterol* 1999;**94**(8):2054–9.

14. Avidan B, Sonnenberg A, Schnell TG, Sontag SJ. Hiatal hernia and acid reflux frequency predict presence and length of Barrett's esophagus. *Dig Dis Sci* 2002;**47**(2): 256–64.

15. Avidan B, Sonnenberg A, Schnell TG *et al*. Hiatal hernia size, Barrett's length, and severity of acid reflux are all risk factors for esophageal adenocarcinoma. *Am J Gastroenterol* 2002;**97**(8):1930–6.

16. Wakelin DE, Al-Mutawa T, Wendel C *et al*. A predictive model for length of Barrett's esophagus with hiatal hernia length and duration of esophageal acid exposure. *Gastrointest Endosc* 2003;**58**(3):350–5.

17. Dent J, Dodds WJ, Friedman RH *et al*. Mechanism of gastroesophageal reflux in recumbent asymptomatic human subjects. *J Clin Invest* 1980;**65**(2):256–67.

18. Goyal RK, Rattan S. Genesis of basal sphincter pressure: effect of tetrodotoxin on lower esophageal sphincter pressure in opossum *in vivo. Gastroenterology* 1976;**71**(1):62–7.

19. Heitmann P, Csendes A, Strauszer T. Esophageal strictures and lower esophagus lined with columnar epithelium. Functional and morphologic studies. *Am J Dig Dis* 1971;**16**(4):307–20.

20. Parrilla P, Ortiz A, Martinez de Haro LF, Aguayo JL, Ramirez P. Evaluation of the magnitude of gastro-oesophageal reflux in Barrett's oesophagus. *Gut* 1990;**31**(9):964–7.

21. Kahrilas PJ. Anatomy and physiology of the gastro-esophageal junction. *Gastroenterol Clin North Am* 1997;**26**(3):467–86.

22. van Herwaarden MA, Samsom M, Smout AJ. Excess gastroesophageal reflux in patients with hiatus hernia is caused by mechanisms other than transient LES relaxations. *Gastroenterology* 2000;**119**(6):1439–46.

23. Holloway RH, Penagini R, Ireland AC. Criteria for objective definition of transient lower esophageal sphincter relaxation. *Am J Physiol* 1995;**268**(1 Pt 1):G128–33.

24. Mittal RK, Holloway RH, Penagini R, Blackshaw LA, Dent J. Transient lower esophageal sphincter relaxation. *Gastroenterology* 1995;**109**(2):601–10.

25. Sifrim D, Holloway R. Transient lower esophageal sphincter relaxations: how many or how harmful? *Am J Gastroenterol* 2001;**96**(9):2529–32.

26. Sifrim D, Holloway R, Silny J *et al*. Acid, nonacid, and gas reflux in patients with gastroesophageal reflux disease during ambulatory 24-hour pH-impedance recordings. *Gastroenterology* 2001;**120**(7):1588–98.

27. Patel GK, Clift SA, Read RC. Mechanisms of gastroesophageal reflux in patients with Barrett's esophagus. *Gastroenterology* 1982;**82**:A1146.

28. Dent J, Holloway RH, Toouli J, Dodds WJ. Mechanisms of lower oesophageal sphincter incompetence in patients with symptomatic gastrooesophageal reflux. *Gut* 1988;**29**(8):1020–8.

29. Monges H, Salducci J, Naudy B. Dissociation between the electrical activity of the diaphragmatic dome and crura muscular fibers during esophageal distension, vomiting and eructation. An electromyographic study in the dog. *J Physiol (Paris)* 1978;**74**(6):541–54.

30. Klein WA, Parkman HP, Dempsey DT, Fisher RS. Sphincter like thoracoabdominal high pressure zone after esophagogastrectomy. *Gastroenterology* 1993; **105**(5):1362–9.

31. Friedland GW. Historical review of the changing concepts of the lower esophageal anatomy: 430 BC–1977. *Am J Roentgenol* 1978;**131**:373–88.

32. Kahrilas PJ, Lin S, Manka M, Shi G, Joehl RJ. Esophagogastric junction pressure topography after fundoplication. *Surgery* 2000;**127**(2):200–8.

33. Kahrilas PJ, Lin S, Chen J, Manka M. The effect of hiatus hernia on gastro-oesophageal junction pressure. *Gut* 1999;**44**(4):476–82.

34. Hill LD, Kozarek RA, Kraemer SJ *et al*. The gastroesophageal flap valve: *in vitro* and *in vivo* observations. *Gastrointest Endosc* 1996;**44**(5):541–7.

35. Pandolfino JE, Shi G, Trueworthy B, Kahrilas PJ. Esophagogastric junction opening during relaxation distinguishes nonhernia reflux patients, hernia patients, and normal subjects. *Gastroenterology* 2003;**125**(4):1018–24.

36. Curry J, Shi G, Pandolfino JE *et al*. Mechanical characteristics of the EGJ after fundoplication compared to normal subjects and GERD patients. *Gastroenterology* 2001;**120**:A112.

37. Helm JF. Role of saliva in esophageal function and disease. *Dysphagia* 1989;**4**(2):76–84.

38. Karvelis KC, Drane WE, Johnson DA, Silverman ED. Barrett esophagus: decreased esophageal clearance shown by radionuclide esophageal scintigraphy. *Radiology* 1987;**162**(1 Pt 1):97–9.

39. Singh P, Adamopoulos A, Taylor RH, Colin-Jones DG. Oesophageal motor function before and after healing of oesophagitis. *Gut* 1992;**33**(12):1590–6.

40. Johnson LF. Twenty-four hour pH monitoring in the study of gastroesophageal reflux. *J Clin Gastroenterol* 1980;**2**(4):387–99.

41. Mittal RK, Lange RC, McCallum RW. Identification and mechanism of delayed esophageal acid clearance in subjects with hiatus hernia. *Gastroenterology* 1987;**92**(1):130–5.

42. Sloan S, Kahrilas PJ. Impairment of esophageal emptying with hiatal hernia. *Gastroenterology* 1991;**100**(3):596–605.

43. Lin S, Brasseur JG, Pouderoux P, Kahrilas PJ. The phrenic ampulla: distal esophagus or potential hiatal hernia? *Am J Physiol* 1995;**268**(2 Pt 1):G320–7.

44. Kahrilas PJ, Dodds WJ, Hogan WJ. Effect of peristaltic dysfunction on esophageal volume clearance. *Gastroenterology* 1988;**94**(1):73–80.

45. Kahrilas PJ, Dodds WJ, Hogan WJ *et al*. Esophageal peristaltic dysfunction in peptic esophagitis. *Gastroenterology* 1986;**91**(4):897–904.

46. Leite LP, Johnston BT, Barrett J, Castell JA, Castell DO. Ineffective esophageal motility (IEM): the primary finding in patients with nonspecific esophageal motility disorder. *Dig Dis Sci* 1997;**42**(9):1859–65.

47. Timmer R, Breumelhof R, Nadorp JH, Smout AJ. Oesophageal motility and gastro-oesophageal reflux before and after healing of reflux oesophagitis. A study using 24 hour ambulatory pH and pressure monitoring. *Gut* 1994;**35**(11):1519–22.

48. Rydberg L, Ruth M, Lundell L. Does oesophageal motor function improve with time after successful antireflux surgery? Results of a prospective, randomised clinical study. *Gut* 1997;**41**(1):82–6.

49. Burgess JN, Payne WS, Andersen HA, Weiland LH, Carlson HC. Barrett esophagus: the columnar–epithelial-lined lower esophagus. *Mayo Clin Proc* 1971;**46**(11):728–34.

50. Robbins AH, Hermos JA, Schimmel EM, Friedlander DM, Messian RA. The columnar-lined esophagus—analysis of 26 cases. *Radiology* 1977;**123**(1):1–7.

51. Stein HJ, Eypasch EP, DeMeester TR, Smyrk TC, Attwood SE. Circadian esophageal motor function in patients with gastroesophageal reflux disease. *Surgery* 1990;**108**(4):769–77; discussion 777–8.

52. Mason RJ, Bremner CC. Motility differences between long-segment and short-segment Barrett's esophagus. *Am J Surg* 1993;**165**(6):686–9.

53. Loughney T, Maydonovitch CL, Wong RK. Esophageal manometry and ambulatory 24-hour pH monitoring in patients with short and long segment Barrett's esophagus. *Am J Gastroenterol* 1998;**93**(6):916–9.

54. McCallum RW. Gastric emptying in gastroesophageal reflux and the therapeutic role of prokinetic agents. *Gastroenterol Clin North Am* 1990;**19**(3):551–64.

55. Johnson DA, Winters C, Drane WE *et al*. Solid-phase gastric emptying in patients with Barrett's esophagus. *Dig Dis Sci* 1986;**31**(11):1217–20.

56. Kogan FJ, Kotler J, Sampliner R. Normal gastric emptying in Barrett's esophagus. *Gastroenterology* 1985;**88**:A1451.

57. Fletcher J, Wirz A, Young J, Vallance R, McColl KE. Unbuffered highly acidic gastric juice exists at the gastroesophageal junction after a meal. *Gastroenterology* 2001;**121**(4):775–83.

58. Vaezi MF, Richter JE. Importance of duodeno-gastroesophageal reflux in the medical outpatient practice. *Hepatogastroenterology* 1999;**46**(25):40–7.

59. King PM, Pryde A, Heading RC. Transpyloric fluid movement and antroduodenal motility in patients with gastro-oesophageal reflux. *Gut* 1987;**28**(5):545–8.

60. Pandolfino JE, Howden CW, Kahrilas PJ. Motility-modifying agents and management of disorders of gastrointestinal motility. *Gastroenterology* 2000;**118**(2 Suppl 1):S32–47.

61. DiPalma JA, Perucca PJ, Martin DF, Pierson WP, Meyer GW. Metoclopramide effect on esophageal peristalsis in normal human volunteers. *Am J Gastroenterol* 1987;**82**(4):307–10.

62. Grande L, Lacima G, Ros E *et al*. Lack of effect of meto-clopramide and domperidone on esophageal peristalsis and esophageal acid clearance in reflux esophagitis. A randomized, double-blind study. *Dig Dis Sci* 1992;**37**(4):583–8.

63. McCallum RW, Fink SM, Winnan GR, Avella J, Callachan C. Metoclopramide in gastroesophageal reflux disease: rationale for its use and results of a double-blind trial. *Am J Gastroenterol* 1984;**79**(3):165–72.

64. Sagor G. Hiatus hernia: slip sliding away. *Nurs Mirror* 1982;**154**(13):39–41.

65. Ortiz Escandell A, Martinez de Haro LF, Parrilla Paricio P *et al*. Surgery improves defective oesophageal peristalsis in patients with gastro-oesophageal reflux. *Br J Surg* 1991;**78**(9):1095–7.

66. Wetscher GJ, Glaser K, Gadenstaetter M, Profanter C, Hinder RA. The effect of medical therapy and antire-flux surgery on dysphagia in patients with gastroesophageal reflux disease without esophageal stricture. *Am J Surg* 1999;**177**(3):189–92.

CHAPTER 7

Mucosal Defense in Barrett's Esophagus

Roy C. Orlando

Abstract

Barrett's esophagus is a clinical condition synonymous with the presence of a metaplastic specialized
columnar epithelium (SCE) lining the distal esophagus. It develops within the esophagus in ~10% of
subjects with reflux esophagitis—and this as replacement for the native stratified squamous epithelium
(SSE) that was damaged by exposure to refluxed
acid–pepsin. Though SCE has a high rate of cell
turnover that increases the risk of esophageal adenocarcinoma, SCE remains stable for life in over 90%
of Barrett's subjects—and some of these subjects, in
part because of SCE's acid resistance, are (reflux)
symptom-free. For these reasons, then, SCE can be
viewed in most subjects as a "successful adaptation"
for esophageal protection against more severe reflux
injury—injury capable of extending deeper into the
esophageal wall to produce an ulceration potentially
complicated by life-threatening hemorrhage or perforation. Given the prevalence and stability of SCE in
most subjects, surprisingly little is known about its
biology and particularly about the means by which it
resists reflux injury. Nonetheless, using a variety of
disparate sources and recently published preliminary data, a working model of mucosal defense in
Barrett's esophagus is presented which emphasizes
those features that make SCE uniquely suited for
survival in a reflux setting.

Introduction

Barrett's esophagus is a clinical condition synonymous with the presence of a metaplastic specialized
columnar epithelium (SCE) lining the distal esophagus. It develops within the esophagus in ~10% of
subjects with reflux esophagitis—and this as replacement for the native stratified squamous epithelium
(SSE) that was damaged by exposure to refluxed
acid–pepsin [1]. SCE, histologically, is a single-
layered tissue with villiform architecture whose
cells typically are of three phenotypes: mucus,
pseudoaborptive, and goblet cells [2]. The goblet
cells are particularly distinctive in that they stain
deeply blue for acidic mucins with Alcian blue, pH
2.5, and this feature is of value in establishing the diagnosis of Barrett's esophagus on esophageal biopsy.

The origin of the cells from which SCE emerges remains unclear, although current theories suggest
that they arise by clonal growth of a pluripotential
(stem) cell derived from either esophageal SSE, gastric epithelium, or ducts of esophageal submucosal
glands [3–5]. A "pluripotential" cell, rather than
growth of an adjacent cell type is supported by the
unique structural and functional characteristics of
SCE, which has features more typical of the small
and large intestine. Although some animal models
suggest that the cell of origin is by upward growth of
gastric epithelium or by outward growth of ductular
epithelium from esophageal submucosal glands, the
columnar lining arising from these models has not
been shown to be SCE in type [6,7]; moreover, in the
rodent models that do develop SCE—this by exposure of the esophagus to acid and bile by creation of
an esophagogastroduodenostomy or esophagoduo-
denostomy [8,9]—esophageal submucosal glands
are absent. Consequently, and based largely on the
presence in Barrett's esophagus of a multilayered epithelium with cytokeratin staining representative of
both squamous and columnar phenotypes, the cell

of origin is believed to originate in squamous epithelium [3]. Further, since human and animal data suggest that reflux is critical for the generation of Barrett's esophagus, the outgrowth of these cells appears to be promoted by direct contact with the refluxate or by contact with inflammatory products produced by reflux-induced injury [3–9]. Recent evidence also suggests that the transition from squamous to SCE phenotype may be mediated by activation of CDX1 and/or CDX2, two homeobox proteins known to play a major role in development of the normal intestine. Both proteins are present in Barrett's esophagus and neither are found in normal gastric or esophageal epithelium [10,11]. Further, ectopic expression of CDX1 or CDX2 protein in transgenic mice has been shown to induce intestinal metaplasia in gastric epithelium and esophageal epithelial cells transfected with the *CDX2* gene have been shown to have this gene activated by chronic exposure to acid [12–14]. Additional support for a role of the CDX1/CDX2 proteins in the development of SCE is provided by Wong *et al.* [15]. They observed that exposure to bile salts and inflammation (tumor necrosis factor-α [TNF-α], interleukin 1β [IL-1β]) could activate CDX1 through NF-κB signaling but only in cell lines in which the CDX1 promoter was either unmethylated or partially methylated [15]. In effect the data support demethylation of the CDX1 promoter as one means by which refluxates or reflux-induced inflammatory products can trigger the activation of a homeobox protein—in this case, CDX1—so that it can serve to induce and maintain an intestinal phenotype typical of Barrett's esophagus.

A vital feature of the pluripotential cells is that they survive to form SCE in an environment noxious enough to destroy the cells that give rise to esophageal SSE, and this they do by having superior defensive capabilities against acid, pepsin, and bile within the refluxate. The fact that SCE has greater acid resistance than SSE, is supported by the following observations: (a) esophageal acid perfusion in Barrett's esophagus elicits no symptoms or symptoms less severe than those with reflux uncomplicated by Barrett's esophagus [16]; (b) most subjects with Barrett's esophagus lack sufficient reflux symptoms to seek medical care [17]; (c) ablation of SCE

heals with SSE when acidity is controlled by proton pump inhibitors (PPIs) [18,19]; and (d) ablation of SSE heals with columnar epithelium when esophageal acidity is enhanced by promoting reflux [7]. In one sense then the development of SCE represents a "successful adaptation" for protection against further reflux injury—injury with the capability of extending deeper into the esophageal wall to produce an ulceration potentially complicated by life-threatening hemorrhage or perforation.

Although SCE represents a successful adaptation to a hostile environment, it has a downside in that it is a premalignant lesion that increases the risk of esophageal adenocarcinoma [20–22]. This risk of cancer is estimated at 30–40 times that of the general population or one in 200 (0.5%) patients per year for an overall lifetime cancer risk of ~5% [1,5,23]. Viewed from the opposite perspective, the data indicate that the large majority (95%) with Barrett's esophagus live with stable SCE for a lifetime. Further, stability is maintained whether or not the subject receives antireflux therapy. This is the case since most with Barrett's esophagus lack sufficient symptoms to seek medical help and so remain undiagnosed and effectively untreated [1,24,25]. In addition, the only sure means of preventing malignancy in Barrett's esophagus is its complete eradication through esophagectomy. However, esophagectomy has significant morbidity (~25%) and mortality (~5%) and so its use is reserved for those with high-grade dysplasia or adenocarcinoma [1,26]. Consequently, even after diagnosis, SCE generally remains in place to perform those functions required of an epithelial lining in the lower esophagus—and, even with acid suppressive therapy, it does so in a decidedly inhospitable environment due to ongoing reflux of duodenogastric cotents.

How SCE provides protection under chronic reflux conditions has not been rigorously investigated. Consequently, knowledge of its protective biology remains rudimentary, even though such mechanisms are at the heart of its very existence. Nonetheless, using a variety of disparate sources and recently published preliminary data, a working model of mucosal defense in Barrett's esophagus is presented

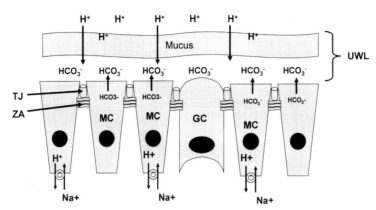

Fig. 7.1 Mucosal defense in Barrett's esophagus. A working model of the mucosal defenses in Barrett's is shown to contain the following components: mucus layer, surface bicarbonate within unstirred water layer, apical cell membrane with capacity for bicarbonate transport, intercellular junctional complex composed of tight junctions and zonula adherens, intracellular buffers, and regulators of intracellular pH such as Na^+/H^+ exchanger. This system is supported by the blood supply, which is not shown. GC, goblet cell; MC, mucus cell; TJ, tight junction; UWL, unstirred water layer; ZA, zonula adherens.

here which emphasizes those features that make SCE uniquely suited for survival in the reflux setting (Fig. 7.1).

Mucosal Defense in Barrett's Esophagus

Mucosal defense is a self-evident term that encompasses those features that enable the mucosa to defend itself against an injurious substance. The major injurious substances for the esophagus are those refluxed into the lumen from the stomach—namely acid, pepsin, and bile salts. How SCE defends against these products is the primary focus of this presentation. For discussion purposes, mucosal defense can be separated into three components based on the relationship to the epithelium proper. They are: (i) the preepithelial (lumen-side); (ii) epithelial (epithelium proper); and (iii) postepithelial (blood-side) components. Individual factors under these components are listed in Table 7.1 and include for SCE a mucus layer, surface bicarbonate, unstirred water layer, apical cell membranes, junctional complex, buffers, ion transporters, blood supply, and repair [27]. Each of these defenses is described below, with the exception of blood flow where data for SCE are notably lacking.

Table 7.1 Mucosal defense in Barrett's esophagus.

Preepithelial components
Mucus layer
Unstirred water layer
Surface bicarbonate
Epithelial components
Apical cell membrane
Membrane ion transporters
Regulators of cell pH
Bicarbonate secretion
Intercellular junctional complex
Tight junctions
Zonula adherens
Cytosolic buffers
Carbonic anhydrase
Intercellular buffers
Epithelial repair
Postepithelial components
Blood supply

A global measure of mucosal health and integrity is the electrical potential difference (PD). The PD follows Ohm's Law in that it is the mathematical product of net current flow across the tissue times the tissue's electrical resistance; and as a mucosal property it is generated almost exclusively by the epithelium. Indeed the PD reflects two characteristic properties of the epithelium—its ion transport and barrier function [28]. Moreover, since each epithelium has a unique set of transporters and barriers, specific epithelial types have characteristic PD values. For instance, *in vivo* esophageal SSE combines high electrical resistance with low current flow to yield a PD that averages ~–15 mV [29]. In contrast, *in vivo* esophageal SCE combines a high current flow with low electrical resistance to yield a PD that averages ~–30 mV [30]. Examples of these differences for SCE and SSE are shown diagrammatically in Fig. 7.2. Moreover, these differences in PD can be detected *in vitro* in biopsies of SCE and SSE when mounted in

mini-Ussing chambers; and consequently this property can be utilized for further investigation of the structures and functions responsible for mucosal defense—for details, see below.

Preepithelial Factors in Mucosal Defense

Among the preepithelial factors for mucosal defense against reflux injury are the surface mucus layer, unstirred water layer, and bicarbonate ions. These factors protect in at least two important ways: (i) surface mucus forms a covering of viscoelastic gel that entraps and prevents large molecules, e.g. pepsin and bile salts, from gaining access to the epithelium; and (ii) bicarbonate ions secreted from surface cells or diffusing from blood via the paracellular pathway are enmeshed within the mucus and unstirred water layer where they serve to neutralize hydrogen ions (H^+) diffusing from lumen to epithelium [27,31] (see Fig. 7.1). The capacity for neutralization of H^+ by the preepithelial factors can be illustrated by recording the lumen-to-surface pH gradient under conditions of varying luminal acidity. When this has been done *in vivo* in humans for gastric or duodenal epithelium, a luminal pH of 2.0 resulted in a pH of 6–7 at the surface of the epithelium—amounting to support of a gradient for H^+ of 100 thousand to 1 million to 1. In contrast, the SSE-lined human esophagus was much less robust yielding at luminal pH 2.0, a surface pH of 2.0–3.0—amounting to at most a gradient of only 10 to 1 [32]. The capacity of Barrett's esophagus to sustain a pH gradient has not been recorded *in vivo*; however, the lumen-to-surface pH gradients for SCE and SSE have been measured and compared *in vitro* using biopsies mounted in mini-Ussing chambers and pH microelectrodes. The results showed that at luminal pH 3.5, SCE maintained a surface pH of ~5 while at luminal pH 3.5, SSE maintained a surface pH of ~4 [33]. This indicates that under similar degrees of luminal acidity SCE has a 10-fold greater capacity to neutralize back diffusing H^+ than SSE—and as such support is provided for the hypothesis that SCE arises in reflux subjects in place of SSE because of its greater acid resistance.

The mechanisms responsible for the greater acid resistance of SCE over SSE have not been fully eluci-

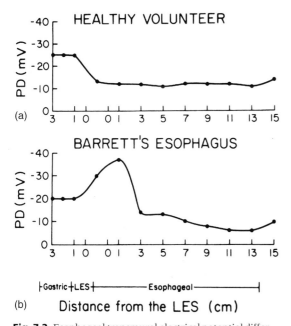

Fig. 7.2 Esophageal transmural electrical potential difference (PD) profiles are shown for a subject with a healthy esophagus lined by stratified squamous epithelium (SSE) and for a subject with a long segment (3 cm) of Barrett's esophagus. The PD values that are recorded were localized to the different regions of esophagus by simultaneous measurements of esophageal pressure so that the values could be referenced as distance above, below, or within the high-pressure zone created by the lower sphincter. LES, lower esophageal sphincter. Modified and reproduced with permission from Herlihy *et al.* [30].

dated. Nonetheless, one factor that likely contributes to the difference is the presence in SCE, but not SSE, of a surface mucus layer [34]. This is illustrated in biopsies of healthy human esophagus and Barrett's esophagus by staining with Alcian blue/periodic acid–Schiff (PAS) (Plate 7.1a,b; color plate section falls between pp. 148–9). Of additional interest is that all cells in SCE secrete mucins and that these mucins are secreted from different areas and have differing biologic properties. For instance, MUC5AC and MUC3 are strongly expressed in the surface epithelium, MUC2 in the goblet cells and MUC6 in the cells of the glands [35–37]. Moreover, MUC5AC and MUC6 are associated with protection of the stomach against acid, and MUC2 and MUC3 are associated with protection of small intestine against bile. Consequently SCE, as producer of all four mucins, appears uniquely suited for defense against a refluxate containing mixtures of both acid and bile salts. As noted above, SSE has no surface mucus layer; but while SSE secretes no mucins, MUC5B is secreted by the esophageal submucosal glands [35,36]. MUC5B, however, is a soluble mucin useful for lubrication but not for surface protection by formation of a gel layer [35]. Consequently, SSE has greater exposure to luminal content, such as pepsin and bile salts, and more limited surface buffering of backdiffusing H^+. Indeed, this weakness of preepithelial defense in SSE-lined esophagus has been suggested as one reason why greater levels of acid suppression are needed for control of symptoms and for lesion healing in reflux esophagitis than in peptic ulcer disease—the former generally requiring PPI therapy and the latter only requiring histamine-2 receptor antagonists [38].

A second factor that likely contributes to the greater acid resistance of SCE over SSE is that SCE secretes significant quantities of bicarbonate ions (see Fig. 7.1). This has been documented by mounting biopsies containing SCE in mini-Ussing chambers and showing that removal of bathing solution bicarbonate reduces its sizable (short–circuit) current by ~6 μAmps/cm^2 while similar experiments with SSE showed a reduction in current by ~0.5 μAmps/cm^2 [39]. This represents a 12-fold greater amount of bicarbonate secreted by SCE compared to SSE. What mechanisms account for bicarbonate secretion in

SCE currently remains under investigation as does the contribution to surface buffering of both SCE and SSE by bicarbonate secreted by the esophageal submucosal glands [40].

Epithelial Defense

The epithelial defense comes into play when surface buffering is exceeded by back diffusing H^+. This occurs, for example, when luminal pH is reduced to 2.0 *in vitro* in both SSE-lined and SCE-lined esophagus [33]. At this point, surface acidity approaches the potentially injurious levels of luminal acidity, and this requires the epithelium proper to revert to another set of defenses for protection against cell injury and death (see Table 7.1). The epithelial defense in SSE has been investigated in both human and rabbit esophagus and is quite robust when it comes to withstanding an attack by luminal H^+. For instance, perfusion of the rabbit esophagus with HCl, pH 2.0, for up to 3 h results in no injury [27,41]—though its vulnerability can be markedly enhanced by the addition of the proteolytic enzyme, pepsin, to the acidic solution [42]. As in the rabbit, the healthy human esophagus is also highly acid resistant. This is illustrated by the lack of symptoms or signs of injury during esophageal perfusion with HCl, pH 1.1, for 30 min (Bernstein test) [43]. The success of this defense is primarily the result of combining two diffusion barriers with two buffering systems. The two diffusion barriers for H^+ are those provided by the apical membrane and intercellular junctional complex [44–46]. The apical membrane resists H^+ penetration by virtue of its lipid bilayers and, though it also possesses cation channels for Na^+ absorption, these channels have been shown to be inhibited at acid pH [45]. Similarly, the intercellular junctions are not aqueous highways for the free diffusion of H^+ into the intercellular space. This is due to the presence of tight junctions (zonula occludens) and adherens junctions (zonula adherens) whose bridging proteins of occludin and claudins and E-cadherin, respectively, limit the rate of H^+ diffusion and to the presence below these junctional bridges of an intercellular glycoprotein matrix with MUC1 and MUC4 containing neutral and sialic acid-rich mucopolysaccharides [47,48]. Nevertheless, circuit analysis of SSE has shown that the paracellular (shunt) pathway is the weak link in the barrier being more permanent than the transcellular pathway to ions and molecules [46].

SCE, as with SSE, also exhibits barrier function, and this is evident both *in vitro* and *in vivo* by the presence of a measurable PD (see Fig. 7.2). Although circuit analysis has not been performed on SCE to date, data from biopsies of SCE mounted in mini-Ussing chambers indicate that SCE has a lower transepithelial resistance than SSE. This suggests that SCE has either greater permeability to ions across its transcellular and/or paracellular pathway than does SSE [39]. Yet details about its structural defense are limited and specifically the capacity to prevent H^+ diffusion from lumen-to-blood have not been examined. What is known, however, is that SCE, like SSE, contains an adherens-type junction—this based on immunohistochemical studies showing the adherens junctional protein E-cadherin complexed to β-catenin within the cell membrane [49,50]. And though Western blots of SCE and SSE indicate that expression of E-cadherin in SCE is significantly lower than SSE from either healthy or reflux subjects, the functional significance of this difference remains unknown [51].

Among the functional components of the epithelial defense are cytosolic and intercellular buffers and ion transporters involved with the regulation of intracellular pH. The former protect by neutralizing H^+ within cytoplasm and intercellular space and the latter by transporting H^+ from cytoplasm into the intercellular space for removal by the blood supply (see Fig. 7.1). The total buffer capacity (B_T) in primary cultures of (rabbit) SSE has been measured by fluorescence microscopy in BCECF-loaded cells—yielding values of 38.6 mmol/pH unit for basal cells at a pHi of 7.1 [52,53]. Similar values for B_T for esophageal cells of human SSE or SCE are unknown. Nonetheless, significant intracellular buffering is likely given that immunohistochemistry has shown that both human esophagus lined by SSE and by SCE contain the enzyme carbonic anhydrase which catalyzes the conversion of CO_2 and H_2O to carbonic acid, and carbonic acid ionizes into bicarbonate and hydrogen ions. Bicarbonate ions are then made available for intracellular buffering by removal of H^+

by a membrane Na^+/H^+ exchanger which removes intracellular H^+ in exchange for extracellular Na^+. Both SSE and SCE have been documented to contain a Na^+/H^+ exchanger of the NHE-1 isotype—this isotype known for its role in regulation of intracellular pH. Further, when cellular buffering capacity is exceeded and pHi falls to acidic levels, cells in SSE are known to raise intracellular pH by a second mechanism—a Na^+-dependent Cl^-/HCO_3^- exchanger [52–55]. The end result is that transporter activity raises low pHi back toward neutrality by dumping H^+ into the intercellular space. Moreover, in SSE activation of acid extruding transporters usually results in an overshoot so that cells transiently become alkaline—a process that activates a cell-acidifying basolateral membrane Na-independent, Cl^-/HCO_3^- exchanger [53]. Details by which SCE regulate pHi are limited; nonetheless, an acid-extruding Na^+/H^+ exchanger of the NHE-1 isotype is known to be present based on identification of its mRNA in SCE and evidence of an amiloride-sensitive acid extrusion process in a Barrett's adenocarcinoma cell line, TE7 [56,57]. Since details regarding the rate of H^+ removal by the Na^+/H^+ exchanger and/or the presence of other mechanisms for regulation of pHi are unknown, it is unclear whether SCE has superior intracellular buffering capacity or acid extruding potency than SSE. Nonetheless, it has been reported that mRNA levels of NHE are significantly higher in SCE than in adjacent SSE [57].

Cell Replication as Mucosal Defense

For preservation of epithelial integrity, cell injury and death in SSE or SCE must be countered by a reparative defense. In SSE two means of repair have been identified—one is through epithelial restitution and the other is through cell replication. Restitution restores epithelial integrity in an area where cells are damaged or lost by senescence through the migration of adjacent, uninjured cells over the exposed basement membrane. The most desirable feature of restitution as protective device is its speed, occurring in 30–60 min due to the lack of need for DNA and protein synthesis [58]. Nonetheless, while shown to occur *in vitro* in cultures of SSE, restitution of barrier function has not been documented to occur following injury to native SSE. This is illustrated *in vitro* by a lack of restoration of electrical resistance in acid-injured SSE whose recovery was monitored for at least 2 h in the Ussing chamber and *in vivo* by the apparent delay in resolution of microscopic injury (dilated intercellular spaces) in SSE following PPI therapy in reflux patients [59,60]. This suggests that replication, not restitution, is the major reparative defense for acid injured SSE-lined esophagus; and this phenomenon detectable by the histopathologic finding of basal cell hyperplasia in esophageal biopsies from subjects with non-erosive reflux disease (NERD) [61]. It is of interest that one stimulus for cell replication in SSE-lined esophagus *in vivo* is exposure to epidermal growth factor (EGF); and the major source of EGF in this setting is saliva. How luminal EGF from saliva gains access to its receptors on the basal cells has been somewhat of a mystery. Yet, recent studies of non-erosive, acid-damaged SSE in Ussing chambers indicates that acid-induced injury, evidenced by dilated intercellular spaces, is associated with changes sufficiently great to permit EGF to access the basal cell layer by diffusion through the paracellular pathway [62].

In SCE studies of repair have been limited to those dealing with cell replication. This is not surprising since, as noted earlier, the high rate of cell turnover in SCE contributes to the increased risk of malignant transformation. High cell turnover involves greater rates of DNA synthesis, and it is during DNA synthesis that the risk is greatest for mutation. Since mutations that confer a survival advantage provide longer cell life, growth-enhancing mutations accumulate so that cells progress toward autonomy. Moreover, the evolution of this process can be identified genomically by the presence of aneuploidy, increased G2 tetraploidy and *p53* mutation, and phenotypically by the presence of dysplasia [63,64]. A coupling then of autonomous cell growth with inhibition of apoptosis provides the ingredients for fulfillment of the metaplasia–dysplasia–carcinoma sequence [65,66].

Cancer risk aside, the high rate of cell turnover in SCE can be viewed in a more positive light—that is, as successful adaptation for maintenance of tissue integrity in the face of repeated injury by contents in the refluxate. It is, therefore, not surprising that Barrett's esophagus contains elevated levels of growth factors and inflammatory products—many of which are known to promote and support cell proliferation (Fig. 7.3). Included among these are: transforming growth factor-α (TGF-α), EGF, EGF receptor, hepatocyte growth factor, vascular endothelial growth factor, cyclooxygenase-2 (COX-2), glutathione peroxidase, *erb*-B2, c-*myc*, TNF-α, IL-6, IL-8, ornithine decarboxylase, nitric oxide synthase, PPARγ, CCK2, gastrin, and metallothionein [23,49,67–73]. TGF-α and EGF, in particular, are potent stimulants for cell proliferation, and their actions mediated via upregulation of such growth-promoting nuclear ongogenes as c-*fos*, c-*jun*, c-*myc* and cyclin D. Transduction of the signal for TGF-α from the cell membrane to the nuclear gene pool has been attributed in Barrett's esophagus to an increase in phosphorylation of β-catenin. When phosphorylated, β-catenin—usually membrane bound in a complex with E-cadherin—can travel to the nucleus and serve as transcription factor for the activation of genes that both promote growth (see above) and angiogenesis [23,49,67,70]. Alternatively, signal transduction for EGF has been associated with activation of membrane phosphatidyl-inositol-3 kinase (PI3)—a pathway whose proliferative signal is mediated by increased phosphorylation of the pro-proliferative protein, Akt (protein kinase B) [74]. This latter pathway will again come to the fore in the discussion of bile salts and most proliferative pathways appear to converge upon COX-2 enzyme activity—see below.

Although proliferative signals for SCE are increased by the products of injury and inflammation, there is also evidence cell proliferation can be stimulated even without injury by components of the refluxate—especially acid and bile salts [75–79] (see Fig. 7.3). For instance, exposure of biopsies from Barrett's esophagus in organ culture to short pulses of acid, pH 3.5 for 1 h are reported to enhance proliferation; and this effect is mediated through prostaglandin E_2 (PGE2) produced by activation of both protein kinase C-ε (PKCε) and COX-2 enzyme [75,76]. PKCε in turn leads to proliferation by activation of a type-1, Na^+/H^+ exchanger (NHE-1)—a process that carries with it both protective (raising intracellular pH) and proliferative benefits. Confirmation of this sequence was further established by showing that the acid-induced proliferative re-

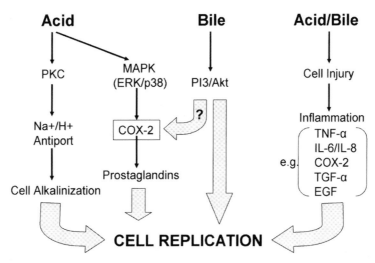

Fig. 7.3 Replication as defense in Barrett's esophagus. This illustration depicts three ways in which exposure to a gastroesophageal refluxate can increase cell proliferation in Barrett's esophagus. More than one may be operative at any point in time and duration of exposure to the refluxate and its components can change a stimulatory effect into an inhibitory effect, attesting to the complexity of the process. A major point of convergence for stimulation by the re-fluxate appears to be through activation of the COX-2 enzyme. See text for discussion of other pathways by which growth factors can increase cell proliferation in Barrett's esophagus. The question mark (?) indicates that this pathway has not been documented in either Barrett's esophagus or a Barrett's cell line. COX-2, cyclooxygenase-2; EGF, epidermal growth factor; ERK, extracellular signal-related kinase; IL, interleukin; MAPK, mitogen activated protein kinase; PI3, phosphatidyl-inositol-3 kinase; PKC, protein kinase C; TGF-α, transforming growth factor-α; TNF-α, tumor necrosis factor-α.

sponse in biopsies of Barrett's esophagus were inhibited by amiloride analogues which are known to block the Na$^+$/H$^+$ exchanger (Fig. 7.4). And the mechanism for NHE-induced proliferation ascribed to an alkaline overshoot induced by NHE following removal of extracellular acidity—the alkaline overshoot documented in TE7 cells, a Barrett's esophagus cancer cell line, using fluorescence microscopy [57].

A second mechanism by which acid may stimulate the proliferative response in Barrett's esophagus is via activation of mitogen activated protein kinase (MAPK) pathways [77,78]. This has been documented to occur *in vivo* by exposing Barrett's esophagus to acid (0.1 N HCl) for 3 min and showing on biopsy that this increased extracellular signal-related kinase (ERK), c-Jun N-terminal kinase (JNK), and *p38* activity, though only *p38* activity reached statistical significance (Fig. 7.5). *In vitro* studies using SEG-1 cells, a Barrett's esophagus cancer cell line, confirmed that acid-induced activation of MAPK pathways results in a proliferative signal mediated

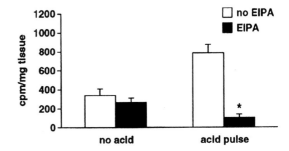

Fig. 7.4 After an acid pulse for 1 h at pH 3.5, proliferation in mucosal biopsies of Barrett's esophagus in organ culture are shown by tritiated thymidine uptake in counts per minute per milligram of tissue (cpm/mg) to be sensitive to inhibition by 5-(N ethyl-NN-isopropyl)-amiloride (EIPA), an inhibitor of Na$^+$/H$^+$ exchange. Modified and reproduced with permission from Fitzgerald *et al.* [57].

through a rapid increase in ERK and *p38* and a delayed increase in JNK. Subsequently, it was shown that the proliferative signals for ERK and *p38* were mediated via an increase in COX-2 protein expres-

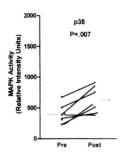
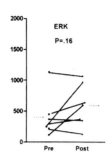
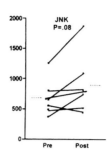

Fig. 7.5 Scatter plots show mitogen activated protein kinase (MAPK) activity in biopsies from Barrett's esophagus before and after acid perfusion for 3 min with 0.1 N HCl. All MAPK pathways were increased by acid exposure but only *p38* levels achieved statistical significance. Modified and reproduced with permission from Souza *et al.* [77].

sion (COX-2 effects mediated by generation of PGE2 [65]) since COX-2 inhibition reduced proliferation and the expression of COX-2 could be abolished by inhibitors to both ERK and *p38*. These findings, coupled with those described above, indicate that acid exposure to Barrett's esophagus can induce proliferation in at least two ways—one injurious and one physiologic—and that both of these pathways lead to increases in COX-2 enzyme (see Fig. 7.3). A key role for COX-2 enzyme in proliferation in Barrett's esophagus is also supported experimentally by showing reductions in proliferation in tissues obtained from an animal model of SCE and from subjects with Barrett's esophagus following treatment with COX-2 inhibitors *in vivo* [80,81]. In addition, there are also *in vivo* data to support the role of acid exposure in the proliferative response in Barrett's esophagus—this by demonstrating reductions in cell turnover using proliferating cell nuclear antigen (PCNA) staining following treatment with PPIs [82]. Notably the reduction in cell turnover in Barrett's esophagus was only evident in those treated with PPIs who could be demonstrated by intraesophageal pH monitoring to have normalized esophageal acidity. Based on these observations, consideration has been given to the use of COX-2 inhibitors and/or PPIs as strategies for chemoprevention of malignancy in Barrett's esophagus [45,83]. The potential benefits of these strategies, however, will have to await additional trials given recent concerns about the cardiac risks associated with long-term use of COX-2 inhibitors and the potential for offsetting influences of hypergastrinemia induced by prolonged hypoacidity with PPIs. Offsetting influences with PPI therapy are suggested by the lack of documented reduction in esophageal adenocarcinoma rates in subjects with

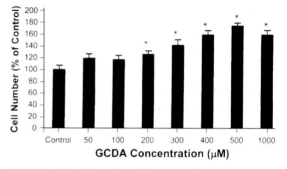

Fig. 7.6 A dose-dependent effect on proliferation is shown for exposure of SEG-1, a Barrett's adenocarcinoma cell line, to the conjugated bile salt, glycochenodeoxycholic acid (GCDA). Values are the mean ± standard error of the mean. Reproduced with permission from Jaiswal *et al.* [79].

Barrett's esophagus treated with PPIs and by the observation that the hormone, gastrin, can also mediate cell proliferation in Barrett's esophagus, this via the presence in Barrett's esophagus of CCK2 receptors [84].

An alternative means of offsetting the benefits of PPI therapy on cell proliferation in Barrett's esophagus is through exposure to bile salts at non-acidic pH within the refluxate. As with brief exposures to acid, brief exposures to bile salts have also been shown to promote PKC and COX-2 dependent proliferation in Barrett's esophagus [85]. And using SEG-1 cells, it was observed that this proliferation is mediated by activation of the PI3/Akt pathway, the same pathway that serves as proliferative signal for EGF [79] (Fig. 7.6). Further, in squamous (not studied for Barrett's esophagus adenocarcinoma) cancer cell lines, bile salt-induced activation of the PI3/Akt pathway was also shown to generate an increase in COX-2 expression [85]. Consequently, acid, bile salts, and the inflammation produced in SCE, all appear to have in common the capacity to generate COX-2 enzyme. COX-2 enzyme then becomes a focal point where diverse signals meet to generate a proliferative response—a response that when contained is protective and when liberated by loss of the apoptotic brake can be harmful (see Fig. 7.3).

Summary

Although esophageal SCE is known as a premalignant lesion, it arose out of necessity as a protective defense against severe reflux injury. In the large majority of subjects, SCE remains in place in the lower esophagus for a lifetime and without signs or symptoms of tissue injury; and as such it can be considered for them a "successful adaptation." How SCE achieves this success in the face of a refluxate capable of destroying the native SSE is not well understood. However, data gathered from a variety of sources and presented here provide an initial working model of SCE as mucosal defense. One component of this mucosal defense is cell replication, an apparent two-edged sword capable of providing a healthy mucosa in most but alternatively in some degenerating into malignancy. Additional research is needed on cell replication and other aspects of the protective biology of SCE—so that armed with new knowledge pharmacologic means can be designed that maintain the obvious benefits of SCE as a reflux-resistant tissue and yet minimize its (cancer) risk.

References

1. Spechler SJ. Barrett's esophagus. In: Orlando RC, ed. *Gastroesophageal Reflux Disease*. New York: Marcel Dekker Inc., 2000: 219–58.
2. Levine DS, Rubin CE, Reid BJ, Haggitt RC. Specialized metaplastic columnar epithelium in Barrett's esophagus. A comparative transmission electron microscopic study. *Lab Invest* 1989;**60**(3):418–32.
3. Boch JA, Shields HM, Antonioli DA *et al*. Distribution of cytokeratin markers in Barrett's specialized columnar epithelium. *Gastroenterology* 1997;**112**:760–5.
4. Gillen P, Keeling P, Byrne PJ, West AB, Hennessey TPJ. Implication of duodenogastric reflux in the pathogenesis of Barrett's oesophagus. *Br J Surg* 1988;**75**:113–5.
5. Spechler SJ, Lee E, Ahnen D *et al*. Long-term outcome of medical and surgical therapies for gastroesophageal reflux disease: follow-up of a randomized controlled trial [see comments]. *JAMA* 2001;**285**:2331–8.
6. Li H, Walsh TN, O'Dowd G *et al*. Mechanisms of columnar metaplasia and squamous regeneration in experimental Barrett's esophagus. *Surgery* 1994;**115**: 176–81.
7. Bremner CG, Lynch VP, Ellis FH, Jr. Barrett's esophagus: congenital or acquired? An experimental study of esophageal mucosal regeneration in the dog. *Surgery* 1970;**68**:209–16.
8. Su Y, Chen X, Klein M *et al*. Phenotype of columnar-lined esophagus in rats with esophagogastroduodenal anastamosis: similarity to human Barrett's esophagus. *Lab Invest* 2004;**84**:753–65.
9. Goldstein SR, Yang GY, Curtis SK *et al*. Development of esophageal metaplasia and adenocarcinoma in a rat surgical model without the use of a carcinogen. *Carcinogenesis* 1997;**18**:2265–70.
10. Eda A, Osawa H, Satoh K *et al*. Aberrant expression of CDX2 in Barrett's epithelium and inflammatory esophageal mucosa. *J Gastroenterol* 2003;**38**:14–22.
11. Phillips RW, Frierson HF, Jr, Moskaluk CA. CDX2 as a marker of epithelial intestinal differentiation in the esophagus. *Am J Surg Pathol* 2003;**27**:1442–7.
12. Mutoh H, Sakurai S, Satoh K *et al*. Cdx1 induced intestinal metaplasia in the transgenic mouse stomach: comparative study with Cdx2 transgenic mice. *Gut* 2004;**53**:1416–23.
13. Silberg DG, Sullivan J, Kang E *et al*. Cdx2 ectopic expression induces gastric intestinal metaplasia in transgenic mice. *Gastroenterology* 2002;**122**:689–96.
14. Marchetti M, Caliot E, Pringault E. Chronic acid exposure leads to activation of the CDX2 intestinal homeobox gene in a long term culture of mouse esophageal keratinocytes. *J Cell Sci* 2003;**116**:1429–36.
15. Wong NA, Wilding J, Barlett S *et al*. CDX1 is an important molecular mediator of Barrett's metaplasia. *Proc Natl Acad Sci U S A* 2005;**102**(21):7565–70.
16. Johnson D, Winters AC, Spurling TJ, Chobanian SJ, Cattau, ELJ. Esophageal acid sensitivity in Barrett's esophagus. *J Clin Gastroenterol* 1987;**9**:23–7.
17. Cameron AJ, Zinsmeister AR, Ballard DJ, Carney JA. Prevalence of columnar-lined (Barrett's) esophagus. Comparison of population-based clinical and autopsy findings. *Gastroenterology* 1990;**99**:918–22.
18. Berenson MM, Johnson TD, Markowitz NR, Buchi KN, Samowitz WS. Restoration of squamous mucosa after

ablation of Barrett's esophageal epithelium. *Gastroenterology* 1993;**104**:1686–91.

19. Overholt BF, Panjehpour M. Photodynamic therapy for Barrett's esophagus: clinical update. *Am J Gastroenterol* 1996;**91**:1719–23.

20. Gray MR. Epithelial proliferation in Barrett's esophagus by proliferating cell nuclear antigen immunolocalization. *Gastroenterology* 1992;**103**:1769–76.

21. Herbst JJ, Berenson MM, McCloskey MD, Wiser WC. Cell proliferation in esophageal columnar epithelium (Barrett's esophagus). *Gastroenterology* 1978;**75**:683–7.

22. Reid BJ, Sanchez CA, Blount PL, Levine DS. Barrett's esophagus: cell cycle abnormalities in advancing stages of neoplastic progression [see comments]. *Gastroenterology* 1993;**105**:119–29.

23. Aldulaimi D, Jankowski J. Barrett's esophagus: an overview of the molecular biology. *Dis Esophagus* 1999;**12**:177–80.

24. Cameron AJ, Zinsmeister AR, Ballard DJ, Carney JA. Prevalence of columnar-lined (Barrett's) esophagus. Comparison of population-based clinical and autopsy findings [see comments]. *Gastroenterology* 1990;**99**: 918–22.

25. Gerson LB, Shetler K, Triadafilopoulos G. Prevalence of Barrett's esophagus in asymptomatic individuals. *Gastroenterology* 2002;**123**:461–7.

26. Goldminc M, Maddern G, Le Prise E *et al.* Oesophagectomy by a transhiatal approach or thoracotomy: a prospective randomized trial. *Br J Surg* 1993;**80**: 367–70.

27. Orlando RC. Pathophysiology of gastroesophageal reflux disease: offensive factors and tissue resistance. In: Orlando RC, ed. *Gastroesophageal Reflux Disease*. New York: Marcel Dekker Inc., 2000: 165–92.

28. Orlando RC. Measurement of esophageal transmural electrical potential difference. In: Scarpignato C, Galmiche J-P, eds. *Frontiers of Gastrointestinal Research, Vol. 22, Functional Investigation of Esophageal Disease*. New York: Karger, 1994: 336–43.

29. Orlando RC, Powell DW, Bryson JC *et al.* Esophageal potential difference measurements in esophageal disease. *Gastroenterology* 1982;**83**:1026–32.

30. Herlihy KJ, Orlando RC, Bryson JC *et al.* Barrett's esophagus: clinical, endoscopic, histologic, manometric, and electrical potential difference characteristics. *Gastroenterology* 1984;**86**:436–43.

31. Silen W. Gastric mucosal defense and repair. In: Johnson LR, ed. *Physiology of the Gastrointestinal Tract*, 2nd edn. New York: Raven Press, 1987: 1055–69.

32. Quigley EM, Turnberg LA. pH of the microclimate lining human gastric and duodenal mucosa *in vivo*. Studies in control subjects and in duodenal ulcer patients. *Gastroenterology* 1987;**92**:1876–84.

33. Abdulnour-Nakhoul S, Orlando RC. Lumen-to-surface pH gradient in Barrett's esophagus. *Gastroenterology* 2004;**126**(4):A235.

34. Dixon J, Strugala V, Griffin SM *et al.* Esophageal mucin: an adherent mucus gel barrier is absent in the normal esophagus but present in columnar-lined Barrett's esophagus. *Am J Gastroenterol* 2001;**96**:2575–83.

35. Arul GS, Moorghen M, Myerscough N *et al.* Mucin gene expression in Barrett's oesophagus: an *in situ* hybridization and immunohistochemical study. *Gut* 2000;**47**(6): 753–61.

36. Flucke U, Steinborn E, Dries V *et al.* Immunoreactivity of cytokeratins (CK7, CK20) and mucin peptide core antigens (MUC1, MuC2, MUC5AC) in adenocarcinomas, normal and metaplastic tissues of the distal oesophagus, oesophagogastric junction and proximal stomach. *Histopathology* 2003;**43**(2):127–34.

37. Van de Bovenkamp JHB, Korteland-Van Male AM, Warson C *et al.* Gastric-type mucin and TFF-peptide expression in Barrett's oesophagus is disturbed during increased expression of MUC2. *Histopathology* 2003; **42**:555–65.

38. Orlando RC. Why is the high grade inhibition of gastric acid secretion afforded by proton pump inhibitors often required for healing of reflux esophagitis? An epithelial perspective. *Am J Gastroenterol* 1996;**91**: 1692–6.

39. Tobey NA, Argote CM, Kav T *et al.* Anion transport in human squamous and Barrett's esophageal epithelium. *Gastroenterology* 2005;**128**:A234.

40. Abdulnour-Nakhoul S, Nakhoul NL, Orlando RC. Lumen-to-surface pH gradients in opossum and rabbit esophagi: role of submucosal glands. *Am J Physiol Gastrointest Liver Physiol* 2000;**278**:G113–20.

41. Salo J, Kivilaakso E. Role of luminal H^+ in the pathogenesis of experimental esophagitis. *Surgery* 1982;**92**: 61–8.

42. Tobey NA, Hosseini SS, Caymaz-Bor C *et al.* The role of pepsin in acid injury to esophageal epithelium. *Am J Gastroenterol* 2001;**96**:3062–70.

43. Orlando RC, Powell DW. Studies of esophageal epithelial electrolyte transport and potential difference in man. In: Allen A, ed. *Mechanisms of Mucosal Protection in the Upper Gastrointestinal Tract*. New York: Raven Press, 1984: 75–9.

44. Khalbuss WE, Marousis CG, Subramanyam M, Orlando RC. Effect of HCl on transmembrane potentials and intracellular pH in rabbit esophageal epithelium. *Gastroenterology* 1995;**108**:662–72.

45. Tobey NA, Hosseini SS, Caymaz-Bor C, Awayda M, Orlando RC. Effect of luminal acidity on the apical membrane Na channel in rabbit esophageal epithelium. *Gastroenterology* 2000;**118**:A883.

46. Tobey NA, Hosseini SS, Argote CM *et al*. Dilated intercellular spaces and shunt permeability in nonerosive acid-damaged esophageal epithelium. *Am J Gastroenterol* 2004;**99**:13–22.

47. Orlando RC, Lacy ER, Tobey NA, Cowart K. Barriers to paracellular permeability in rabbit esophageal epithelium. *Gastroenterology* 1992;**102**:910–23.

48. Tobey NA, Argote CM, Hosseini SS, Orlando RC. Calcium-switch technique and junctional permeability in native rabbit esophageal epithelium. *Am J Physiol Gastrointest Liver Physiol* 2004;**286**:G1042–9.

49. Seery JP, Syrigos KN, Karayiannakis AJ, Valizadeh A, Pignatelli M. Abnormal expression of the E-cadherin–catenin complex in dysplastic Barrett's oesophagus. *Acta Oncologica* 1999;**38**:945–8.

50. Feith M, Stein HJ, Mueller J, Siewert JR. Malignant degeneration of Barrett's esophagus: the role of the Ki-67 proliferation fraction, expression of E-cadherin and *p53*. *Dis Esophagus* 2004;**17**(4):322–7.

51. Swami S, Kumble S, Triadafilopoulos G. E-cadherin expression in gastroesophageal reflux disease, Barrett's esophagus, and esophageal adenocarcinoma: an immunohistochemical and immunoblot study. *Am J Gastroenterol* 1995;**90**:1808–13.

52. Tobey NA, Reddy SP, Keku TO, Cragoe EJ, Jr, Orlando RC. Studies of pHi in rabbit esophageal basal and squamous epithelial cells in culture. *Gastroenterology* 1992;**103**:830–9.

53. Tobey NA, Reddy SP, Khalbuss WE *et al*. Na$^+$-dependent and -independent Cl$^-$/HCO$_3^-$ exchangers in cultured rabbit esophageal epithelial cells. *Gastroenterology* 1993;**104**:185–95 [published erratum appears in *Gastroenterology* 1993;**105**(2):649].

54. Layden TJ, Agnone LM, Schmidt LN, Hakim B, Goldstein JL. Rabbit esophageal cells possess an Na$^+$, H$^+$ antiport. *Gastroenterology* 1990;**99**:909–17.

55. Layden TJ, Schmidt L, Agnone L *et al*. Rabbit esophageal cell cytoplasmic pH regulation: role of Na$^+$-H$^+$ antiport and Na$^+$-dependent HCO$_3^-$ transport systems. *Am J Physiol Gastrointest Liver Physiol* 1992; **263**:G407–13.

56. Carpizo DR. Acute acid exposure increases rabbit esophageal cell proliferation. *Am J Physiol* 1996;**271**: G483–93.

57. Fitzgerald RC, Omary MB, Triadafilopoulos, TG. Altered sodium–hydrogen exchange activity is a mechanism for acid-induced hyperproliferation in Barrett's esophagus. *Am J Physiol Gastrointestinal Liver Physiol* 1998;**275**:G47–55.

58. Jimenez P, Lanas A, Piazuelo E, Esteva F. Effects of extracellular pH on restitution and proliferation of rabbit oesophageal epithelial cells. *Aliment Pharmacol Ther* 1999;**13**(4):545–52.

59. Orlando RC. Pathophysiology of gastroesophageal reflux disease: esophageal epithelial resistance. In: Castell DO, Richter JE, eds. *The Esophagus*, 4th edn. Philadelphia: Lippincott Williams & Wilkins, 2004: 421–33.

60. Calabrese C, Bortolotti M, Fabbri A *et al*. Reversibility of GERD ultrastructural alterations and relief of symptoms after omeprazole treatment. *Am J Gastroenterol* 2005;**100**:537–42.

61. Ismail-Beigi F, Pope CE, II. Distribution of the histological changes of gastroesophageal reflux in the distal esophagus of man. *Gastroenterology* 1974;**66**:1109–13.

62. Tobey NA, Hosseini SS, Argote CM *et al*. Dilated intercellular spaces and shunt permeability in nonerosive acid-damaged esophageal epithelium. *Am J Gastroenterol* 2004;**99**:13–22.

63. Reid BJ, Haggitt RC, Rubin CE, Rabinovitch PS. Barrett's esophagus. Correlation between flow cytometry and histology in detection of patients at risk for adenocarcinoma. *Gastroenterology* 1987;**93**:1–11.

64. Maley CC, Galipeau PC, Li X *et al*. The combination of genetic instability and clonal expansion predicts progression to esophageal adenocarcinoma. *Cancer Res* 2004;**64**(20):7629–33.

65. Gray MR. Epithelial proliferation in Barrett's esophagus by proliferating cell nuclear antigen immunolocalization. *Gastroenterology* 1992;**103**:1769–76.

66. Herbst JJ, Berenson MM, McCloskey MD, Wiser WC. Cell proliferation in esophageal columnar epithelium (Barrett's esophagus). *Gastroenterology* 1978;**75**:683–7.

67. Harrison RF, Perry I, Jankowski JA. Barrett's mucosa: remodeling by the microenvironment. *J Pathol* 2000; **192**(1):1–3.

68. Tselepis C, Perry I, Dawson C *et al*. Tumour necrosis factor-α in Barrett's oesophagus: a potential novel mechanism of action. *Oncogene* 2002;**21**(39):6071–81.

69. Dvorakova K, Payne CM, Ramsey L *et al*. Increased expression and secretion of interleukin-6 in patients with Barrett's esophagus. *Clin Cancer Res* 2004;**10**(6): 2020–8.

70. Jankowski J, Hopwood D, Wormsley KG. Expression of epidermal growth factor, transforming growth factor α and their receptor in gastro-oesophageal diseases. *Dig Dis* 1993;**11**(1):1–11.

71. Tselepis C, Morris CD, Wakelin D *et al*. Upregulation of the oncogene c-*myc* in Barrett's adenocarcinoma: induction of c-*myc* by acidified bile acid *in vitro*. *Gut* 2003;**52**(2):174–80.

72. Konturek PC, Nikiforuk A, Kania J *et al*. Activation of NFκB represents the central event in the neoplastic progression associated with Barrett's esophagus: a possible link to the inflammation and over expression of COX-2, PPARγ and growth factors. *Dig Dis Sci* 2004; **49**(7–8):1075–83.

73. Li Y, Wo JM, Cai L *et al*. Association of metallothionein expression and lack of apoptosis with progression of carcinogenesis in Barrett's esophagus. *Exp Biol Med (Maywood)* 2003;**228**(3):286–92.

74. Okano J, Gaslightwala I, Birnbaum MJ, Rustgi AK, Nakagawa H. Akt/protein kinase B isoforms are differentially regulated by epidermal growth factor stimulation. *J Biol Chem* 2000;**275**:30 934–42.

75. Kaur BS, Triadafilopoulos G. Acid- and bile-induced PGE2 release and hyperproliferation in Barrett's esophagus are COX-2 and PKC-ε dependent. *Am J Physiol Gastrointest Liver Physiol* 2002;**283**(2):G327–34.

76. Fitzgerald RC, Omary MB, Triadafilopolous G. Dynamic effects of acid on Barrett's esophagus. An *ex vivo* proliferation and differentiation model. *J Clin Invest* 1996;**98**:2120–8.

77. Souza RF, Shewmake K, Terada LS, Spechler SJ. Acid exposure activates the mitogen-activated protein kinase pathways in Barrett's esophagus. *Gastroenterology* 2002;**122**:299–307.

78. Souza RF, Shewmake K, Pearson S, Sarosi GA, Jr. Acid increases proliferation via ERK and *p38* MAPK-mediated increases in cyclooxygenase-2 in Barrett's adenocarcinoma cells. *Am J Physiol Gastrointest Liver Physiol* 2004;**287**:G743–8.

79. Jaiswal K, Tello V, Lopez-Guzman C *et al*. Bile salt exposure causes phosphatidyl-inositol-3-kinase-mediated proliferation in a Barrett's adenocarcinoma cell line. *Surgery* 2004;**136**:160–8.

80. Buttar NS, Wang KK, Leontovich O *et al*. Chemoprevention of esophageal adenocarcinoma by COX-2 inhibitors in an animal model of Barrett's esophagus. *Gastroenterology* 2002;**122**(4):1101–12.

81. Kaur BS, Khamnehei N, Iravani M *et al*. Rofecoxib inhibits cyclooxygenase 2 expression and activity and reduces cell proliferation in Barrett's esophagus. *Gastroenterology* 2002;**123**:60–7.

82. Ouatu-Lascar R, Fitzgerald R, Triadafilopolous G. Differentiation and proliferation in Barrett's esophagus and the effects of acid suppression. *Gastroenterology* 1999;**117**:327–35.

83. Fennerty MB, Triadafilopolous G. Barrett's-related esophageal adenocarcinoma: is chemoprevention a potential option? *Am J Gastroenterol* 2001;**96**:2302–5.

84. Haigh CR, Attwood SE, Thompson DG *et al*. Gastrin induces proliferation in Barrett's metaplasia through activation of the CCK2 receptor. *Gastroenterology* 2003;**124**:615–25.

85. Zhang F, Altorki NK, Wu YC *et al*. Duodenal reflux induces cycooxygenase-2 in the esophageal mucosa of rats: evidence for involvement of bile acids. *Gastroenterology* 2001;**121**:1391–9.

CHAPTER 8

The Role of *Helicobacter pylori* in Barrett's Esophagus

Peter Malfertheiner and Ulrich Peitz

The relationship of *Helicobacter pylori* infection with gastroesophageal reflux disease (GERD) is complex and intriguing. Studies with different degrees of scientific strength provide evidence for an ambiguous role of *H. pylori* infection in GERD and its complications, Barrett's esophagus, and esophageal adenocarcinoma. However, the range of this relationship is from causative, with no reciprocal influence, to even protective. At present, there is no unequivocal evidence as to whether *H. pylori* infection can be considered causative or protective in the development of Barrett's esophagus or esophageal adenocarcinoma. To further elucidate the relationship, we attempt to apply the criteria of Hill in a simplified version with considerations to [1]:

- biological plausibility (pathophysiology);
- association (epidemiology);
- effect of clinical intervention.

We will consider non-erosive reflux disease, erosive reflux disease, and Barrett's esophagus as distinct entities, although at present there is still uncertainty whether all these manifestations of GERD may be linked by a temporal continuum. Different etiologic and pathophysiologic traits, and a different magnitude and composition of the refluxate in the esophagus have been reported in patients with Barrett's esophagus.

Pathophysiology

H. pylori infection is mostly acquired in childhood, usually persistent, and invariably induces chronic active gastritis. At least one out of 10 infected subjects will experience one of the following diseases during their lifetime: gastroduodenal ulcer, gastric MALT lymphoma, or gastric cancer. Patients with duodenal ulcer are unlikely to develop gastric cancer. Pathophysiological data show that the phenotype of gastritis and acid output are key determinants for these different outcomes of *H. pylori* infection. Duodenal ulcer occurs in patients with antral-predominant gastritis associated with a high acid output, whereas gastric cancer (confined to intestinal type, which is predominant) is mainly linked to corpus-predominant gastritis and multifocal atrophic gastritis with low acid output. *H. pylori* infection exerts a variable influence on gastric acid output [1–4]. The mechanisms by which *H. pylori* exerts its effect on acid secretion are becoming increasingly elucidated. It appears obvious that the interplay between *H. pylori* infection and acid output can also have a bearing on the pathogenesis of Barrett's esophagus.

Conceivable mechanisms that might mediate the influence of *H. pylori* infection on the development of Barrett's esophagus can be categorized as follows:

(a) composition of the gastroesophageal refluxate;
(b) esophagogastric motor function;
(c) inflammation of the esophagogastric junction.

Composition of the Gastroesophageal Refluxate Bacterial cytotoxins of *H. pylori* are unlikely to be active in the refluxate. Cytotoxins like Vac A and CagA proteins exert their effect only through a close contact of the bacterium with the epithelial cell. Ammonium, by contrast, is likely to be an important component of the refluxate. It is produced by *H. pylori* in such amounts that it slightly reduces the gastric juice acidity [5,6]. The strongest influence of *H.*

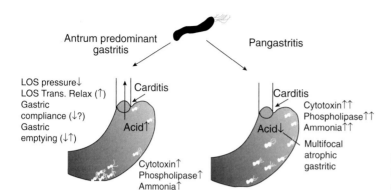

Fig. 8.1 Impact of the pattern of gastritis: antrum predominant gastritis versus pangastritis.

pylori on gastric acid secretion, however, is mediated through gastric mucosal inflammation (Fig. 8.1). The inflammation of the gastric mucosa may either increase or decrease acid secretion depending on the topographical distribution of the inflammation. The antrum-predominant gastritis leads to a high acid output [2,4]. Pangastritis or, in particular, the corpus-predominant gastritis is linked with acid hyposecretion [3]. The mechanisms leading to hypersecretion are an elevated serum level of gastrin which is universally found in *H. pylori* infection and the disruption of negative feedback during neural connections, but requires a functioning corpus mucosa [7]. If the corpus mucosa is severly inflamed, acid secretion is inhibited despite an elevated gastrin level. This inhibition is mediated by cytokines, in particular interleukin-1β which is abundantly released in the inflamed mucosa. Recent data indicate that genetic host factors, in particular polymorphisms of interleukin-1β, have an important effect on gastric acid suppression [8,9].

The relationship between distribution of *H. pylori* gastritis and acid output is also reciprocal. The topographic pattern of *H. pylori* gastritis determines acid output, but also the acid secretion impacts on the bacterial distribution. This has been well demonstrated through therapeutic interventions. If acid secretion is inhibited with a proton pump inhibitor, then an antrum predominant gastritis shifts to a corpus-predominant gastritis. *H. pylori* eradication in a patient with antrum predominant gastritis on the contrary reduces acid hypersection because it lowers gastrin and restores the neural feedback system. *H. pylori* eradication in pangastritis or corpus-

predominant gastritis may lead to normalization of acid secretion in those cases, in which atrophic changes of gastric mucosa can be reversed. In advanced atrophy of the corpus mucosa, low acid secretion is an irreversible condition [3,10]. With the return to normal acid output following eradication several authors have reported an increase in GERD. However this apparently requires that the gastro-esophageal reflux barrier is impaired and, therefore, becomes permissive for acid reflux [11–14]. This is currently the best acceptable explanation for how *H. pylori* infection in certain selected cases may exert a "protective effect" against GERD.

Esophagogastric Motor Function Incompetence of the lower esophagus sphincter is considered to be one of the critical disorders responsible for GERD. *H. pylori* infection induces the production of nitric oxide known to decrease the pressure of the lower esophagus sphincter [15]; however, it is as yet not clear whether nitric oxide reaches the lower esophagus in relevant amounts. On the other hand, *H. pylori* infection is also linked to increased gastrin release [2,4,15] and gastrin enhances the lower esophageal sphincter pressure. Clinical data on the influence of *H. pylori* status on motor functions of the esophagus and lower esophageal sphincter are scarce and conflicting [16–18]. From current data we conclude that *H. pylori* exerts, if any, only a minor influence on lower esophagus sphincter function in healthy volunteers or patients with GERD. In patients with Barrett's esophagus, the influence of *H. pylori* on esophagogastric motor function has not yet been investigated.

Duodenogastroesophageal reflux is also involved in the development of Barrett's esophagus. Two mechanisms contribute to duodenogastric reflux: retrograde movement of duodenal contents and impaired gastric emptying. A number of studies on the effect of *H. pylori* on gastric emptying, using scintigraphy, ^{13}C-octanoic acid breath test and ultrasound measurement of the antral area [19–25], and studies on antroduodenal motility using antroduodenal manometry [22,25], and electric gastric activity by electrogastrography [26,27] have not shown a significant role. Duodenogastric reflux has not appeared to be influenced by *H. pylori* infection according to three small studies using biliary scintigraphy [28,29] and Bilitec 2000 bilirubin monitoring [30]. Indirect evidence for duodenogastric reflux can be obtained from histopathology, as duodenogastric reflux induces reflux gastritis, also defined as reactive gastritis [31,32]. There is a minor association between duodenogastric reflux and intestinal metaplasia of the stomach [33,34], and also between reactive gastritis and the presence of intestinal metaplasia of the esophagogastric junction [32]. However, the dominant cause of intestinal metaplasia in both the distal stomach and the gastric cardia is *H. pylori* infection [35]. In the presence of *H. pylori* infection, it becomes difficult to attribute the inflammation to abnormal duodenogastric reflux. In *H. pylori*-negative patients, the association of reactive gastritis with intestinal metaplasia of the esophagogastric junction awaits confirmation by further studies.

Inflammation of the Esophagogastric Junction

Inflammation of the cardia contributes to the development of intestinal metaplasia in that area. It is also well established that Barrett's carcinoma is the final step in a sequence of inflammation, metaplasia, dysplasia (intraepithelial neoplasia), and neoplasia of the distal esophagus [36]. However, it is difficult to assess the relative contribution of *H. pylori* infection and GERD to the development of intestinal metaplasia and eventually cancer progression. In an endoscopically normal esophagogastric junction, some authors report inflammation and intestinal metaplasia associated with *H. pylori* infection, others demonstrate a close association with GERD (reviews:

[35,37]). Some of these discrepancies may be due to the different definitions of the normal anatomy of the esophagogastric junction in this region. Cardia-type mucosa may either represent normal gastric cardia or columnar lined epithelium as metaplasia of the distal esophagus [38–40]. The extent of cardia-type mucosa in the distal esophagus and the severity of GERD are correlated [41], and there is controversy if cardia-type mucosa may precede the development of intestinal metaplasia [40,42]. However only specialized intestinal metaplasia of the esophagus bears the increased risk of adenocarcinoma, and fulfills the most recent definition of Barrett's esophagus [43]. Numerous studies have shown that the gastric cardia can be colonized by *H. pylori* [44], although its colonization in this area is lower than that in the gastric antrum [45]. Also cardia-type metaplasia of the lower esophagus can be colonized, whereas intestinal metaplasia cannot [46,47]. Since *H. pylori* cannot colonize the intestinalized columnar epithelium in the esophagus, the bacterium is unlikely to promote the transition from Barrett's mucosa to carcinoma by mechanisms known for the stomach, like adhesion and intraepithelial injection of cytokines [48].

Epidemiology

Both, *H. pylori* infection and GERD are common conditions and the prevalence of both conditions increases with age. Therefore, correlation of *H. pylori* infection and GERD should be expected by chance, due to age as a confounder. However, two systematic reviews reported an inverse association of GERD with the prevalence of *H. pylori* infection, being 10% lower in GERD patients than in controls [44,49]. Of note, a significant lower *H. pylori* prevalence in GERD was found mainly in studies from the Far East [49].

Barrett's Esophagus

Few data are available with regard to the association of *H. pylori* infection and Barrett's. The systematic review of O'Connor summarized the small-size studies published up to 1999 and revealed no difference of the *H. pylori* prevalence between patients with Barrett (29%) and controls (30%) [44]. More recent

Table 8.1 *Helicobacter pylori* prevalence (determined with histology, rapid urease test and/or serology) in patients with Barrett's esophagus, reflux esophagitis, and control subjects, presented as percentage (number of cases).

	Barrett's esophagus %	Reflux esophagitis %	Controls %
Loffeld *et al.* 2000 [53]	39 (14/36)	35 (41/118)	55 (248/454)
Laheij *et al.* 2002 [52]	39 (9/23)	46 (57/125)	57 (300/528)
Ackermark *et al.* 2003 [51]	41 (21/51)	No data	63 (39/62)
Abe *et al.* 2004 [50]	9 (3/32)	30 (24/80)	71 (57/80)

	Barrett's esophagus %	Controls %
Vaezi *et al.* 2000 [55]	7 (2/28)	44 (11/25)
Loffeld *et al.* 2000* [53]	15 (2/13)	59 (130/222)
Ackermark *et al.* 2003† [51]	10 (10/51)	36 (22/62)
Kudo *et al.* 2005* [54]	35 (8/23)	79 (19/24)

Table 8.2 Prevalence of positive CagA status (serum immunoglobulin G [IgG] antibodies assessed by enzyme immuno assay or immunoblot) among patients with Barrett's esophagus and control subjects presented as percentage (number of cases).

* CagA status determined only in patients with positive *Helicobacter pylori* whole cell IgG antibodies.
† CagA status determined in all patients.

results are presented in Table 8.1 [50–53]. In these studies, the *H. pylori* prevalence was lower than in controls, but all studies included a rather small number of Barrett's patients. Another drawback is that the control groups comprised referred patients (not population-based studies).

Studies that have addressed the prevalence of antibodies against the CagA cytotoxin are shown in Table 8.2 [51,53–55]. The importance of CagA antibodies for epidemiological studies is twofold. First, *H. pylori* bacteria with the CagA virulence factor exert a more pronounced effect on the severity of gastritis and subsequent diseases like gastroduodenal ulcer or gastric cancer. Therefore, their impact on acid secretion is stronger. Also, corpus-predominant gastritis induced by CagA-positive strains leads to stronger acid suppression than does corpus gastritis by CagA-negative strains [56]. Moreover, the immune response against the CagA protein is stronger and longer lasting than the immune response against other bacterial antigens [57]. This is of interest in epidemiological studies as CagA determination permits to identify patients, who were infected with *H. pylori* in the remote past, but have cleared their infection.

Probably due to hypochlohydria, these patients have a high risk of gastric cancer [58,59] (Table 8.3). In case-control studies positive *H. pylori* tests from serum samples, that were obtained more than 10 years before the manifestation of gastric cancer, indicated a higher risk (odds ratio) of gastric cancer than in patients in whom serum samples were taken more recently. Therefore, some investigators have evaluated for the CagA status in patients with negative serology status, i.e. negative results of serum immunoglobulin G (IgG) enzyme linked immunosorbent assay (ELISA) detecting antibodies against whole cell *H. pylori* bacteria. However, the proportion of patients with negative *H. pylori* serology but positive CagA serology is rather small (<5% of the study population) (see Tables 8.2 & 8.4). Patients with Barrett's esophagus have a considerable lower prevalence of CagA antibodies than controls, but numbers are small.

Esophageal Adenocarcinoma

More important than the data on Barrett's esophagus are those on esophageal adenocarcinoma [60]. Among 550 patients with Barrett's esophagus, those

Table 8.3 Meta-analysis of 12 nested case-control studies on the risk of gastric adenocarcinoma dependent on *Helicobacter pylori* serology (*H. pylori* whole-cell immunoglobulin G [IgG] antibodies by enzyme immono assay). Odds ratios were stratified according to the subsite of adenocarcinoma and the time interval between serum sampling and tumor manifestation.

		Odds ratio of positive IgG *H. pylori status* (number of cases)	
Author	Subsite of adenocarcinoma	Serum obtained < 10 years ago	Serum obtained > 10 years ago
Heliocobacter and Cancer Collaborative Group, 2001 [58]	Gastric cardia Gastric non-cardia	1.2 ($n = 226$) 2.4 ($n = 539$)	0.5 ($n = 48$) 5.9 ($n = 223$)

Table 8.4 Cross-sectional case-control studies on the prevalence of *Helicobacter pylori* infection in patients with adenocarcinoma of the esophagus and/or the gastric cardia. *H. pylori* infection status was assessed by serum enzyme immuno assay on immunoglobulin G (IgG) antibodies against whole cell *H. pylori* antigens. In addition, CagA status was determined by serum IgG antibodies against CagA (enzyme immuno assay or immunoblot). Results are presented as odds ratios of a respective positive status. All odds ratios were adjusted for age, sex, race, and further socioeconomic and cancer risk variables including smoking.

				Odds ratio	
Author	Country	Site of adenocarcinoma	n	Positive *H. Pylori* status	Positive CagA status
Chow *et al.* 1998 [61]	USA	Esophagus/gastric cardia Distal stomach (non-cardia)	129 67	0.7 1.3	0.4† 1.4†
Limburg *et al.* 2001 [62]	China	Gastric cardia Distal stomach (non-cardia)	99 82	1.6 1.7	1.8* 1.8*
Wu *et al.* 2003 [63]	USA	Esophagus/gastric cardia Distal stomach (non-cardia)	167 127	1.3 1.9	0.9* 2.2*
Ye *et al.* 2004 [64]	Sweden	Esophagus Gastric cardia	97 133	0.3 0.8	0.5* 1.0*

* CagA status determined in all patients.
† CagA status determined only in patients with positive *H. pylori* whole cell IgG antibodies.

with high-grade dysplasia (intraepithelial neoplasia) or carcinoma had a lower prevalence of *H. pylori* than those without dysplasia. During follow-up, patients with *H. pylori* had less progression towards dysplasia or cancer. Particularly intriguing are the results of four large-scale case-control studies, presented in Table 8.4 [61–64]. Controls were population-based and the number of cases exceeded 100. In addition to esophageal adenocarcinoma, cases of gastric cardia carcinoma were also analysed, since these tumors often involve the esophagogastric junction and may, originate from Barrett's metaplasia. Furthermore, it is also conceivable that the gastric cardia is involved in reflux induced carcinogenesis.

The first study by Chow *et al.*, in a US population, demonstrated that the *H. pylori* prevalence was lower in patients with esophageal or gastric cardia adenocarcinoma than in controls [61]. In particular, antibodies against CagA were inversely associated with these tumor entities. In contrast, in a Chinese population, patients with cardia carcinoma were more likely to be *H. pylori* infected and having CagA antibodies than controls [62]. The explanation for the discrepancy between the US and Chinese studies is that Barrett's carcinoma is virtually non-existent in the Chinese population, while gastric carcinoma is more common than in Western countries. Therefore, the cardia cancers could represent true gastric cancers in China, whereas in regions with a higher incidence of Barrett's carcinoma (like Western countries), cancers ascribed to the cardia are more likely to originate from Barrett's metaplasia.

The large study by Wu *et al.*, again a US-population based study, contradicted the inverse association between *H. pylori* infection and adenocarcinoma of the gastric cardia or esophagus and instead revealed a slight positive association [63]. Interestingly, also in this study, *H. pylori* infected patients with junctional carcinoma (esophagus and gastric cardia combined) less frequently had antibodies against CagA than controls.

The most recent study from Sweden corroborated the inverse association between *H. pylori* and CagA status on one hand and esophageal adenocarcinoma on the other [64]. There was no correlation with gastric cardia carcinoma. In this study, pepsinogen I was assessed in the serum since a low serum pepsinogen is an indicator of gastric corpus atrophy. The hypothesis that the reduced risk of esophageal carcinoma in *H. pylori*-positive patients could be due to gastric atrophy could not however be confirmed. A possible explanation is that corpus-predominant *H. pylori* gastritis may inhibit gastric acid output even in the absence of atrophy.

Furthermore, a meta-analysis of nested case-control studies on gastric cancer demonstrates a reduced risk of gastric cardia cancer in cases with positive *H. pylori* serum tests, but only if serum samples were obtained more than 10 years ago [58] (see Table 8.3). A possible explanation is that those patients who have lost their *H. pylori* infection as a consequence of hypochlorhydria may have a lower risk of cancer.

Clinical Intervention

The most robust evidence for a causal relation would come from clinical intervention trials. There are, however, no data substantiating any change of the incidence of Barrett's carcinoma after *H. pylori* eradication. As the influence of eradication may evolve several years after the intervention, long-term data can be expected in the future. Therefore, surrogate markers for the risk of Barrett's carcinoma, like the development of GERD or Barrett's mucosa, need special consideration. Data on the alteration of GERD after *H. pylori* eradication are conflicting. GERD may be induced or exacerbated after eradication, but may also decline or disappear [65,66]. With respect to post-therapeutic time intervals evaluated at present (up to 5 years), there is no clear trend for the preponderance of a positive or negative effect [67]. However, the majority of data allow, the conclusion that *H. pylori* eradication is not a threat for developing GERD and its complications.

Conclusions

There is epidemiological data indicating that a subset of *H. pylori*-infected patients may experience a reduced risk of Barrett's carcinoma. However, there is substantial controversy about this. Pathophysiological considerations suggest that gastric acid hyposecretion is caused by gastric corpus gastritis and may reduce the risk of Barrett's esophagus and esophageal adenocarcinoma. Acid hyposecretion and corpus-predominant gastritis, however, are important risk factors for distal gastric (non-cardia) carcinoma, a condition that is still ten times more frequent than Barrett's carcinoma in most populations. Therefore, in clinical terms, it is not justified to assign *H. pylori* infection to a "protective role" against the development of esophageal adenocarcinoma [68].

References

1. Hill AB. The environment and disease: association or causation? *Proc R Soc Med* 1965;**58**:295–300.

2. Calam J, Gibbons A, Healey ZV *et al*. How does *Helicobacter pylori* cause mucosal damage? Its effect on acid and gastrin physiology. *Gastroenterology* 1997;**113**(6 Suppl):S43–9.

3. El Omar EM, Oien K, El Nujumi A *et al*. *Helicobacter pylori* infection and chronic gastric acid hyposecretion. *Gastroenterology* 1997;**113**(1):15–24.

4. McColl KE, El Omar E, Gillen D. *Helicobacter pylori* gastritis and gastric physiology. *Gastroenterol Clin North Am* 2000;**29**(3):687–703.

5. Bercik P, Verdu EF, Armstrong D *et al*. The effect of ammonia on omeprazole-induced reduction of gastric acidity in subjects with *Helicobacter pylori* infection. *Am J Gastroenterol* 2000;**95**(4):947–55.

6. Verdu EF, Armstrong D, Sabovcikova L *et al*. High concentrations of ammonia, but not volatile amines, in gastric juice of subjects with *Helicobacter pylori* infection. *Helicobacter* 1998;**3**(2):97–102.

7. Hamlet A, Olbe L. The influence of *Helicobacter pylori* infection on postprandial duodenal acid load and duodenal bulb pH in humans. *Gastroenterology* 1996;**111**(2):391–400.

8. El Omar EM, Carrington M, Chow WH *et al*. Interleukin-1 polymorphisms associated with increased risk of gastric cancer. *Nature* 2000;**404**(6776):398–402.

9. El Omar EM, Rabkin CS, Gammon MD *et al*. Increased risk of noncardia gastric cancer associated with proinflammatory cytokine gene polymorphisms. *Gastroenterology* 2003;**124**(5):1193–201.

10. Iijima K, Sekine H, Koike T *et al*. Long-term effect of *Helicobacter pylori* eradication on the reversibility of acid secretion in profound hypochlorhydria. *Aliment Pharmacol Ther* 2004;**19**(11):1181–8.

11. El Serag HB, Sonnenberg A, Jamal MM *et al*. Corpus gastritis is protective against reflux oesophagitis. *Gut* 1999;**45**(2):181–5.

12. Hamada H, Haruma K, Mihara M *et al*. High incidence of reflux oesophagitis after eradication therapy for *Helicobacter pylori*: impacts of hiatal hernia and corpus gastritis. *Aliment Pharmacol Ther* 2000;**14**(6):729–35.

13. Koike T, Ohara S, Sekine H *et al*. *Helicobacter pylori* infection prevents erosive reflux oesophagitis by decreasing gastric acid secretion. *Gut* 2001;**49**(3):330–4.

14. Koike T, Ohara S, Sekine H *et al*. Increased gastric acid secretion after *Helicobacter pylori* eradication may be a factor for developing reflux oesophagitis. *Aliment Pharmacol Ther* 2001;**15**(6):813–20.

15. Obonyo M, Guiney DG, Fierer J, Cole SP. Interactions between inducible nitric oxide and other inflammatory mediators during *Helicobacter pylori* infection. *Helicobacter* 2003;**8**(5):495–502.

16. Tefera S, Hatlebakk JG, Berstad AE, Berstad A. Eradication of *Helicobacter pylori* does not increase acid reflux in patients with mild to moderate reflux oesophagitis. *Scand J Gastroenterol* 2002;**37**(8):877–83.

17. Wu JC, Lai AC, Wong SK *et al*. Dysfunction of oesophageal motility in *Helicobacter pylori*-infected patients with reflux oesophagitis. *Aliment Pharmacol Ther* 2001;**15**(12):1913–9.

18. Zerbib F, Bicheler V, Leray V *et al*. *H. pylori* and transient lower esophageal sphincter relaxations induced by gastric distension in healthy humans. *Am J Physiol Gastrointest Liver Physiol* 2001;**281**(2):G350–6.

19. Manes G, Malfertheiner P. Relationship of *Helicobacter pylori* infection with gastrointestinal motility. *Ital J Gastroenterol Hepatol* 1999;**31**(8):705–12.

20. Thumshirn M, Camilleri M, Saslow SB *et al*. Gastric accommodation in non-ulcer dyspepsia and the roles of *Helicobacter pylori* infection and vagal function. *Gut* 1999;**44**(1):55–64.

21. Chiloiro M, Russo F, Riezzo G *et al*. Effect of *Helicobacter pylori* infection on gastric emptying and gastrointestinal hormones in dyspeptic and healthy subjects. *Dig Dis Sci* 2001;**46**(1):46–53.

22. Dominguez-Munoz JE, Malfertheiner P. Effect of *Helicobacter pylori* infection on gastrointestinal motility, pancreatic secretion and hormone release in asymptomatic humans. *Scand J Gastroenterol* 2001;**36**(11):1141–7.

23. Koskenpato J, Farkkila M, Sipponen P. *Helicobacter pylori* and different topographic types of gastritis: treatment response after successful eradication therapy in functional dyspepsia. *Scand J Gastroenterol* 2002;**37**(7):778–84.

24. Saslow SB, Thumshirn M, Camilleri M *et al*. Influence of *H. pylori* infection on gastric motor and sensory function in asymptomatic volunteers. *Dig Dis Sci* 1998;**43**(2):258–64.

25. Testoni PA, Bagnolo F. In dyspeptic patients without gastric phase III of the migrating motor complex, *Helicobacter pylori* eradication produces no short-term changes in interdigestive motility pattern. *Scand J Gastroenterol* 2000;**35**(8):808–13.

26. Lin Z, Chen JD, Parolisi S *et al*. Prevalence of gastric myoelectrical abnormalities in patients with nonulcer dyspepsia and *H. pylori* infection: resolution after *H. pylori* eradication. *Dig Dis Sci* 2001;**46**(4):739–45.

27. Miyaji H, Azuma T, Ito S *et al*. The effect of *helicobacter pylori* eradication therapy on gastric antral myoelectrical activity and gastric emptying in patients with non-ulcer dyspepsia. *Aliment Pharmacol Ther* 1999;**13**(11):1473–80.

28. Ladas SD, Katsogridakis J, Malamou H *et al*. *Helicobacter pylori* may induce bile reflux: link between *H. pylori* and bile induced injury to gastric epithelium. *Gut* 1996;**38**(1):15–8.

29. Artiko VM, Chebib HY, Ugljesic MB *et al*. Relationship between enterogastric reflux estimated by scintigraphy and the presence of *Helicobacter pylori*. *Hepatogastroenterology* 1999;**46**(26):1234–7.

30. Manifold DK, Anggiansah A, Rowe I *et al*. Gastro-oesophageal reflux and duodenogastric reflux before and after eradication in *Helicobacter pylori* gastritis. *Eur J Gastroenterol Hepatol* 2001;**13**(5):535–9.

31. Dixon MF, Neville PM, Mapstone NP *et al*. Bile reflux gastritis and Barrett's oesophagus: further evidence of a role for duodenogastro-oesophageal reflux? *Gut* 2001;**49**(3):359–63.

32. Dixon MF, Mapstone NP, Neville PM *et al*. Bile reflux gastritis and intestinal metaplasia at the cardia. *Gut* 2002;**51**(3):351–5.

33. Nakamura M, Haruma K, Kamada T *et al*. Duodenogastric reflux is associated with antral metaplastic gastritis. *Gastrointest Endosc* 2001;**53**(1):53–9.

34. Zullo A, Rinaldi V, Hassan C *et al*. Gastric pathology in cholecystectomy patients: role of *Helicobacter pylori* and bile reflux. *J Clin Gastroenterol* 1998;**27**(4): 335–8.

35. Malfertheiner P, Peitz U. The interplay between *Helicobacter pylori*, gastro-oesophageal reflux disease, and intestinal metaplasia. *Gut* 2005;**54**(suppl 1):i13–20.

36. Jankowski JA, Harrison RF, Perry I *et al*. Barrett's metaplasia. *Lancet* 2000;**356**(9247):2079–85.

37. Peitz U, Vieth M, Malfertheiner P. Carditis at the interface between GERD and *Helicobacter pylori* infection. *Dig Dis* 2004;**22**(2):120–5.

38. Chandrasoma PT, Der R, Dalton P *et al*. Distribution and significance of epithelial types in columnar-lined esophagus. *Am J Surg Pathol* 2001;**25**(9):1188–93.

39. Chandrasoma PT, Der R, Ma Y *et al*. Histologic classification of patients based on mapping biopsies of the gastroesophageal junction. *Am J Surg Pathol* 2003;**27**(7): 929–36.

40. Peitz U, Vieth M, Pross M *et al*. Cardia-type metaplasia arising in the remnant esophagus after cardia resection. *Gastrointest Endosc* 2004;**59**(7):810–7.

41. Chandrasoma PT, Lokuhetty DM, DeMeester TR *et al*. Definition of histopathologic changes in gastro-esophageal reflux disease. *Am J Surg Pathol* 2000; **24**(3):344–51.

42. Oberg S, Johansson J, Wenner J, Walther B. Metaplastic columnar mucosa in the cervical esophagus after esophagectomy. *Ann Surg* 2002;**235**(3):338–45.

43. Sampliner RE. Updated guidelines for the diagnosis, surveillance, and therapy of Barrett's esophagus. *Am J Gastroenterol* 2002;**97**(8):1888–95.

44. O'Connor HJ. Review article: *Helicobacter pylori* and gastro-oesophageal reflux disease—clinical implications and management. *Aliment Pharmacol Ther* 1999;**13**(2):117–27.

45. Hackelsberger A, Gunther T, Schultze V *et al*. Prevalence and pattern of *Helicobacter pylori* gastritis in the gastric cardia. *Am J Gastroenterol* 1997;**92**(12):2220–4.

46. Henihan RD, Stuart RC, Nolan N *et al*. Barrett's esophagus and the presence of *Helicobacter pylori*. *Am J Gastroenterol* 1998;**93**(4):542–6.

47. Sharma VK, Demian SE, Taillon D *et al*. Examination of tissue distribution of *Helicobacter pylori* within columnar-lined esophagus. *Dig Dis Sci* 1999;**44**(6):1165–8.

48. Naumann M, Crabtree JE. *Helicobacter pylori*-induced epithelial cell signalling in gastric carcinogenesis. *Trends Microbiol* 2004;**12**(1):29–36.

49. Raghunath A, Hungin AP, Wooff D, Childs S. Prevalence of *Helicobacter pylori* in patients with gastro-oesophageal reflux disease: systematic review. *BMJ* 2003;**326**(7392):737–43.

50. Abe Y, Ohara S, Koike T *et al*. The prevalence of *Helicobacter pylori* infection and the status of gastric acid secretion in patients with Barrett's esophagus in Japan. *Am J Gastroenterol* 2004;**99**(7):1213–21.

51. Ackermark P, Kuipers EJ, Wolf C *et al*. Colonization with CagA-positive *Helicobacter pylori* strains in intestinal metaplasia of the esophagus and the esophagogastric junction. *Am J Gastroenterol* 2003;**98**(8):1719–24.

52. Laheij RJ, Van Rossum LG, De Boer WA, Jansen JB. Corpus gastritis in patients with endoscopic diagnosis of reflux oesophagitis and Barrett's oesophagus. *Aliment Pharmacol Ther* 2002;**16**(5):887–91.

53. Loffeld RJ, Werdmuller BF, Kuster JG *et al*. Colonization with CagA-positive *Helicobacter pylori* strains inversely associated with reflux esophagitis and Barrett's esophagus. *Digestion* 2000;**62**(2–3):95–9.

54. Kudo M, Gutierrez O, El Zimaity HM *et al*. CagA in Barrett's oesophagus in Colombia, a country with a high prevalence of gastric cancer. *J Clin Pathol* 2005;**58**(3): 259–62.

55. Vaezi MF, Falk GW, Peek RM *et al.* CagA-positive strains of *Helicobacter pylori* may protect against Barrett's esophagus. *Am J Gastroenterol* 2000;**95**(9):2206–11.

56. Kuipers EJ, Perez-Perez GI, Meuwissen SG, Blaser MJ. *Helicobacter pylori* and atrophic gastritis: importance of the CagA status. *J Natl Cancer Inst* 1995;**87**(23):1777–80.

57. Klaamas K, Held M, Wadstrom T *et al.* IgG immune response to *Helicobacter pylori* antigens in patients with gastric cancer as defined by ELISA and immunoblotting. *Int J Cancer* 1996;**67**(1):1–5.

58. Helicobacter and Cancer Collaborative Group. Gastric cancer and *Helicobacter pylori*: a combined analysis of 12 case control studies nested within prospective cohorts. *Gut* 2001;**49**(3):347–53.

59. Yamaji Y, Mitsushima T, Ikuma H *et al.* Inverse background of *Helicobacter pylori* antibody and pepsinogen in reflux oesophagitis compared with gastric cancer: analysis of 5732 Japanese subjects. *Gut* 2001;**49**(3):335–40.

60. Weston AP, Sharma P, Mathur S *et al.* Risk stratification of Barrett's esophagus: updated prospective multivariate analysis. *Am J Gastroenterol* 2004;**99**(9):1657–66.

61. Chow WH, Blaser MJ, Blot WJ *et al.* An inverse relation between CagA+ strains of *Helicobacter pylori* infection and risk of esophageal and gastric cardia adenocarcinoma. *Cancer Res* 1998;**58**(4):588–90.

62. Limburg P, Qiao Y, Mark S *et al. Helicobacter pylori* seropositivity and subsite-specific gastric cancer risks in Linxian, China. *J Natl Cancer Inst* 2001;**93**(3):226–33.

63. Wu AH, Crabtree JE, Bernstein L *et al.* Role of *Helicobacter pylori* CagA+ strains and risk of adenocarcinoma of the stomach and esophagus. *Int J Cancer* 2003;**103**(6):815–21.

64. Ye W, Held M, Lagergren J *et al. Helicobacter pylori* infection and gastric atrophy: risk of adenocarcinoma and squamous-cell carcinoma of the esophagus and adenocarcinoma of the gastric cardia. *J Natl Cancer Inst* 2004;**96**(5):388–96.

65. McColl KE, Dickson A, El Nujumi A *et al.* Symptomatic benefit 1–3 years after *H. pylori* eradication in ulcer patients: impact of gastroesophageal reflux disease. *Am J Gastroenterol* 2000;**95**(1):101–5.

66. Malfertheiner P, Dent J, Zeijlon L *et al.* Impact of *Helicobacter pylori* eradication on heartburn in patients with gastric or duodenal ulcer disease—results from a randomized trial programme. *Aliment Pharmacol Ther* 2002;**16**(8):1431–42.

67. Sharma P, Vakil N. Review article: *Helicobacter pylori* and reflux disease. *Aliment Pharmacol Ther* 2003;**17**(3):297–305.

68. Graham DY. *Helicobacter pylori* is not and never was "protective" against anything, including GERD. *Dig Dis Sci* 2003;**48**(4):629–30.

CHAPTER 9

Molecular Biology of Barrett's Esophagus

Linda A. Feagins and Rhonda F. Souza

Introduction

The current strategy to reduce the risk of cancer in patients with Barrett's esophagus relies on periodic endoscopic surveillance. However, recent studies suggest this strategy is ineffective because the majority of patients diagnosed with esophageal adenocarcinoma are unaware that they have Barrett's esophagus and therefore are not being screened [1]. Another problem with our current strategy is that it is targeted at the detection of dysplasia in the Barrett's mucosa, an imperfect predictor of cancer risk for a variety of reasons [2]. Since dysplasia is essentially the histologic manifestation of genomic damage that precedes malignancy, an earlier indicator of cancer risk would be detection of the genetic damage itself. With the recent advances in molecular biology, efforts to characterize the specific molecular events that occur during the evolution of esophageal adenocarcinoma have intensified. The identification of molecular biomarkers may offer easy reproducibility and standardization in addition to the truly early detection of neoplastic progression. These molecular biomarkers may also serve as targets at which to direct therapeutic agents. Therefore, it has become increasingly important to understand the pathogenesis of Barrett's esophagus and esophageal adenocarcinoma at the molecular level in order to improve the diagnosis and therapy of this deadly disease.

Genetic Instability

The spontaneous mutation rate of DNA is so low that during an individual's lifespan cells do not have a chance to acquire the full array of mutations essential for cancer formation [3]. Therefore, preneoplastic cells must have unstable genomes in order for tumor progression to proceed. Genomic instability can manifest as mutations in particular DNA sequences, or by abnormalities in chromosomal content. Aneuploidy refers to an alteration in chromosomal content other than the normal diploid (2N) or tetraploid (4n) (where n equals chromosomal number). Aneuploidy reflects widespread DNA damage rather than any single mutation and has been associated with an increased risk of neoplastic progression.

Aneuploidy can be detected by flow cytometry. In combination with histology, aneuploidy has been used to predict neoplastic progression of Barrett's esophagus in a large prospective study [4]. In addition to aneuploidy, the number of tetraploid (4N) cell populations was examined as an indicator of neoplastic progression. Tetraploid cell populations can be normal, but if tissues contain more than 6% of the total cell population as tetraploid cells there is an increased risk to progress to aneuploidy [4]. Patients with aneuploidy in their biopsies of Barrett's mucosa had a 5-year incidence of cancer progression of 64%; in patients with elevated (> 6%) 4N fractions, the 5-year cancer incidence was 57%; and in patients with both aneuploidy and elevated 4N, the 5-year cancer incidence was 75% [4]. In contrast, the rate of cancer incidence in patients whose biopsies did not demonstrate aneuploidy or tetraploidy was only 5.2% and all of these patients had high-grade dysplasia histologically. The use of aneuploidy or tetraploidy as an adjunct to histologic assessment was most helpful in predicting cancer progression in patient biopsies demonstrating no dysplasia, indefinite, or low-grade dysplasia. The presence of either aneuploidy or tetraploidy in biopsies from these patients heralded a 5-year cancer incidence of 39% compared to 0% in patients with neither of these flow cytometric abnormalities [4]. Determining aneuploidy and tetraploidy in Barrett's patients without high-grade dysplasia may be useful to select a subset of patients who may require more frequent endoscopic surveillance. As yet, this strategy has not been tested in large, prospective clinical trials to determine if more frequent endoscopic surveillance will increase the rate of detection of high-grade dysplasia leading to therapeutic interventions that ultimately will decrease mortality from cancer in patients with Barrett's esophagus.

Cell Cycle

Many of the genes targeted for damage regulate the cell cycle clock apparatus, the central mechanism that controls whether a cell will proliferate, differentiate, or die. The cell cycle is divided into four phases: (i) G1 (first gap); (ii) S (DNA synthesis); (iii) G2 (second gap); and (iv) M (mitosis). Near the end of G1, there is a key regulatory point termed the restriction or R point where the cell decides if it will enter S phase and complete the cycle, or exit the cell cycle into the quiescent G0 phase. The retinoblastoma (Rb) protein appears to be the molecular switch in control of the R point. In non-dividing cells, Rb is hypo-phosphorylated and blocks progression through the cell cycle. Following phosphorylation, Rb becomes inactive, thereby allowing the cell to pass through the R-point into the remainder of the cell cycle.

Multiple studies suggest that Barrett's esophagus has an increased rate of proliferation and hence an increased proportion of cells entering into the cell cycle. Multiple techniques to measure cellular proliferation have been used to evaluate biopsy samples of Barrett's esophagus [5,6]. Using these various techniques, the specialized intestinal metaplasia of Barrett's esophagus demonstrated increased proliferation compared to gastric fundic and junctional-type epithelia. Moroever, using these same techniques, episodic acid exposure has been shown to increase proliferation in Barrett's esophagus *in vivo*, in *ex vivo* cultures, and *in vitro* in adenocarcinoma cells [7–10].

Clinical Implications

One potential strategy to decrease the cancer risk in patients with Barrett's esophagus may be to prevent exposure of the esophageal mucosa to acidic gastric refluxate by the administration of potent antisecretory agents. This approach has been supported by clinical studies showing decreased proliferation, increased differentiation, and fewer pro-proliferative cell cycle abnormalities after normalization of intraesophageal pH using proton pump inhibitors (PPIs) compared to patients with continued abnormal esophageal acid exposure [11–12]. A recent study also showed a significant reduction in the risk of developing dysplasia in Barrett's mucosa in patients treated symptomatically with PPIs versus those not treated or treated only with H2-blockers [13]. However, some controversy still remains over this treatment as it is well known that PPI therapy leads to elevations in serum gastrin levels which, according to one study, may be linked to increased proliferation in Barrett's biopsies *in vitro* [14]. In light of these findings, well-designed, controlled prospective clinical trials are needed before aggressive acid suppression (i.e. more than that required to eliminate symptoms and heal esophagitis) can be recommended for widespread clinical application.

Oncogenes

Proto-oncogenes are normal cellular genes that promote cell growth. When these proto-oncogenes become mutated in such a way that they become overactive, they are called oncogenes. Several examples of oncogenes implicated in Barrett's esophagus are cyclins D1, E, and B1. Cyclins D1 and E along with cyclin-dependent kinases (cdks) regulate the phosphorylation of Rb whereas cyclin B1 acts to control the G2 to M transition. Phosphorylation of Rb occurs by interactions of cyclins with cdks. Increased nuclear expression of cyclin D1 protein has been detected in biopsy specimens of non-dysplastic Barrett's metaplasia compared to normal squamous controls [15]. In contrast, overexpression of cyclin E has been found in both low-grade and high-grade dysplastic areas of Barrett's esophagus as well as in adenocarcinomas, but not in non-dysplastic Barrett's samples [16]. Expression of cyclin B1 has been detected in non-dysplastic and dysplastic samples of Barrett's esophagus and in adenocarcinomas [17]. Unfortunately, the expression of cyclin B1 in control tissues such as normal esophageal or intestinal-type tissue was not examined, making the role of cyclin B1 expression in the neoplastic progression of Barrett's esophagus questionable [17].

Clinical Implications

Given the integral relationship between cyclins and cdks in allowing cell cycle progression to proceed, cdks would appear to be logical targets at which to direct therapies to inhibit cell proliferation. Flavopiridol, a synthetic flavone, is a potent inhibitor of cdk-2 and cdk-4, which are the enzymes primarily responsible for Rb phosphorylation. In a phase I clinical trial, patients with esophageal adenocarcinoma treated with flavopiridol in combination with paclitaxel demonstrated either a complete or partial response to this combined therapy [18]. Given these encouraging results, phase II studies using the combination of flavopiridol and paclitaxel are currently in progress.

Growth Factors, Growth Factor Receptors, and Signal Transduction Pathways

Epidermal growth factor (EGF) and transforming growth factor-α (TGF-α), have been found to be increased in metaplastic Barrett's esophagus and have been implicated in neoplastic progression [19,20]. The growth factor receptor, EGF receptor (also called ErbB-1), has been detected at increased levels in intestinal metaplasia and in esophageal adenocarcinomas and is thought to play a role in neoplastic progression of Barrett's esophagus [19,20]. However, the role of an oncogenic form of the normal EGF receptor family member *erb*B-2 (also called HER2 or Neu) in the development of Barrett's-associated adenocarcinomas is not clear [21,22]. The binding of growth factors to receptors that are members of the tyrosine kinase family often activates Ras/Raf pro-

teins which in turn activate the mitogen activated protein kinase (MAPK) signal transduction cascade to promote cell proliferation [23,24]. In a number of extra-esophageal tumors, ras proteins (including H-ras and K-ras,) and recently the B-raf protein have been identified as important human oncogenes [25,26]. However, available data do not support an important role for oncogenic ras or B-raf in Barrett's-associated cancers [26,27]. Activation of the MAPK pathways by acid exposure has been associated with an increased rate of cell proliferation and a decreased rate of apoptosis in a human Barrett's-associated adenocarcinoma cell line [10].

Clinical Implications

Blocking growth factors, growth factor receptors, or their signaling cascades are potential directions for future treatments in Barrett's esophagus and esophageal adenocarcinoma. For example, a potential therapeutic strategy in Barrett's esophagus may be to inhibit activation of the EGF receptor, an approach which is already under investigation in other cancers [28]. Alternatively, inhibitors of the MAPK pathway may prove to be successful therapies as they are already showing promise and appear safe in early clinical trials in Crohn's disease [29].

Tumor Suppressor Genes

Tumor suppressor genes (TSGs) are normal genes that restrain the cells ability to proliferate by preventing phosphorylation of Rb. Therefore, it is advantageous to cancer cells to inactivate TSGs, which can be done by at least three mechanisms, including mutation, deletion of the chromosomal region containing the gene (called loss of heterozygosity [LOH]), or by attachment of methyl groups to the promoter region of genes (called promoter methylation).

Since the Rb protein is the central regulator of cell cycle progression, it would be a logical target for inactivation. Although mutation of the *Rb* gene itself in Barrett's esophagus or in esophageal adenocarcinomas has not yet been demonstrated, multiple studies have identified alterations in genes that eliminate Rb function such as *p53* and *p16* [30,31]. Inactivation of *p53* by LOH of 17p, the *p53* locus, and mutation of the remaining allele have been found in approximately 50–90% of esophageal adenocarcinomas [32,33]. LOH of 17p also has been detected in metaplastic Barrett's esophagus, suggesting that inactivation of *p53* is an early step in carcinogenesis [34]. Barrett's-associated adenocarcinomas frequently demonstrate allelic loss of 9p21, the chromosomal locus for *p16* [35]. In addition, LOH of 9p21 has been found in 90% of metaplastic Barrett's epithelium demonstrating aneuploidy [36]. Methylation of the *p16* promoter, an alternative mechanism for silencing a TSG, has been found in 45% of esophageal adenocarcinomas and in non-dysplastic, specialized intestinal metaplasia suggesting that *p16* methylation is the earliest event in the neoplastic progression of Barrett's esophagus [36,37]. *p27*, an inhibitor of cdk-2 and cyclin E, has also been implicated as a TSG in Barrett's-associated adenocarcinomas. Loss of *p27* protein expression has been demonstrated in 83% of esophageal adenocarcinomas, but as yet no mutations have been identified. Furthermore, loss of expression of this protein correlated with an increase in aggressive behavior of the tumor and poor patient outcome [38,39].

Other TSGs such as the adenomatous polyposis coli (*APC*) gene block cell proliferation by inhibiting proteins that are involved in proliferative signaling. Inactivation of *APC* has been implicated in the neoplastic progression of Barrett's esophagus. Esophageal adenocarcinomas commonly demonstrate LOH of 5q21, the *APC* locus, but only rare mutation in *APC* [40]. *APC* promoter methylation is more common, with 83–92% of Barrett's high-grade dysplasia and esophageal adenocarcinomas and 40–50% of Barrett's metaplasias without dysplasia demonstrating *APC* inactivation by this mechanism [41].

Clinical Implications

In the future, risk stratification for neoplastic progression in patients with Barrett's esophagus may include assaying for alterations in TSGs. For example, in a large prospective study, LOH of 17p was found to be a significant predictor of cancer progression at 5 years [42]. Additionally, antibodies to *p53* have been detected in the serum of Barrett's patients who later progressed to dysplasia and cancer [43]. Finally,

methylated *APC* DNA has been found in the plasma in 25% of patients with esophageal adenocarcinoma, and has been associated with a significantly shortened patient survival [44]. Although results such as these are promising, large-scale prospective studies are needed to validate the utility of these markers to predict neoplastic progression before their widespread clinical use.

Apoptosis

Apoptosis is an innate, cellular self-destruct mechanism encoded in all normal cells. In normal cells, apoptosis is beneficial in that it prevents a cell with damaged, mutated DNA from undergoing replication. However, apoptosis is detrimental to cancer cells, and cells must find ways to overcome this suicide program. The apoptotic machinery comprises of several death-commitment signaling pathways that can be activated by DNA damage, metabolic abnormalities, and death receptor activation. Once activated, the death-commitment pathways converge on a common executioner pathway which ultimately leads to cell destruction [45].

Barrett's-associated adenocarcinomas have found ways in which to overcome triggering apoptosis. As already discussed, inactivation of *p53* is one way in which Barrett's cancer cells avoid inducing apoptosis initiated by DNA damage or mutation. The expression of 13-*S*-hydroxyoctadecadienoic acid (13-*S*-HODE), a fatty acid that is formed from linoleic acid through the action of 15-lipoxygenase-1 (15-LOX-1), normally activates the apoptotic machinery. Decreased expression of 15-LOX-1 has been found in 75% of esophageal adenocarcinomas [46].

Interfering with the activation of the Fas death receptor by its death promoting ligand, Fas-ligand (FasL) is another way which Barrett's cells avoid apoptosis [47]. Normally, the Fas receptor is found on the surface of both lymphocytes and gut epithelial cells, whereas FasL is expressed only by activated lymphocytes. When FasL binds to the Fas receptor, apoptosis is induced in the cell expressing the Fas receptor. By expressing FasL, tumor cells would be capable of binding the Fas receptor on the surface of attacking lymphocytes, thereby destroying the tumor killing immune cells. FasL expression has been found in one study of 13 esophageal adenocarcinomas [48].

Finally, another mechanism whereby Barrett's cancer cells might avoid apoptosis is by increasing the synthesis of an agent that normally blocks the death-commitment signaling pathways. For example, overexpression of cyclooxygenase-2 (COX-2) reduces the rate of apoptosis *in vitro* [49], and COX-2 overexpression has been detected both in esophageal adenocarcinomas and in the metaplastic epithelium of Barrett's esophagus [49,50].

Clinical Implications

Understanding the mechanisms whereby Barrett's cancer cells avoid apoptosis has guided investigations into potential therapeutic interventions. Antibodies to Fas and the Fas ligand itself have been tested in animal models, however these therapies have been met with limited success so far [51,52]. Selective inhibition of COX-2 has also gained a lot of attention as a chemopreventive strategy in Barrett's esophagus. Although data appears to support a possible role for COX-2 inhibitors in altering the rate of neoplastic progression in Barrett's esophagus, the exact mechanism underlying the potential benefits of these non-steroidal anti-inflammatory drugs (NSAIDs) remains controversial [53].

Telomeres and Telomerase

In contrast to normal cells, cancer cells have unlimited replicative potential and have achieved immortalization. Immortalization requires that tumor cells overcome autonomous, intrinsic mechanisms, which involve shortening of telomeres that limit the proliferative capacity of normal cells. Telomeres are long stretches of simple, non-coding DNA repeats located on the ends of chromosomes. With each successive round of cell replication, telomeric DNA is lost. Eventually, short telomeres trigger an exit from the cell cycle at G1 and entry into senescence, characterized by permanent growth arrest. Therefore, in order for cells to become immortal, they must prevent telomere shortening. Telomerase is the enzyme responsible for the synthesis of new telomeres [54]. Telomerase is a protein-RNA complex composed of hTERT (human telomerase reverse transcriptase

protein) and hTR (human telomerase RNA) that uses its RNA as a template for the addition of telomeric sequences to the ends of chromosomes. Most normal esophageal cells and tissues lack telomerase. Barrett's esophagus expresses low levels of telomerase which appears to increase as the metaplastic cells progress to high-grade dysplasia; esophageal adenocarcinomas demonstrate high levels of telomerase expression [55,56].

Clinical Implications

Anticancer therapies that target telomerase expression are appealing for several reasons. First, by targeting telomerase, such anticancer therapies become more selective for cancer cells over normal cells since cancer cells primarily express telomerase. Also, antitelomerase therapies in Barrett's esophagus have the potential to limit progression of early cancers since the expression level of telomerase progressively increases from metaplasia to high-grade dysplasia. Preclinical data suggest such therapies may be promising for Barrett's cancers [57]. Current phase I and II clinical trials evaluating inhibitors of telomerase do not yet involve patients with esophageal adenocarcinoma.

Vascular Endothelial Growth Factors

Vascular endothelial growth factors (VEGFs) and their receptors, the VEGF receptors (VEGFRs), are potent inducers of endothelial cell proliferation and migration. The VEGF family consists of VEGF-A, B, C, D, E and the placenta growth factor (PIGF), with VEGF-A being the most potent and well studied. There are three known VEGFRs (VEGFR-1–3) and all are tyrosine kinase receptors [58].

The expression of VEGF-A and its corresponding receptor, the VEGFR-2, has been found in the epithelial cells and in the blood vessels of metaplastic Barrett's esophagus, but not in normal squamous esophagus [59]. VEGF-C expression has been found in metaplastic Barrett's epithelium whereas neoplastic Barrett's tissues demonstrate expression of VEGFR-3 [60]. Compared to dysplastic and metaplastic Barrett's esophagus and normal esophageal mucosa, esophageal adenocarcinomas express significantly increased levels of VEGF mRNA and protein [61]. There is speculation that the infiltrating vascular network is responsible for the salmon color characteristic of the specialized, intestinal metaplasia of Barrett's esophagus [59].

Clinical Implications

The use of anti-VEGF agents is currently under study as a first-line combination chemotherapy agent in colon cancer [62]. However, no current trials have investigated VEGF inhibitors in Barrett's esophagus or esophageal adenocarcinoma. Recombinant human VEGF has been shown to enhance angiogenesis and ulcer healing in an animal model of reflux induced esophageal ulceration [63]. The ability of recombinant human VEGF to promote healing of reflux damaged squamous mucosa suggests such therapy may play a role in the preventing the development of Barrett's esophagus in patients with erosive esophagitis.

Cadherins and Catenins

Cadherins and catenins are involved in maintaining cell–cell interaction. Cadherins, a large family of cell adhesion molecules, bind to cytoplasmic proteins called catenins that are linked to the cell's actin cytoskeleton [64]. Processes that prevent the interaction of cadherins and catenins can impair cell adhesion and predispose to invasion and metastasis. E-cadherin and β-catenin are found primarily in the cell membrane in normal esophageal squamous mucosa and the non-dysplastic, specialized intestinal metaplasia of Barrett's esophagus [65,66]. In dysplastic Barrett's esophagus, membrane associated E-cadherin and β-catenin protein expression has been found to decrease while cytoplasmic and nuclear staining for these proteins has been found to increase [67]. Furthermore, membrane associated E-cadherin and β-catenin expression appears to fall as the degree of dysplasia increases [68].

Clinical Implications

A number of synthetic and naturally occurring agents have been evaluated for their ability to interfere with β-catenin. *In vitro* data suggest that enhancing membrane associated and decreasing nuclear associated β-catenin protein expression could be

a promising strategy for early chemopreventive intervention as well as delaying tumor progression [69]. Unfortunately, so far none of these studies has been directed at Barrett's associated adenocarcinomas.

Matrix Metaloproteinases

Matrix metaloproteinases (MMPs) play an important role in the process of invasion and metastasis [70]. MMPs are a family of zinc-dependent proteolytic enzymes that destroy the extracellular matrix, an early process during invasion and metastasis. The MMPs are divided into five groups: (i) stromelysins; (ii) collagenases; (iii) gelatinises; (iv) membrane types; and (v) others. MMPs, mainly matrilysin (MMP-7), have been detected in Barrett's esophagus, esophageal adenocarcinoma, and lymph node metastases. The detection of MMP-7 expression correlated with aggressiveness of the tumor as determined by histologic criteria [71].

Clinical Implications

Recent understanding of the role of MMPs in tumor invasion and metastasis has spurred efforts to generate clinically useful inhibitors for cancer treatment. Thus far, the major types of MMP inhibitors (MMPIs) investigated include pseudopeptides that mimic MMP substrates, non-peptide molecules that bind Zn which is needed for enzyme function, and AE-941, an extract from shark cartilage with an unknown MMPI function [70,72]. To date, MMPIs have not been investigated in Barrett's esophagus or in esophageal adenocarcinoma. However, clinical trials investigating the role of MMPIs in other tumor types have been unsuccessful, making MMPI therapy unlikely in the management of Barrett's esophagus [70].

Conclusion

The genetic abnormalities described have been identified during the neoplastic progression of Barrett's esophagus. However, it is almost certain that these genetic alterations represent only a fraction of the abnormalities acquired by a benign cell as it progresses to cancer. Nevertheless, understanding the basic

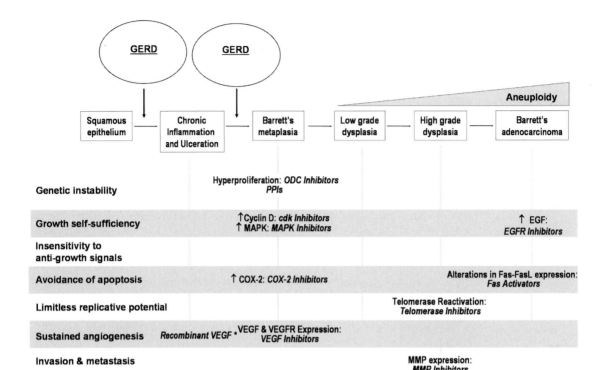

Fig 9.1 Potential therapies targeting molecular alterations in the neoplastic progression in Barrett's esophagus. Not all the genetic alterations identified in Barrett's esophagus are depicted. The alterations represented are the ones targeted by potential therapies. The potential therapies are in italics. * The use of recombinant VEGF to enhance angiogenesis may promote healing of reflux-damaged squamous epithelium and prevent the development of Barrett's esophagus. cdk, cyclin-dependent kinase; COX-2, cyclooxygenase-2; EGF, epidermal growth factor; EGFR, epidermal growth factor receptor; FasL, Fas-ligand; MAPK, mitogen activated protein kinase; MMP, matrix metaloproteinase; ODC, ornithine decarboxylase; PPIs, proton pump inhibitors; VEGF, vascular endothelial growth factor; VEGFR, vascular endothelial growth factor receptor. Reproduced with permission from Feagins and Souza [73].

mechanisms underlying carcinogenesis in Barrett's esophagus has lead to the identification of potentially useful clinical biomarkers and therapeutic targets. Although the routine clinical use of these biomarkers and targeted molecular therapies (Fig. 9.1 [73]) is not yet recommended, it is reasonable to assume that diagnostic and therapeutic strategies based on molecular composition will lead to clinical advances and improved outcomes for patients with adenocarcinoma in Barrett's esophagus.

References

1. Dulai GS, Guha S, Kahn KL, Gornbein J, Weinstein WM. Preoperative prevalence of Barrett's esophagus in esophageal adenocarcinoma: a systematic review. *Gastroenterology* 2002;**122**:26–33.

2. Reid BJ, Haggitt RC, Rubin CE *et al.* Observer variation in the diagnosis of dysplasia in Barrett's esophagus. *Hum Pathol* 1988;**19**:166–78.

3. Hahn WC, Weinberg RA. Rules for making human tumor cells. *N Engl J Med* 2002;**347**:1593–603.

4. Rabinovitch PS, Longton G, Blount PL, Levine DS, Reid BJ. Predictors of progression in Barrett's esophagus III: baseline flow cytometric variables. *Am J Gastroenterol* 2001;**96**:3071–83.

5. Gray MR, Hall PA, Nash J *et al.* Epithelial proliferation in Barrett's esophagus by proliferating cell nuclear antigen immunolocalization. *Gastroenterology* 1992;**103**:1769–76.

6. Hong MK, Laskin WB, Herman BE *et al.* Expansion of the Ki-67 proliferative compartment correlates with degree of dysplasia in Barrett's esophagus. *Cancer* 1995;**75**:423–9.

7. Ouatu-Lascar R, Fitzgerald RC, Triadafilopoulos G. Differentiation and proliferation in Barrett's esophagus and the effects of acid suppression. *Gastroenterology* 1999;**117**:327–35.

8. Fitzgerald RC, Omary MB, Triadafilopoulos G. Dynamic effects of acid on Barrett's esophagus. An *ex vivo* proliferation and differentiation model. *J Clin Invest* 1996;**98**:2120–8.

9. Fitzgerald RC, Omary MB, Triadafilopoulos G. Altered sodium–hydrogen exchange activity is a mechanism for acid-induced hyperproliferation in Barrett's esophagus. *Am J Physiol* 1998;**275**:G47–55.

10. Souza RF, Shewmake K, Terada LS, Spechler SJ. Acid exposure activates the mitogen-activated protein kinase pathways in Barrett's esophagus. *Gastroenterology* 2002;**122**:299–307.

11. Peters FT, Ganesh S, Kuipers EJ *et al.* Effect of elimination of acid reflux on epithelial cell proliferative activity of Barrett esophagus. *Scand J Gastroenterol* 2000;**35**:1238–44.

12. Umansky M, Yasui W, Hallak A *et al.* Proton pump inhibitors reduce cell cycle abnormalities in Barrett's esophagus. *Oncogene* 2001;**20**:7987–91.

13. El Serag HB, Aguirre TV, Davis S *et al.* Proton pump inhibitors are associated with reduced incidence of dysplasia in Barrett's esophagus. *Am J Gastroenterol* 2004;**99**:1877–83.

14. Haigh CR, Attwood SE, Thompson DG *et al.* Gastrin induces proliferation in Barrett's metaplasia through activation of the CCK2 receptor. *Gastroenterology* 2003;**124**:615–25.

15. Arber N, Lightdale C, Rotterdam H *et al.* Increased expression of the cyclin D1 gene in Barrett's esophagus. *Cancer Epidemiol Biomarkers Prev* 1996;**5**:457–9.

16. Sarbia M, Bektas N, Muller W *et al.* Expression of cyclin E in dysplasia, carcinoma, and nonmalignant lesions of Barrett esophagus. *Cancer* 1999;**86**:2597–601.

17. Geddert H, Heep HJ, Gabbert HE, Sarbia M. Expression of cyclin B1 in the metaplasia–dysplasia–carcinoma sequence of Barrett esophagus. *Cancer* 2002;**94**:212–8.

18. Schwartz GK, O'Reilly E, Ilson D *et al.* Phase I study of the cyclin-dependent kinase inhibitor flavopiridol in combination with paclitaxel in patients with advanced solid tumors. *J Clin Oncol* 2002;**20**:2157–70.

19. Jankowski J, Hopwood D, Wormsley KG. Flow-cytometric analysis of growth-regulatory peptides and their receptors in Barrett's oesophagus and oesophageal adenocarcinoma. *Scand J Gastroenterol* 1992;**27**:147–54.

20. Brito MJ, Filipe MI, Linehan J, Jankowski J. Association of transforming growth factor α (TGFα) and its precursors with malignant change in Barrett's epithelium: biological and clinical variables. *Int J Cancer* 1995;**60**:27–32.

21. Flejou JF, Paraf F, Muzeau F *et al.* Expression of c-erbB-2 oncogene product in Barrett's adenocarcinoma: pathological and prognostic correlations. *J Clin Pathol* 1994;**47**:23–6.

22. Brien TP, Odze RD, Sheehan CE, McKenna BJ, Ross JS. *HER-2/neu* gene amplification by FISH predicts poor survival in Barrett's esophagus-associated adenocarcinoma. *Hum Pathol* 2000;**31**:35–9.

23. Lundberg AS, Weinberg RA. Control of the cell cycle and apoptosis. *Eur J Cancer* 1999;**35**:531–9.

24. Liu JJ, Chao JR, Jiang MC *et al.* Ras transformation results in an elevated level of cyclin D1 and acceleration of G1 progression in NIH 3T3 cells. *Mol Cell Biol* 1995;**15**:3654–63.

25. Cooper GM. Cellular transforming genes. *Science* 1982;**217**:801–6.

26. Sommerer F, Vieth M, Markwarth A *et al.* Mutations of BRAF and KRAS2 in the development of Barrett's adenocarcinoma. *Oncogene* 2004;**23**:554–8.

27. Meltzer SJ, Mane SM, Wood PK *et al.* Activation of c-Ki-ras in human gastrointestinal dysplasias determined by direct sequencing of polymerase chain reaction products. *Cancer Res* 1990;**50**:3627–30.

28. El Rayes BF, LoRusso PM. Targeting the epidermal growth factor receptor. *Br J Cancer* 2004;**91**:418–24.

29. Hommes D, van den BB, Plasse T *et al.* Inhibition of stress-activated MAP kinases induces clinical improvement in moderate to severe Crohn's disease. *Gastroenterology* 2002;**122**:7–14.

30. Boynton RF, Huang Y, Blount PL *et al.* Frequent loss of heterozygosity at the retinoblastoma locus in human esophageal cancers. *Cancer Res* 1991;**51**:5766–9.

31. Huang Y, Meltzer SJ, Yin J *et al.* Altered messenger RNA and unique mutational profiles of p53 and Rb in human esophageal carcinomas. *Cancer Res* 1993;**53**:1889–94.

32. Hamelin R, Flejou JF, Muzeau F *et al.* TP53 gene mutations and p53 protein immunoreactivity in malignant and premalignant Barrett's esophagus. *Gastroenterology* 1994;**107**:1012–8.

33. Galipeau PC, Prevo LJ, Sanchez CA, Longton GM, Reid BJ. Clonal expansion and loss of heterozygosity at chromosomes 9p and 17p in premalignant esophageal (Barrett's) tissue. *J Natl Cancer Inst* 1999;**91**:2087–95.

34. Blount PL, Galipeau PC, Sanchez CA *et al.* 17p allelic losses in diploid cells of patients with Barrett's esophagus who develop aneuploidy. *Cancer Res* 1994;**54**: 2292–5.

35. Barrett MT, Sanchez CA, Galipeau PC *et al.* Allelic loss of 9p21 and mutation of the *CDKN2/p16* gene develop as early lesions during neoplastic progression in Barrett's esophagus. *Oncogene* 1996;**13**:1867–73.

36. Wong DJ, Barrett MT, Stoger R, Emond MJ, Reid BJ. *p16INK4a* promoter is hypermethylated at a high frequency in esophageal adenocarcinomas. *Cancer Res* 1997;**57**:2619–22.

37. Klump B, Hsieh CJ, Holzmann K, Gregor M, Porschen R. Hypermethylation of the *CDKN2/p16* promoter during neoplastic progression in Barrett's esophagus. *Gastroenterology* 1998;**115**:1381–6.

38. Kawamata N, Morosetti R, Miller CW *et al.* Molecular analysis of the cyclin-dependent kinase inhibitor gene *p27/Kip1* in human malignancies. *Cancer Res* 1995;**55**: 2266–9.

39. Singh SP, Lipman J, Goldman H *et al.* Loss or altered subcellular localization of *p27* in Barrett's associated adenocarcinoma. *Cancer Res* 1998;**58**:1730–5.

40. Dolan K, Garde J, Walker SJ *et al.* LOH at the sites of the *DCC, APC,* and *TP53* tumor suppressor genes occurs in Barrett's metaplasia and dysplasia adjacent to adenocarcinoma of the esophagus. *Hum Pathol* 1999;**30**: 1508–14.

41. Eads CA, Lord RV, Kurumboor SK *et al.* Fields of aberrant CpG island hypermethylation in Barrett's esophagus and associated adenocarcinoma. *Cancer Res* 2000; **60**:5021–6.

42. Reid BJ, Prevo LJ, Galipeau PC *et al.* Predictors of progression in Barrett's esophagus II: baseline 17p (*p53*) loss of heterozygosity identifies a patient subset at increased risk for neoplastic progression. *Am J Gastroenterol* 2001;**96**:2839–48.

43. Cawley HM, Meltzer SJ, De Benedetti VM *et al.* Anti-*p53* antibodies in patients with Barrett's esophagus or esophageal carcinoma can predate cancer diagnosis. *Gastroenterology* 1998;**115**:19–27.

44. Kawakami K, Brabender J, Lord RV *et al.* Hypermethylated *APC* DNA in plasma and prognosis of patients with esophageal adenocarcinoma. *J Natl Cancer Inst* 2000; **92**:1805–11.

45. Hetts SW. To die or not to die: an overview of apoptosis and its role in disease. *JAMA* 1998;**279**:300–7.

46. Shureiqi I, Xu X, Chen D *et al.* Nonsteroidal anti-inflammatory drugs induce apoptosis in esophageal cancer cells by restoring 15-lipoxygenase-1 expression. *Cancer Res* 2001;**61**:4879–84.

47. Suda T, Takahashi T, Golstein P, Nagata S. Molecular cloning and expression of the Fas ligand, a novel member of the tumor necrosis factor family. *Cell* 1993;**75**:1169–78.

48. Younes M, Schwartz MR, Ertan A, Finnie D, Younes A. Fas ligand expression in esophageal carcinomas and their lymph node metastases. *Cancer* 2000;**88**:524–8.

49. Tsujii M, DuBois RN. Alterations in cellular adhesion and apoptosis in epithelial cells overexpressing prostaglandin endoperoxide synthase 2. *Cell* 1995;**83**: 493–501.

50. Wilson KT, Fu S, Ramanujam KS, Meltzer SJ. Increased expression of inducible nitric oxide synthase and cyclooxygenase-2 in Barrett's esophagus and associated adenocarcinomas. *Cancer Res* 1998;**58**:2929–34.

51. Lacronique V, Mignon A, Fabre M *et al.* Bcl-2 protects from lethal hepatic apoptosis induced by an anti-Fas antibody in mice. *Nat Med* 1996;**2**:80–6.

52. Aoki K, Akyurek LM, San H *et al.* Restricted expression of an adenoviral vector encoding Fas ligand (CD95L) enhances safety for cancer gene therapy. *Mol Ther* 2000;**1**:555–65.

53. Souza RF, Shewmake K, Beer DG, Cryer B, Spechler SJ. Selective inhibition of cyclooxygenase-2 suppresses growth and induces apoptosis in human esophageal adenocarcinoma cells. *Cancer Res* 2000;**60**:5767–72.

54. Shay JW, Bacchetti S. A survey of telomerase activity in human cancer. *Eur J Cancer* 1997;**33**:787–91.

55. Lord RV, Salonga D, Danenberg KD *et al.* Telomerase reverse transcriptase expression is increased early in the Barrett's metaplasia, dysplasia, adenocarcinoma sequence. *J Gastrointest Surg* 2000;**4**:135–42.

56. Morales CP, Lee EL, Shay JW. *In situ* hybridization for the detection of telomerase RNA in the progression from Barrett's esophagus to esophageal adenocarcinoma. *Cancer* 1998;**83**:652–9.

57. Shammas MA, Koley H, Beer DG *et al.* Growth arrest, apoptosis, and telomere shortening of Barrett's-associated adenocarcinoma cells by a telomerase inhibitor. *Gastroenterology* 2004;**126**:1337–46.

58. Kleespies A, Guba M, Jauch KW, Bruns CJ. Vascular endothelial growth factor in esophageal cancer. *J Surg Oncol* 2004;**87**:95–104.

59. Auvinen MI, Sihvo EI, Ruohtula T *et al.* Incipient angiogenesis in Barrett's epithelium and lymphangiogenesis in Barrett's adenocarcinoma. *J Clin Oncol* 2002;**20**: 2971–9.

60. Achen MG, Jeltsch M, Kukk E *et al.* Vascular endothelial growth factor D (VEGF-D) is a ligand for the tyrosine kinases VEGF receptor 2 (Flk1) and VEGF receptor 3 (Flt4). *Proc Natl Acad Sci U S A* 1998;**95**:548–53.

61. Lord RV, Park JM, Wickramasinghe K *et al*. Vascular endothelial growth factor and basic fibroblast growth factor expression in esophageal adenocarcinoma and Barrett esophagus. *J Thorac Cardiovasc Surg* 2003;**125**:246–53.

62. Hurwitz H, Fehrenbacher L, Novotny W *et al*. Bevacizumab plus irinotecan, fluorouracil, and leucovorin for metastatic colorectal cancer. *N Engl J Med* 2004;**350**:2335–42.

63. Baatar D, Jones MK, Tsugawa K *et al*. Esophageal ulceration triggers expression of hypoxia-inducible factor-1α and activates vascular endothelial growth factor gene: implications for angiogenesis and ulcer healing. *Am J Pathol* 2002;**161**:1449–57.

64. Aberle H, Schwartz H, Kemler R. Cadherin–catenin complex: protein interactions and their implications for cadherin function. *J Cell Biochem* 1996;**61**:514–23.

65. Swami S, Kumble S, Triadafilopoulos G. E-cadherin expression in gastroesophageal reflux disease, Barrett's esophagus, and esophageal adenocarcinoma: an immunohistochemical and immunoblot study. *Am J Gastroenterol* 1995;**90**:1808–13.

66. Washington K, Chiappori A, Hamilton K *et al*. Expression of β-catenin, α-catenin, and E-cadherin in Barrett's esophagus and esophageal adenocarcinomas. *Mod Pathol* 1998;**11**:805–13.

67. Seery JP, Syrigos KN, Karayiannakis AJ, Valizadeh A, Pignatelli M. Abnormal expression of the E-cadherin–catenin complex in dysplastic Barrett's oesophagus. *Acta Oncol* 1999;**38**:945–8.

68. Bailey T, Biddlestone L, Shepherd N *et al*. Altered cadherin and catenin complexes in the Barrett's esophagus–dysplasia–adenocarcinoma sequence: correlation with disease progression and dedifferentiation. *Am J Pathol* 1998;**152**:135–44.

69. Clapper ML, Coudry J, Chang WC. β-catenin-mediated signaling: a molecular target for early chemopreventive intervention. *Mutat Res* 2004;**555**:97–105.

70. Coussens LM, Fingleton B, Matrisian LM. Matrix metalloproteinase inhibitors and cancer: trials and tribulations. *Science* 2002;**295**:2387–92.

71. Salmela MT, Karjalainen-Lindsberg ML, Puolakkainen P, Saarialho-Kere U. Upregulation and differential expression of matrilysin (MMP-7) and metalloelastase (MMP-12) and their inhibitors TIMP-1 and TIMP-3 in Barrett's oesophageal adenocarcinoma. *Br J Cancer* 2001;**85**:383–92.

72. Wagenaar-Miller RA, Gorden L, Matrisian LM. Matrix metalloproteinases in colorectal cancer: is it worth talking about? *Cancer Metastasis Rev* 2004;**23**:119–35.

73. Feagins LA, Souza RF. Molecular targets for treatment of Barrett's esophagus. In: *Diseases of the Esophagus*. 2005; **18**(2):75–86.

CHAPTER 10

Histology of Barrett's Esophagus: Metaplasia and Dysplasia

Joel E. Mendelin and John R. Goldblum

Introduction

Although there have been several definitions of Barrett's esophagus since its original description almost 100 years ago [1], all have shared two features in common—an alteration of the esophageal mucosa visible without a microscope and a corresponding histologic abnormality. The endoscopic landmarks used to identify the esophagogastric junction (EGJ) are reviewed in greater detail elsewhere in this book, but given that the definition of Barrett's esophagus depends upon this anatomic landmark, a brief review of the macroscopic and microscopic anatomy of this region is in order.

Normal Anatomy and Histology

In the region where the esophagus joins the stomach, two anatomic landmarks are visible at the time of endoscopy—the muscular EGJ and the mucosal EGJ also known as the squamocolumnar junction (SCJ), Z line or ora serrata. The muscular EGJ is the point at which the distal most portion of the tubular esophagus meets the saccular stomach [2]. Although the EGJ may be approximated by the most proximal extent of the gastric folds, precise anatomic localization remains difficult in many cases, particularly in the setting of a hiatal hernia [3]. The mucosal EGJ is also identifiable at endoscopy by differences in color and texture of the mucosal lining. Normally, the mucosal and muscular EGJ coincide, but in many adult patients, the SCJ lies 1–2 cm proximal to the muscular EGJ, presumably seconady to reflux of gastric contents into the distal most esophagus.

Traditionally, the narrow segment of mucus-secreting columnar mucosa distal to the squamous esophageal mucosa but proximal to acid-secreting oxyntic gastric mucosa has been termed the gastric cardia. In recent years, the existence of the gastric cardia as a native structure has been called into question by some authors who believe that cardiac-type mucosa is always metaplastic, likely in response to gastroesophageal reflux [4,5]. While metaplastic cardiac-type mucosa undoubtedly is frequently identified in the distal esophagus, evidence from a detailed studies of the anatomy and histology of the EGJ, including pediatric autopsy series, supports the notion that the gastric cardia is a native structure [6–8]. Thus, there is sufficient evidence to support the presence of a small zone of native cardiac mucosa in the most proximal stomach, and in many individuals, metaplastic cardiac-type mucosa of variable length in the distal esophagus.

Histology of Barrett's Esophagus

Although the existence of a columnar-lined organ within the thorax had been documented for nearly 50 years prior to Dr. Norman Barrett's influential paper in 1957 [9], his description affirmed that this structure was indeed the esophagus and not the stomach [3]. Until 1976, histologic descriptions of what had by then become known as Barrett's esophagus included several epithelial types, including mucus-secreting cardiac-type glands, acid-secreting fundic-type glands, and intestinal-type epithelium with goblet cells. In 1976, Paull more fully described the metaplastic columnar epithelium lining the esophagus, separating them into three different subtypes: (i) fundic-type; (ii) cardiac-type (junctional); and (iii) specialized columnar epithelium [10]. Subsequently, several studies have found that only patients with metaplastic columnar epithelium containing goblet cells (i.e. specialized columnar epithelium or intestinal metaplasia) are at an increased risk of developing esophageal adenocarcinoma [11–13], and as such the identification of intestinal metaplasia has become one part of the currently accepted two-pronged definition of Barrett's esophagus published by the American College of Gastroenterology and its Practice Parameters Committee [14].

Architecturally, specialized columnar epithelium most closely resembles slightly distorted gastric mucosa with glands and foveolae, but it may take on a more villiform appearance in some cases. In addition to goblet cells, the specialized columnar epithelium may also contain gastric foveolar-type cells (incomplete intestinal metaplasia) or intestinal absorptive-type cells (complete intestinal metaplasia), the former being more common. Less frequently, other specialized cell types may be present including Paneth cells, neuroendocrine cells, and even pancreatic acinar metaplasia. The lamina propria surrounding the glands contains variable numbers of inflammatory cells and fibroblasts.

Goblet cells are best identified by virtue of their shape and the chemical makeup of their cytoplasmic mucin contents. Abundant cytoplasmic mucin distends the cell, imparting its characteristic "goblet" shape, which at times may also appear more barrel-shaped. Goblet cell mucin is acidic and composed predominantly of sialomucins admixed with lesser quantities of sulfated mucins [15]. Histochemical stains for acidic mucins, such as Alcian blue at pH 2.5, show intense dark-blue staining for this combination of sialomucins and sulfated mucins which contrasts with the predominantly periodic acid–Schiff (PAS)-positive neutral mucins found within the adjacent gastric foveolar-type cells (Fig. 10.1: see also Plate 10.1; color plate section falls between pp. 148–9). Because of their acidic mucin content, goblet cells may also have a basophilic cytoplasmic blush which is recognizable in well-stained hematoxylin and eosin (H&E) stained tissue sections.

On occasion, confusion may arise when interpreting a special stain for acidic mucin as the columnar cells intervening between the goblet cells take on the appearance of goblet cells and may show some Alcian blue positivity (so-called "columnar blues") due to the presence of small quantities of acidic mucin in their cytoplasm. Without the use of special stains, metaplastic cardiac-type epithelium may also

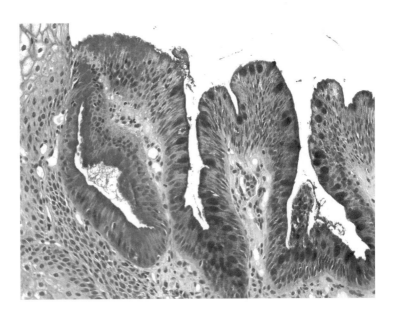

Fig. 10.1 Periodic acid–Schiff (PAS)/Alcian blue at pH 2.5 demonstrates incomplete intestinal metaplasia. Goblet cells containing acid mucin stain intensely blue with Alcian blue (right), while the adjacent columnar cells containing neutral mucin stain with PAS (left).

contain cells with a markedly distended cytoplasm, thereby resembling goblet cells (so-called "pseudo-goblet cells"). These cells, however, contain neutral mucin that does not react with Alcian blue at pH 2.5. In the absence of goblet cell metaplasia, the identification of these cells does not meet the criteria for a definitive diagnosis of Barrett's esophagus.

If the endoscopic impression is clearly that of Barrett's esophagus, then the absence of intestinal metaplasia may simply be a function of sampling error. Thus, although the pathologist may not be able to make a definitive diagnosis of Barrett's esophagus in this situation, the endoscopic impression may still strongly suggest this diagnosis. Fortunately, this problem is relatively rare, as Weinstein *et al.* found non-intestinal tongues of columnar epithelium extending greater than 2 cm into the lower esophagus in less than 1% of 250 cases of Barrett's esophagus studied [16].

Intestinal Metaplasia of the EGJ

Although it is by far the most common method of identifying intestinal metaplasia in biopsies taken near the EGJ, examination of paired H&E and Alcian blue stained tissue sections does not allow one to accurately distinguish between intestinal metaplasia of the gastric cardia (cardia intestinal metaplasia [CIM]) and short segment Barrett's esophagus. Some of the data are conflicting, but it appears as though CIM is more strongly associated with *Helicobacter pylori* chronic gastritis than with gastroesophageal reflux [17–19] and that CIM carries a lower risk of neoplastic progression than either short or long segment Barrett's esophagus [20–22]. If prospective studies corroborate these initial findings, then given the inconsistent endoscopic landmarks in this region and lack of precision regarding the location of a biopsy with intestinal metaplasia taken near the EGJ, it would be useful to have an ancillary means of accurately distinguishing CIM from short segment Barrett's esophagus.

To date, most studies have used immunohistochemistry to focus on different patterns of protein expression in CIM and short segment Barrett's esophagus. Ormsby *et al.* compared the cytokeratin 7 and 20 expression patterns in resected long segments

of Barrett's esophagus to gastric resections with intestinal metaplasia of the distal stomach and found that each had a distinctive cytokeratin pattern [23]. Virtually all cases of long segment Barrett's esophagus were characterized by superficial and deep CK7 immunoreactivity in the intestinalized mucosa with only superficial CK20 staining ("Barrett's CK 7/20 pattern"). In contrast, distal gastric intestinal metaplasia was characterized by patchy, superficial and deep CK20 staining in areas of incomplete intestinal metaplasia, strong, superficial and deep CK20 staining in areas of complete intestinal metaplasia and patchy or absent CK7 staining in either type of gastric intestinal metaplasia. As an extension of this study, the same group was also able to demonstrate that these patterns were also capable to distinguishing CIM from short segment Barrett's esophagus in biopsy specimens [24], a finding that was corroborated by some authors [25,26] but not others [27–29].

The expression of *CDX2*, a caudal homeobox gene expressed during development, is specific evidence of intestinal differentiation [30] and several studies have shown that *CDX2* is expressed in Barrett's esophagus-related intestinal metaplasia [31–33]. To date, no direct comparisons have been published with regard to potential expression differences between CIM and short segment Barrett's esophagus. Several other markers have been evaluated in an attempt to distinguish CIM from short segment Barrett's esophagus, including the monoclonal antibody Das1, various mucin proteins (i.e. MUC1, MUC2, MUC 5AC and MUC6), as well as mucin histochemistry. These studies are hampered by differences in endoscopic biopsy protocols and study populations that contribute to apparent discrepancies in their results and lack of reproducibility. Thus, the clinical utility of evaluating intestinal metaplasia of the EGJ using these various biomarkers has not yet been established and requires additional study.

Barrett's Esophagus-Related Dysplasia

All patients with Barrett's esophagus are at risk of developing esophageal adenocarcinoma [34]. However, among Barrett's esophagus patients, certain epidemiological and pathologic characteristics are associated with an even greater risk of malignancy. Increased risk is associated with increased age, male gender and being Caucasian [35,36]. Data from retrospective mapping studies [11], as well as few prospective studies [37,38], support the notion that adenocarcinoma only arises in a background of intestinal metaplasia, and thus, the identification of goblet cells has become part of the definition of Barrett's esophagus [14]. Although adenocarcinoma does occur in short segments of Barrett's esophagus [39], there is evidence that patients with longer segments are at a higher risk [19,40]. Mapping studies have also documented epithelial dysplasia in mucosa adjacent to adenocarcinoma in resection specimens, supporting a dysplasia-carcinoma sequence [35]. In addition, there are also studies that have reported patients progressing from dysplasia to adenocarcinoma in serial endoscopies with biopsies [13,37]. Epithelial dysplasia, particularly high-grade dysplasia, has come to be considered one of the most important risk factors for both synchronous and metachronous esophageal adenocarcinoma [38,42,43] and its identification is an integral part of cancer screening and surveillance programs for Barrett's esophagus patients.

Dysplasia can be defined as neoplastic change of the epithelium that remains confined within the basement membrane of the gland from which it arises (i.e. intraepithelial neoplasia) [44]. Dysplastic epithelium may form an endoscopically visible mass (e.g. adenoma) or it may not be distinguishable from adjacent non-dysplastic mucosa. Histologically, there are two morphologic characteristics used to identify dysplastic glandular epithelium in routine stained sections, architecture, and cytology.

At low magnification, dysplastic epithelium typically appears darker (hyperchromatic) than non-dysplastic epithelium and this appearance is principally due to changes within the individual cells lining the dysplastic glands. Dysplastic cells characteristically have less cytoplasmic mucin and the mucin that is present is more basophilic than normal. Nuclear enlargement, hyperchromasia and crowding that extend out from the crypts onto the mucosal surface are characteristic of dysplastic epithelium. Not all of these nuclear changes are required; in some cases, the nuclei are not necessarily crowded,

but rather are large, hyperchromatic and have lost their polarity with their long axes no longer being perpendicular to the underlying basement membrane. Although more complex glandular architecture (glandular crowding, branching, and cribriform glands) usually accompanies more severe cytologic alterations, this is not always the case. Occasionally, mild architectural alterations accompany severe cytologic atypia and, as such, cytologic changes are generally more important than architecture in grading the severity of dysplasia. The most widely accepted grading scheme for Barrett's-related dysplasia mirrors the classification of dysplasia first applied from idiopathic inflammatory bowel disease [44].

Low-Grade Dysplasia

The glandular architecture is at most mildly distorted in low-grade dysplasia, as the crypts remain parallel with one another with minimal crypt branching or budding. Cytologically, the basal nuclei are enlarged, hyperchromatic and crowded with overlapping nuclear membranes. The nuclear abnormalities extend out from the crypts to involve the mucosal surface (Fig. 10.2). Goblet cells are often decreased in number and so-called dystrophic goblet cells, where the nucleus is located at the apical aspect of the cell, may also be present.

High-Grade Dysplasia

In high-grade dysplasia, both the cytologic atypia and the architectural distortion are more pronounced. The crypts are markedly distorted with branching, "back-to-back" glands and cribriform intraglandular growth. The nuclear changes of low-grade dysplasia persist, but in addition, the nuclei become stratified and are no longer situated at the basilar aspects of the cells. There may also be a loss of nuclear polarity, where the long axis of the nucleus no longer is perpendicular to the basement membrane. These alterations extend onto the mucosal surface (Fig. 10.3).

There are cases where the degree of glandular architectural distortion becomes so severe that it becomes exceedingly difficult to exclude the possibility of intramucosal adenocarcinoma, especially in biopsy specimens. These cases are often characterized by extensive back-to-back glandular growth

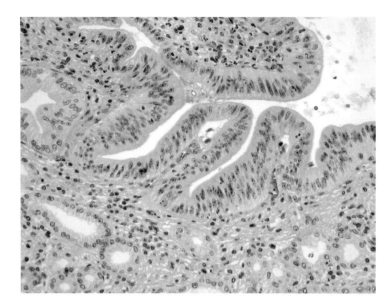

Fig. 10.2 Barrett's esophagus with low-grade dysplasia. The dysplastic cells contain enlarged hyperchromatic nuclei with slightly irregular contours. The nuclear changes extend out from the base of the glands onto the mucosal surface where there is also significant overlapping and crowding. Note the small round nuclei of the non-dysplastic glands beneath the dysplastic epithelium.

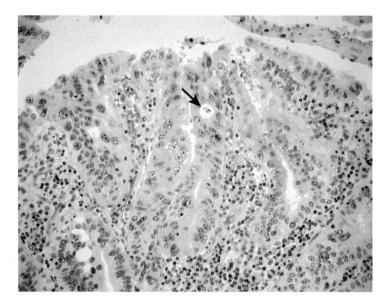

Fig. 10.3 Barrett's esophagus with high-grade dysplasia. This focus of high-grade dysplasia is characterized by severe cytologic atypia, including markedly enlarged, irregular nuclei with coarse chromatin and small nucleoli. There is also an area of cribriform growth (arrowhead).

with little, if any, intervening stroma between the neoplastic glands, or by ill-defined abortive glands within the lamina propria. Although not always possible in practice [45,46], this distinction is important because there is a small but definite risk of lymph node metastases in patients with intramucosal adenocarcinoma of the esophagus given the presence of lymphatic channels within the esophageal mucosa

[47,48]. In most cases, intramucosal adenocarcinoma can only be diagnosed with confidence when unequivocal single cell invasion into the lamina propria is identified.

Indefinite for Dysplasia

The diagnosis of indefinite for dysplasia should be reserved for cases where: (i) the cytologic and glandular architectural changes exceed the so-called "base-line atypia" of metaplastic specialized columnar epithelium, but fall short of low-grade dysplasia; (ii) when co-existing inflammation or ulceration is associated with striking cytologic nuclear atypia precluding a definitive distinction between regenerative atypia and dysplasia; or (iii) there is marked glandular distortion in the absence of surface nuclear changes which would be diagnostic of dysplasia.

One the unique features of metaplastic Barrett's mucosa is that there is a certain degree of "baseline atypia" present in the specialized columnar epithelium that is neither dysplastic nor inflamed. This atypia is most pronounced within the regenerative glandular compartment at the base of the mucosa, where the nuclei are typically slightly enlarged and hyperchromatic. Importantly, these nuclear changes do not involve the surface epithelial cells, as the cells demonstrate normal surface maturation.

Active inflammation, and its attendant neutrophil-mediated epithelial cell injury, is capable of producing profound cytologic alterations that overlap with those of Barrett's esophagus-related dysplasia. Distinguishing reactive cytologic atypia from dysplasia is frequently very difficult, if not impossible. The appearance from low-magnification is critical in this evaluation, because truly dysplastic epithelium usually appears darker than normal at this power. Confirmation of these changes is required at higher magnification that reveals nuclear enlargement, hyperchromasia, crowding, and irregular nuclear contours. In addition, inspection at higher power enables one to determine whether these changes extend onto the mucosal surface. Accurate assessment of the changes involving the mucosal surface is more difficult when faced with a tangentially sectioned biopsy specimen.

In contrast to dysplasia, reactive atypia has a more uniform appearance among the cells in question, whereas dysplastic nuclei are pleomorphic and thus vary more considerably from one cell to the next. While cell size does not discriminate between a reactive cell and a dysplastic cell, the nuclear : cytoplasmic (N : C) ratio is increased in the setting of dysplasia when compared with reactive cells. The chromatin distribution pattern is also helpful, as reactive nuclei have a more open chromatin pattern with prominent nucleoli, which contrast with the more condensed chromatin pattern seen in dysplastic nuclei. In practice, one needs to weigh all of these features together when deciding whether or not the changes qualify as dysplasia.

Sampling Error and Observer Variation in Barrett's Esophagus-Related Dysplasia

Dysplasia may extend diffusely throughout a Barrett's esophagus segment, or the changes may be focal and limited to a small area of one fragment in a patient with multiple biopsy specimens. When dysplasia is diffuse, there is a high likelihood that a rigorous biopsy protocol will detect foci of dysplasia at a high frequency; however, small foci may go unsampled. The need for thorough biopsy sampling is further emphasized by the fact that high-grade dysplasia and even early adenocarcinoma may not be associated with an endoscopically visible lesion [38,49]. Given this potential for sampling error, subsequent biopsies that are negative for dysplasia following earlier biopsies with dysplasia should not lull the gastroenterologist into a false sense of security.

Another problem facing the pathologist and the gastroenterologist, thoracic surgeon and ultimately the patient is both the intra and interobserver variation in the diagnosis of dysplasia. Given the spectrum of changes from baseline atypia to low-grade to high-grade dysplasia, it is not surprising that this variation exists. Reid et al. found this variation to be most significant at the low end of the spectrum—that is, in distinguishing negative for dysplasia from low-grade dysplasia or indefinite for dysplasia [50]. This study described overall agreement in terms of a percentage, which does not take into account agreement that may occur by chance alone. A more recent study by Montgomery et al. using kappa statistical analysis (which accounts for agreement occurring by chance alone) confirmed a high degree of intra and interobserver variation among these same diagnostic categories, even among pathologists with a special interest in gastrointestinal pathology [51]. This variation underscores the need to obtain multiple opinions in challenging cases.

Surrogate Biomarkers for Assessing Risk of Esophageal Adenocarcinoma

Given the limitations of light microscopy, several adjunctive techniques have been proposed as having a possible role in the screening or surveillance of patients with Barrett's esophagus. For virtually every marker tested, there is an increased probability of finding an abnormality as one progresses along the dysplasia–carcinoma sequence. Certain markers are detectable early in the sequence, whereas others are found at later stages. The ideal marker would be detectable early in the metaplasia–dysplasia–carcinoma sequence, even before there is morphologic evidence of dysplasia, and capable of discriminating those patients who will progress along this sequence from those who will not.

Numerous studies have evaluated p53 expression by immunohistochemistry, most of which attempt to correlate the degree of p53 expression with the grade of dysplasia or solely as a marker of increased risk of progressing to adenocarcinoma. p53 overexpression has been observed in 9–60% of cases with low-grade dysplasia and 55–100% of cases with high-grade dysplasia [52–55]. Although some have advocated the use of p53 immunohistochemistry to confirm a diagnosis of dysplasia and/or assist in grading of dysplasia, its use has not been widely accepted [56,57]. There is some discrepancy between p53 expression as detected by immunohistochemistry and molecular alterations detectable at the gene level [58,59]. Also, the lack of a standardized immunohistochemical technique likely accounts for some of the discrepant data reported in the literature.

DNA content, as measured by flow cytometry, has also been evaluated in patients with Barrett's esophagus, but the results are conflicting. In 1987, Reid *et al.* found an increased prevalence of DNA aneuploidy and elevated S-phase fraction with increasing severity of the histologic grade of dysplasia [60]. In a subsequent prospective study of 62 patients with Barrett's esophagus without dysplasia [61] and mean follow-up of 34 months, nine of 13 patients with aneuploid or increased G2/tetraploid populations in their initial biopsy specimens developed high-grade dysplasia or esophageal adenocarcinoma. A more recent prospective study found that patients with negative, indefinite, or low-grade dysplasia histology and no evidence of aneuploidy or increased 4N fractions by flow cytometry had a cumulative 0% 5-year cancer risk, compared with a 28% risk for patients with either aneuploidy or increased 4N fractions [62]. Patients with baseline increased 4N, aneuploidy, and high-grade dysplasia had 5-year cancer rates of 56%, 43%, and 59%, respectively. In contrast to the results of Reid *et al.*, Fennerty *et al.* found discordance between flow cytometric abnormalities and dysplasia in Barrett's esophagus patients [63].

Although numerous others potential individual biomarkers of neoplastic progression in Barrett's esophagus patients have also been evaluated with variable results (e.g. Ki-67, *bcl*-2, cyclin D1, *p16*, EGFR, c-*erb*B-2), microarray-based technologies are well suited for surveying genomic abnormalities on a much broader scale. These methods allow for the rapid comparison of chromosomal copy numbers or relative expression of thousands of genes in a single assay, creating genomic profiles for the tissues tested. Not surprisingly, initial studies [64–66] have identified a long list of chromosomal abnormalities and genes that are up or downregulated as one proceeds along the metaplasia–dysplasia–carcinoma sequence in Barrett's esophagus. However, additional prospective studies are needed to determine the significance of these initial findings and whether or not they have a potential role in distinguishing those patients who are very unlikely to have their disease progress from those at greatest risk of progression.

References

1. Tileston W. Peptic ulcer of the oesophagus. *Am J Med Sci* 1906;**132**:240–65.
2. Hayward J. The lower end of the oesophagus. *Thorax* 1961;**16**:36–41.
3. Spechler SJ. The columnar-lined esophagus, intestinal metaplasia, and Norman Barrett. *Gastroenterology* 1996;**110**:614–21.
4. Chandrasoma PT *et al.* Definition of histopathologic changes in gastroesophageal reflux disease. *Am J Surg Pathol* 2000;**24**:344–51.
5. Chandrasoma PT *et al.* Histology of the gastroesophageal junction: an autopsy study. *Am J Surg Pathol* 2000;**24**:402–9.

6. Kilgore SP *et al*. The gastric cardia: fact or fiction? *Am J Gastroenterol* 2000;**95**:921–4.

7. Zhou H *et al*. Origin of cardiac mucosa: ontogenic consideration. *Pediatr Dev Pathol* 2001;**4**:358–63.

8. Derdoy JJ *et al*. The gastric cardia: to be or not to be? *Am J Surg Path* 2003;**27**:499–504.

9. Barrett NR. The lower esophagus lined by columnar epithelium. *Surgery* 1957;**41**:881–94.

10. Paull A. The histologic spectrum of Barrett's esophagus. *N Engl J Med* 1976;**29**:476–80.

11. Hamilton SR *et al*. The relationship between columnar epithelial dysplasia and invasive adenocarcinoma arising in Barrett's esophagus. *Am J Clin Pathol* 1987;**87**:301–12.

12. Lee DG *et al*. Dysplasia in Barrett's esophagus. A clinicopathologic study of six patients. *Am J Surg Path* 1985;**9**:845–52.

13. Reid BJ *et al*. Flow-cytometric and histological progression to malignancy in Barrett's esophagus: prospective endoscopic surveillance of a cohort. *Gastroenterology* 1992;**102**:1212–9.

14. Sampliner RE. Updated guidelines for the diagnosis, surveillance, and therapy of Barrett's esophagus. *Am J Gastroenterol* 2002;**97**:1888–95.

15. Haggitt RC *et al*. Barrett's esophagus. Correlation between mucin histochemistry, flow cytometry, and histologic diagnosis for predicting increased cancer risk. *Am J Pathol* 1988;**13**:53–61.

16. Weinstein WM *et al*. The diagnosis of Barrett's esophagus. Goblets, goblets, goblets. *Gastrointest Endosc* 1996;**44**:91–4.

17. Hackelsberger A *et al*. Intestinal metaplasia at the gastroesophageal junction: *Helicobacter pylori* gastritis or gastro-esophageal refluz disease? *Gut* 1998;**43**:17–21.

18. Goldblum JR *et al*. Inflammation and intestinal metaplasia of the gastric cardia: The role of the gastroesophageal reflux and *H. Pylori* infection. *Gastroenterology* 1998;**114**:633–9.

19. Hirota WK *et al*. Specialized intestinal metaplasia, dysplasia and cancer of the esophagus and esophagogastric junction: prevalence and clinical data. *Gastroenterology* 1999;**116**: 277–85.

20. Sharma P *et al*. Relative risk of dysplasia for patients with intestinal metaplasia in the distal oesophagus and in the gastric cardia. *Gut* 2000;**46**:9–13.

21. Morales TG *et al*. Long-term follow-up of intestinal metaplasia of the gastric cardia. *Am J Gastroenterol* 2000;**95**:1677–80.

22. Goldstein NS *et al*. Gastric cardia intestinal metaplasia: Biopsy and follow-up of 85 patients. *Mod Pathol* 2000;**13**:1072–9.

23. Ormsby AH *et al*. Cytokeratin subsets can reliably distinguish Barrett's esophagus from intestinal metaplasia of the stomach. *Hum Pathol* 1990;**30**:288–94.

24. Ormsby AH *et al*. Cytokeratin immunoreactivity patterns in the diagnosis of short-segment Barrett's esophagus. *Gastroenterology* 2000;**119**:683–90.

25. Couvelard A *et al*. Cytokertain immunoreactivity of intestinal metaplasia at normal oesophagogastric junction indicates its aetiology. *Gut* 2001;**49**:761–6.

26. Wallner B *et al*. Immunohistochemical markers for Barrett's esophagus and associations to esophageal Z-line appearance. *Scand J Gastroenterol* 2001;**9**:910–5.

27. Mohammed IA *et al*. Utilization of cytokeratins 7 and 20 does not differentiate between Barrett's esophagus and gastric cardiac intestinal metaplasia. *Mod Pathol* 2002;**15**:611–6.

28. El-Zimaity HM *et al*. Cytokeratin subsets for distinguishing Barrett's esophagus from intestinal metaplasia in the cardia using endoscopic biopsy specimens. *Am J Gastroenterol* 2001;**96**:1378–82.

29. Gulmann C *et al*. Cytokeratin 7/20 and MUC1, 2, 5AC, and 6 expression patterns in Barrett's esophagus and intestinal metaplasia of the stomach: intestinal metaplasia of the cardia is related to Barrett's esophagus. *Appl Immunohistochem Mol Morphol* 2004; **12**:142–7.

30. Suh E *et al*. An intestine-specific homeobox gene regulates proliferation and differentiation. *Mol Cell Biol* 1996;**16**:619–25.

31. Groisman GM *et al*. Expression of the intestinal marker *CDX2* in the columnar-lined esophagus with and without intestinal (Barrett's) metaplasia. *Mod Pathol* 2004;**17**:1282–8.

32. Phillips RW *et al*. *CDX2* as a marker of epithelial intestinal differentiation in the esophagus. *Am J Surg Pathol* 2003;**27**:1442–7.

33. Moons LM *et al*. The homeodomain protein CDX2 is an early marker of Barrett's oesophagus. *J Clin Pathol* 2004;**57**:1063–8.

34. Haggitt RC *et al*. Adenocarcinoma complicating columnar epithelium-lined (Barrett's) esophagus. *Am J Clin Pathol* 1978;**70**:1–5.

35. Splechler SJ. Barrett's esophagus. *N Engl J Med* 1986;**315**:362–71.

36. Sjogren RW. Barrett's esophagus: a review. *Am J Med* 1983;**74**:313–21.

37. Hameeteman W *et al*. Barrett's esophagus: development of dysplasia and adenocarcinoma. *Gastroenterology* 1989;**96**:1249–56.

38. Reid BJ *et al*. Endoscopic biopsies diagnose high-grade dysplasia or early operable adenocarcinoma in Bar-

rett's esophagus without grossly recognizable neoplastic lesions. *Gastroenterology* 1988;**94**:81–90.

39. Schnell TG *et al*. Adenocarcinoma arising in tongues or short segments of Barrett's esophagus. *Dig Dis Sci* 1992;**37**:137–43.

40. Menke-Pluymers MBE *et al*. Risk factors for the development of an adenocarcinoma in columnar lined (Barrett's) esophagus. *Cancer* 1993;**72**:1155–8.

41. Haggitt RC. Barrett's esophagus, dysplasia, and adenocarcinoma. *Hum Pathol* 1994;**25**:982–93.

42. Schmidt HG *et al*. Dysplasia in Barrett's esophagus. *J Cancer Res Clin Oncol* 1985;**110**:145–52.

43. Smith RRL *et al*. The spectrum of carcinoma arising in Barrett's esophagus: a clincopathologic study of 26 patients. *Am J Surg Path* 1984;**8**:562–73.

44. Riddell RH *et al*. Dysplasia in inflammatory bowel disease: standard classification with provisional clinical implications. *Hum Pathol* 1983;**14**:931–68.

45. Mendelin JE *et al*. Interobserver agreement in the evaluation of pre-resection biopsies with at least high-grade dysplasia in 163 Barrett's esophagus patients. *Mod Pathol* 2005;**18**:A112.

46. Ormsby AH *et al*. Observer variation in the diagnosis of superficial oesophageal adenocarcinoma. *Gut* 2002;**51**:671–6.

47. Goseki M *et al*. Histopathologic characteristics of early stage esophgeal adenocarcinoma. A comparative study with gastric carcinoma. *Cancer* 1992;**69**:1088–93.

48. Sabik JF *et al*. Superficial esophageal carcinoma. *Ann Thorac Surg* 1995;**60**:896–901.

49. Falk GW *et al*. Jumbo biopsy forceps protocol still misses unsuspected cancer in Barrett's esophagus with high-grade dysplasia. *Gastrointest Endosc* 1999;**49**:170–6.

50. Reid BJ *et al*. Observer variation in the diagnosis of dysplasia in Barrett's esophagus. *Hum Pathol* 1998;**19**:166–78.

51. Montgomery E *et al*. Reproducibility of the diagnosis of dysplasia in Barrett'esophagus: a reaffirmation. *Hum Pathol* 2001;**32**:368–78.

52. Younes M *et al*. p53 protein accumulation in Barrett's metaplasia, dysplasia and carcinoma: a follow-up study. *Gastroenterology* 1993;**105**:1637–42.

53. Krishnadath KK *et al*. Accumulation of p53 protein in normal, dysplastic and neoplastic Barrett's esophagus. *J Pathol* 1995;**175**:175–80.

54. Jones DR *et al*. Potential applications of p53 as an intermediate biomarker in Barrett's esophagus. *Ann Thorac Surg* 1994;**57**:598–603.

55. Ramel S *et al*. Evaluation of p53 protein expression in Barrett's esophagus by two-parameter flow cytometry. *Gastroenterology* 1992;**102**:1220–8.

56. Klump B *et al*. Diagnostic significance of nuclear p53 expression in the surveillance of Barrett's esophagus: a longitudinal study. *Z Gastroenterol* 1999;**37**:1005–11.

57. Khan S *et al*. Diagnostic value of p53 immunohistochemistry in Barrett's esophagus: an endoscopic study. *Pathology* 1998;**30**:136–40.

58. Hamelin R *et al*. TP53 gene mutations and p53 protein immunoreactivity in malignant and premalignant Barrett's esophagus. *Gastroenterology* 1994;**107**:1012–8.

59. Coggi G *et al*. p53 protein accumulation and *p53* gene mutation in esophegeal carcinoma. A molecular and immunohistolochemical study with clinicopathologic correlations. *Cancer* 1997;**79**:425–32.

60. Reid BJ *et al*. Flow cytometry complements histology in detecting patients at risk for Barrett's adenocarcinoma. *Gastroenterology* 1987;**93**:1–11.

61. Reid BJ *et al*. Barrett's esophagus: cell cycle abnormalities in advancing stages of neoplastic progression. *Gastroenterology* 1993;**105**:119–29.

62. Reid BJ *et al*. Predictors of progression to cancer in Barrett's esophagus: baseline histology and flow cytometry identify low- and high-risk patient subsets. *Am J Gastroenterol* 2000;**95**:1669–76.

63. Fennerty MB *et al*. Discordance between flow cytometric abnormalities and dysplasia in Barrett's esophagus. *Gastroenterology* 1989;**97**:815–20.

64. Xu Y *et al*. Artificial neural networks and gene filtering distinguish between global gene expression profiles of Barrett's esophagus and esophageal cancer. *Cancer Res* 2002;**62**:3493–7.

65. Brabender J *et al*. A multigene expression panel for the molecular diagnosis of Barrett's esophagus and Barrett's adenocarcinoma of the esophagus. *Oncogene* 2004;**23**:4780–8.

66. Selaru FM *et al*. Global gene expression profiling in Barrett's esophagus and esophageal cancer: a comparative analysis using cDNA microarrays. *Oncogene* 2002;**21**:475–8.

CHAPTER 11

Screening for Barrett's Esophagus: Targeting High-Risk Patients

Richard E. Sampliner

Background

Barrett's esophagus is the premalignant lesion for esophageal adenocarcinoma, the most rapidly rising incidence cancer in the Western world [1]. In Barrett's esophagus the squamous epithelium has been replaced with a metaplastic lining with goblet cells—intestinal metaplasia. The incidence of esophageal adenocarcinoma has continued to rise through 1998 [2] and the prognosis remains poor. With all of the advances in medical care from 1973 to 1997, the 5-year survival for histologically proven esophageal adenocarcinoma only improved from 5% to 13% [3]. More than 95% of patients undergoing resection for esophageal adenocarcinoma have not had Barrett's esophagus recognized prior to the diagnosis of cancer [4]. In these unidentified Barrett's esophagus patients, the opportunity for detecting earlier stage disease was missed, highlighting the rationale for screening for Barrett's esophagus.

Definition of Screening

Screening is usually defined as testing individuals for a disease in the absence of symptoms. For screening to be effective the test must be sensitive, specific, acceptable to "patients," and affordable to society. However, Barrett's esophagus is usually recognized in the clinical context of gastroesophageal reflux disease (GERD). Therefore, screening for Barrett's esophagus is commonly done in patients with GERD symptoms to look for the premalignant disease. A recently highlighted challenge to screening for Barrett's esophagus is the asymptomatic patient. Two studies of patients undergoing colon screening who also had endoscopy revealed Barrett's esophagus in patients lacking GERD symptoms. In a predominantly Veteran group of 110 patients, 7% had long segment and 17% short segment Barrett's esophagus [5]. In contrast, another study of 556 subjects showed 0.36% long segment and 5.2% short segment Barrett's esophagus in patients lacking GERD symptoms [6].

The goal of screening for Barrett's esophagus is not only the detection of intestinal metaplasia, but also the recognition of high-grade dysplasia and esophageal adenocarcinoma. The early detection of dysplasia and cancer provides the opportunity to improve patient outcome with early intervention.

Prevalence of Barrett's Esophagus

The prevalence of Barrett's esophagus in patients undergoing endoscopy is 1.5% [7]. The prevalence of Barrett's esophagus in patients with GERD ranges from 5% to 12% [8,9]. Assessing the frequency of Barrett's esophagus in an autopsy study [10] and applying it to a population prevalence, only about one in five cases are clinically detected [11]. In spite of the increased application of endoscopy only the minority of patients with Barrett's esophagus are diagnosed emphasizing the potential for screening.

Who to Screen for Barrett's Esophagus

In the absence of large-scale population based trails to identify risk factors for Barrett's esophagus, attempts have been made to predict Barrett's esophagus from clinical and demographic features. Patients with Barrett's esophagus have been compared to GERD patients lacking Barrett's esophagus. A Veterans Affairs (VA) Medical Center study found age greater than 40 years, heartburn or acid regurgitation, and heartburn more than once a week were independent predictors of Barrett's esophagus by multivariate logistic regression (88 patients with Barrett's esophagus compared to 88 with GERD) [12]. Another study evaluated seven questions relating to GERD symptoms. Male gender, heartburn, nocturnal pain, and dysphagia were significant predictors of Barrett's esophagus (99 patients with Barrett's esophagus compared to 48 with GERD) [13]. A nomogram was developed for screening patients for Barrett's esophagus with a sensitivity of 77% and specificity of 63%. Another VA study found no symptoms were reliable in predicting Barrett's esophagus (235 patients with Barrett's esophagus, 306 with erosive esophagitis) [14]. GERD symptoms longer than 13 years were a risk factor for Barrett's esophagus in eight departments of gastroenterology in Italy (149 patients with Barrett's esophagus, 143 with esophagitis) [15]. To summarize these prospective studies, the only associated risk factor in common is heartburn.

The epidemiology of esophageal adenocarcinoma, the ultimate complication, also provides clear risk factors for Barrett's esophagus, the premalignant lesion. In the USA the annual incidence of esophageal adenocarcinoma in Caucasian men is 3.6/100 000, in African American men 0.8, and in Caucasian women 0.3 [2]. In series of surgically resected patients with esophageal adenocarcinoma and Barrett's esophagus from the USA and Western Europe, 85% of the patients are Caucasian men [16–20].

A Swedish population-bases study demonstrated that more frequent (≥three times per week, odds ratio [OR] 16.7), more severe (as judged by patients, OR 20), and longer duration (≥20 years, OR 16) reflux symptoms were associated with a significantly greater risk of esophageal adenocarcinoma [21]. Duration and severity of GERD symptoms have also been documented to relate to the likelihood of finding Barrett's esophagus at endoscopy in patients with GERD [22,23].

Barrett's esophagus is uncommon in younger patients undergoing endoscopy. In one study in which 3634 patients lacking alarm symptoms under the age of 45 years were endoscoped, only one in 363 patients had Barrett's esophagus [24]. Olmstead County data suggest the median age of onset of Barrett's esophagus is 40 years, although the mean age of diagnosing Barrett's esophagus was not until 63 years [25]. While the onset of symptomatic GERD is readily identified, the onset of Barrett's esophagus can only be identified when endoscopy is performed. Therefore the recognition of Barrett's esophagus occurs in the clinical context without relation to the indeterminable onset of the disease.

The information from the clinical and population based studies has led to the recommendation of screening older patients with chronic GERD symptoms. The highest yield of Barrett's esophagus is in Caucasian men [26] (Table 11.1). The specific age to initiate screening as well as the specific duration of reflux symptoms at which to screen are not evidence based.

An additional risk factor for Barrett's esophagus is a family history of GERD or Barrett's esophagus. Familial aggregation of GERD in patients with Barrett's esophagus but not in patients with reflux esophagitis has been documented [27,28]. Familial aggregation of Barrett's esophagus and esophageal adenocarcinoma has been demonstrated compared to controls—a positive family history in a Barrett's esophagus/adenocarcinoma family is 12 times more likely, 95% confidence interval (CI) 3.34–44.76 than in GERD controls lacking Barrett's esophagus [29]. Preliminary trials of endoscopy in first-degree relatives of patients with Barrett's esophagus also

Table 11.1 High-risk candidates for screening.

Chronic GERD symptoms
Older age
Male
Caucasian

GERD, gastroesophageal reflux disease.

Table 11.2 Challenges for screening.

Barrett's patients lacking GERD symptoms
Cost/risk of endoscopy
Accuracy of endoscopy and histology
Lack of predictors to increase yield of screening
Benefits unproven

GERD, gastroesophageal reflux disease.

Table 11.3 Screening endoscopy alternatives.

Brush cytology
Unsedated endoscopy
Esophageal capsule endoscopy

suggests a higher frequency of Barrett's esophagus [30,31].

How to Screen for Barrett's Esophagus

The current definition of Barrett's esophagus has criteria necessitating endoscopy and biopsy—a columnar appearing distal esophagus with intestinal metaplasia by biopsy. The issues related to screening endoscopy include the invasiveness and therefore the risk, the accuracy, the cost, and the lack of proven benefit (Table 11.2).

Even though Barrett's esophagus is the only known premalignant precursor of esophageal adenocarcinoma and is a complication of GERD, not all patients with Barrett's esophagus have apparent GERD-related symptoms. In a prospective multi-center Italian study, 40% of patients with Barrett's esophagus lacked reflux symptoms [15]. Similarly, 40% of patients in a Swedish population-based study of esophageal adenocarcinoma lacked GERD symptoms [21].

The accuracy of endoscopy and histologic interpretation are important issues. The lack of standardization of criteria and practice are highlighted by process of care problems. Endoscopists often fail to identify the critical landmarks for the recognition of Barrett's esophagus—the squamocolumnar junction, the esophagogastric junction, and the diaphragmatic pinch [32,33]. At an academic and a community hospital, the location of the esophagogastric junction was identified in only 72%, the length of Barrett's esophagus in 74%, and the presence or absence of an hiatal hernia in 60% of endoscopy reports [34]. The location of the biopsies, critical in separating intestinal metaplasia of the

esophagus (Barrett's esophagus) from cardia intestinal metaplasia, is often neglected—59% of endoscopic reports in this study. Additionally, pathologists do not always identify key criteria for the documentation of intestinal metaplasia—"specialized" or "intestinalized" was mentioned in 61%, and the presence or lack of goblet cells in only 16% of pathology reports [32,35].

Alternatives to screening endoscopy are necessary (Table 11.3). Balloon cytology independent of endoscopy has been performed with a disappointing yield of diagnostic goblet cells in 24% of 63 patients [36]. A more abrasive balloon may give a higher yield. Unsedated endoscopy has been performed by the peroral and transnasal route, typically with smaller caliber endoscopes. A multicenter randomized trial compared unsedated ultrathin endoscopy (5–6 mm diameter endoscopes) versus conventional sedated endoscopy (8–11 mm). The unsedated patients were as satisfied and just as willing to repeat the procedure [37]. The procedure was faster and less costly than the sedated endoscopy. Even with unsedated small caliber endoscopy, biopsies can be performed enabling recognition of Barrett's esophagus and dysplasia [38]. The lack of sedation can eliminate monitoring, recovery time, loss of work time, and the need for an accompanying driver, all further reducing the expense. However, in two US studies 31% and 37% of patients declined to undergo unsedated endoscopy [37,39]. Patients often desire a procedure totally lacking any potential discomfort. Additionally, in spite of published studies over a span of 9 years, unsedated procedures are not being widely utilized.

The latest non-endoscopic technologic development is esophageal capsule endoscopy [40]. The most recent US Food and Drug Administration (FDA) approved capsule acquires video images from both ends of the capsule at 14 frames per second and the capsule study is completed within 20 min. With validation of the ability to diagnosis columnar lining, this technique could be administered by non-physicians and the video read by experts to readily screen a larger segment of the population at risk for Barrett's esophagus. Patients may well prefer this screening technique to any form of endoscopy. High-risk patients for Barrett's esophagus, as identified by interpretation of the video recording, would still need to undergo conventional endoscopy and biopsy for the definitive diagnosis of Barrett's esophagus.

Effectiveness and Cost of Screening

There is suggestive evidence that performance of endoscopy is associated with earlier stage adenocarcinoma and better survival. In a cohort of 777 patients with esophageal adenocarcinoma from the Surveillance, Epidemiology and End Results Program, a prior endoscopy was associated with earlier stage disease—62% of patients early stage versus 35% not undergoing endoscopy—and a reduced risk of death—relative hazard 0.73, 95% CI 0.57–0.93 [41]. A case-control study of 245 incident deaths from adenocarcinoma of the esophagus in which reflux was present was performed using Veterans Administration databases. Cases were less likely to have an endoscopy than controls—OR 0.66, 95% CI 0.45–0.96 [42].

In the absence of large-scale clinical studies of screening endoscopy, modeling studies have been reported. For screening to be cost-effective by decision analysis, the patients evaluated have to have a high prevalence of Barrett's esophagus, high-grade dysplasia, and esophageal adenocarcinoma; the endoscopic recognition of Barrett's esophagus and histologic diagnosis of dysplasia need to be accurate and health-related quality of life needs to be maintained post-therapeutic intervention [43]. These criteria are difficult to meet given endoscopic and pathologic quality of care issues and variable pathologic interpretation in the community [35]. In a cost–utility analysis of both screening and surveillance, the benefit of screening is greater because the prevalence of esophageal adenocarcinoma in patients presenting for endoscopy with symptoms of GERD is greater than the subsequent annual incidence of esophageal adenocarcinoma in patients with known

Barrett's esophagus [44]. The higher prevalence of esophageal adenocarcinoma is well documented in a multicenter cohort study with a 6.6% prevalence compared to an annual incidence of 0.5% [45]. At these ratios, it would take 13 years of surveillance endoscopy in Barrett's esophagus patients lacking esophageal adenocarcinoma within the first year to equal the prevalence figure.

Although a separate chapter will deal with surveillance endoscopy of patients found to have Barrett's esophagus by screening, it is difficult to separate screening and surveillance. In the USA, once Barrett's esophagus is recognized, 98% of endoscopists perform surveillance endoscopy [46,47]. As demonstrated above, the prevalence of esophageal adenocarcinoma found within the first year is usually 10 times the incidence of adenocarcinoma found with ongoing surveillance. When high-grade dysplasia is added to adenocarcinoma then the prevalence of neoplasia is even greater, providing the rationale for screening. The recognition that more than 95% of patients undergoing resection for esophageal adenocarcinoma with Barrett's esophagus have not had Barrett's esophagus recognized prior to the diagnosis of cancer adds another reason for screening [4].

Future Screening

The future offers developments that will make screening feasible (Table 11.4). The availability of evidence-based risk criteria for patients with Barrett's esophagus and at high risk of esophageal adenocarcinoma will enable focusing of screening. This will require larger scale screening trials, ideally of a random sample of the adult population with utilization of a validated GERD questionnaire and a standardized endoscopy and biopsy protocol. Less invasive technology may soon lead to cheaper, safer,

Table 11.4 The future of screening.

Specific evidence-based risk criteria
Less invasive technology
Non-subspecialty performed
More broadly targeted

more widely applied, and acceptable screening. Potentially, this could be accomplished with capsule endoscopy and/or balloon cytology. Such advances would enable cost-effective screening targeting high-risk patients for Barrett's esophagus.

References

1. Blot W, Devesa SS, Kneller RW, Fraumeni JF. Rising incidence of adenocarcinoma of the esophagus and gastric cardia. *JAMA* 1991;**265**:1287–9.

2. Brown LM, Devesa SS. Epidemiologic trends in esophageal and gastric cancer in the United States. *Surg Oncol Clin N Am* 2002;**11**:235–56.

3. Eloubeide MA, Mason AC, Desmond RA, El-Serag HB. Temporal trends (1973–1997) in survival of patients with esophageal adenocarcinoma in the United States: a glimmer of hope? *Am J Gastroenterol* 2003;**98**: 1627–33.

4. Dulai GS, Guha S, Kahn KL, Gornbein J, Weinstein WM. Preoperative prevalence of Barrett's esophagus in esophageal adenocarcinoma: a systematic review. *Gastroenterology* 2002;**122**:26–33.

5. Gerson LB, Sheltler K, Triadafilopoloulos G. Prevalence of Barrett's esophagus in asymptomatic individuals. *Gastroenterology* 2002;**123**:461–7.

6. Rex DK, Cummings OW, Shaw M *et al.* Screening for Barrett's esophagus in colonoscopy patients with and without heartburn. *Gastroenterology* 2003;**125**:1670–7.

7. Cameron AJ. Epidemiology of Barrett's esophagus and adenocarcinoma. *Dis Esophagus* 2002;**15**:106–8.

8. Cameron AJ, Kamath PS, Carpenter HA. Prevalence of Barrett's esophagus and intestinal metaplasia at the esophagogastric junction. *Gastroenterology* 1997; **112**:A82.

9. Winters C, Spurling TJ, Chobanian S *et al.* Barrett's esophagus. A prevalent occult complication of gastroesophageal reflux disease. *Gastroenterology* 1987;**92**: 118–24.

10. Cameron AJ, Zinsmeister AR, Ballard DJ, Carney JA. Prevalence of columnar-lined (Barrett's) esophagus. Comparison of population based clinical and autopsy findings. *Gastroenterology* 1990;**99**:918–27.

11. Conio M, Cameron AJ, Romero Y *et al.* Secular trends in the epidemiology and outcome of Barrett's oesophagus in Olmsted County, Minnesota. *Gut* 2001;**48**:304–9.

12. Eloubeide MA, Provenzale D. Clinical and demographic predictors of Barrett's esophagus among patients with gastroesophageal reflux disease. *J Clin Gastroenterol* 2001;**33**:306–9.

13. Gerson LB, Edson R, Lavori PW, Triadafilopoloulos G. Use of a simple symptom questionnaire to predict Barrett's esophagus in patients with symptoms of gastroesophageal reflux. *Am J Gastroenterol* 2001;**96**: 2005–12.

14. Avidan B, Sonnenberg A, Schnell TG, Sontag SJ. There are no reliable symptoms for erosive oesophagitis and Barrett's oesophagus: endoscopic diagnosis is still essential. *Aliment Pharmacol* 2002;**16**:735–42.

15. Conio M, Filiberti R, Blanchi S *et al.* Risk factors for Barrett's esophagus: a case-control study. *Int J Cancer* 2002;**97**:225–9.

16. Haggitt RC, Tryzelaar J, Ellis FH, Colcher H. Adenocarcinoma complicating columnar epithelium lined (Barrett's) esophagus. *Am J Clin Pathol* 1978;**70**:1–5.

17. Skinner DB, Walther BC, Riddell RH *et al.* Barrett's esophagus: comparison of benign and malignant cases. *Ann Surg* 1983;**198**:554–66.

18. Smith RRL, Hamilton SO, Boitnott JK, Rogers EL. The spectrum of carcinoma arising in Barrett's esophagus. *Am J Burg Pathol* 1984;**8**:563–73.

19. Rosenberg JO, Budev H, Edwards RC *et al.* Analysis of adenocarcinoma in Barrett's esophagus utilizing a staging system. *Cancer* 1985;**55**:1353–60.

20. Paraf F, Flejou JF, Pignon JP, Fekete F, Potet F. Surgical pathology of adenocarcinoma arising in Barrett's esophagus. *Am J Surg Pathol* 1995;**19**:183–91.

21. Lagergren J, Bergstrom R, Lindgren A, Nyren O. Symptomatic gastroesophageal reflux as a risk factor for esophageal adenocarcinoma. *N Engl J Med* 1999;**340**: 825–31.

22. Lieberman DA, Oehlke M, Helfand M. Risk factors for Barrett's esophagus in community-based practice. GORGE consortium. *Am J Gastroenterol* 1997;**92**:1293–7.

23. Eisen GM, Sandier IS, Murray S, Gottfried M. The relationship between gastroesophageal reflux disease and its complications with Barrett's esophagus. *Am J Gastroenterol* 1997;**92**:27–31.

24. Breslin NP, Thompson ABR, Bailey RJ *et al.* Gastric cancer and other endoscopic diagnoses in patients with benign dyspepsia. *Gut* 2000;**46**:93–7.

25. Cameron AJ, Lomboy CT. Barrett's esophagus: age, prevalence and extent of columnar epithelium. *Gastroenterology* 1992;**103**:1241–5.

26. Sampliner RE, Practice Parameters Committee ACG. Updated guidelines for the diagnosis, surveillance, and therapy of Barrett's esophagus. *Am J Gastroenterol* 2002;**97**:1888–95.

27. Romero Y, Cameron AJ, Locke GR *et al.* Familial aggregation of gastroesophageal reflux in patients with

Barrett's esophagus and esophageal adenocarcinoma. *Gastroenterology* 1997;**113**:1449–56.

28. Trudgill NJ, Kapur KC, Riley SA. Familial clustering of reflux symptoms. *Am J Gastroenterol* 1999;**94**:1172–8.

29. Chak A, Lee T, Kinnard MF *et al*. Familial aggregation of Barrett's oesophagus, oesophageal adenocarcinoma, and oesophagogastric junctional adenocarcinoma in Caucasian adults. *Gut* 2002;**51**:323–8.

30. Romero Y, Cameron AJ, Schaid DJ *et al*. Barrett's esophagus: prevalence in symptomatic relatives. *Am J Gastroenterol* 2002;**97**:1127–32.

31. Chak A, Faulx A, Kinnard MF *et al*. Identification of Barrett's esophagus in relatives by endoscopic screening. *Am J Gastroenterol* 2004;**99**:2107–14.

32. Ofman JJ, Shaheen NJ, Desai AA *et al*. The quality of care in Barrett's esophagus: endoscopist and pathologist practices. *Am J Gastroenterol* 2001;**96**:876–81.

33. Sampliner RE. Detecting, measuring, and managing Barrett's esophagus—the complete endoscopist. *Gastrointest Endosc* 1997;**45**:533–5.

34. Ballinger PJ, Hogan WJ, Bohorfoush AG *et al*. Short segment Barrett's epithelium: prevalence and accuracy of endoscopic detection. *Gastrointest Endosc* 1993;**39**:A93.

35. Alikhan M, Rex D, Khan A *et al*. Variable pathologic interpretation of columnar lined esophagus by general pathologists in community practice. *Gastrointest Endosc* 1999;**50**:23–6.

36. Falk GA, Chittajallu R, Goldblum JR *et al*. Surveillance of patients with Barrett's esophagus for dysplasia and cancer with balloon cytology. *Gastroenterology* 1997;**112**:1787–97.

37. Garcia RT, Cello JP, Nguyen MH *et al*. Unsedated ultrathin EGD is well accepted when compared with conventional sedated EGD: a multicenter randomized trial. *Gastroenterology* 2003;**125**:1606–12.

38. Saeian K, Staff DM, Vasilopoulos S *et al*. Unsedated transnasal endoscopy accurately detects Barrett's metaplasia and dysplasia. *Gastrintest Endosc* 2002;**56**:472–8.

39. Zaman A, Hapke R, Sahagun G, Katon RM. Unsedated peroral endoscopy with a video ultrathin endoscope: patient acceptance, tolerance, and diagnostic accuracy. *Am J Gastroenterol* 1998;**93**:1260–3.

40. Eliakim R, Yassin K, Shlomi I, Suissa A, Eisen GM. A novel diagnostic tool for detecting oesophageal pathology: the PillCam oesophageal video capsule. *Aliment Pharmacol Ther* 2004;**20**:1083–9.

41. Cooper GS, Yuan Z, Chak A, Rimm AA. Association of prediagnosis endoscopy with stage and survival in adenocarcinoma of the esophagus and gastric cardia. *Cancer* 2002;**95**:32–8.

42. Kearney DJ, Crump C, Maynard C, Boyko EJ. A case-controlled study of endoscopy and mortality from adenocarcinoma of the esophagus or gastric cardia in persons with GERD. *Gastrointest Endosc* 2003;**57**:823–9.

43. Soni A, Sampliner RE, Sonnenberg A. Screening for high grade dysplasia in gastroesophageal reflux disease: is it cost effective? *Am J Gastroenterol* 2000;**95**:2086–93.

44. Inadomi JM, Sampliner RE, Lagergren J *et al*. Screening and surveillance for Barrett's esophagus in high-risk groups: a cost–utility analysis. *Ann Intern Med* 2003;**138**:176–86.

45. Sharma P, Reker D, Falk GW *et al*. Progression of Barrett's esophagus to high grade dysplasia and cancer: preliminary results of the BEST (Barrett's esophagus study) trial. *Gastroenterology* 2001;**120**:A16–7.

46. Falk GW, Ours TM, Richter J. Practice patterns for surveillance of Barrett's esophagus in the United States. *Gastrointest Endosc* 2000;**52**:197–203.

47. Gross GP, Canto MI, Hixson J, Powe NR. Management of Barrett's esophagus: a national study of practice patterns and their cost implications. *Am J Gastroenterol* 1999;**94**:3440–7.

CHAPTER 12
Surveillance of Barrett's Esophagus

Gary W. Falk

Introduction

Barrett's esophagus is the most severe complication of chronic gastroesophageal reflux disease (GERD). The importance of Barrett's esophagus is due to its well-recognized association with adenocarcinoma of the esophagus. The incidence of adenocarcinoma of the esophagus continues to increase and the 5-year survival rate for this cancer remains dismal. Barrett's esophagus and its associated dysplasia are well-recognized risk factors for esophageal adenocarcinoma. Currently, the best hope for improved survival of patients with esophageal adenocarcinoma is detection of cancer at an early and potentially curable stage. This chapter summarizes current issues in endoscopic surveillance of Barrett's esophagus.

The Increasing Incidence of Esophageal Adenocarcinoma

Adenocarcinoma of the esophagus was previously recognized as an uncommon disorder. Studies now show that the incidence of this cancer has increased approximately 400% among White men since the mid-1970s [1]. In the USA, the incidence of adenocarcinoma of the esophagus in White men has increased by 21% per year, a rate greater than that for any other cancer in White men [2]. Similar trends are seen in other Western countries. However, the overall burden of esophageal adenocarcinoma remains relatively low. Approximately 14 250 new cases of esophageal carcinoma were diagnosed in the USA in 2004, of which approximately 60% were adenocarcinoma [3,4].

The age-specific incidence rate of esophageal adenocarcinoma increases until ages 75–79 years after which it declines [5] (Fig. 12.1). Recent studies indicate a disturbing increase in the incidence of esophageal cancer among younger patients: there are higher incidence rates in cohorts born more recently [5]. El-Serag *et al.* estimated that the odds of developing adenocarcinoma increases by 37.6% for each 5-year increase in year of birth and 6.6% for each 5-year increase in age [5]. This birth cohort effect strongly suggests the possibility that an exposure or set of exposures is contributing to the changing epidemiology of esophageal adenocarcinoma. However, the exposure or exposures resulting in the increase in the incidence of esophageal adenocarcinoma remains unknown.

Barrett's esophagus is clearly a risk factor for adenocarcinoma of the esophagus. Epidemiologic studies have identified a variety of other risk factors for the development of esophageal adenocarcinoma. Work from Lagergren *et al.* showed that the more frequent, severe and long-lasting the symptoms of reflux, the greater the risk for esophageal adenocarcinoma [6]. There is increasing evidence of an association between increasing body mass index (BMI) and esophageal adenocarcinoma [7,8]. Dietary and environmental issues implicated include a diet low in fresh fruit and smoking [9,10] whereas *Helicobacter pylori* infection, especially with *cagA*+ strains, may protect against the development of esophageal adenocarcinoma [11]. There are conflicting data on the role of drugs that relax the lower esophageal sphincter as a risk factor for esophageal adenocarcinoma [12].

Esophageal adenocarcinoma is a lethal disease. The median 5-year survival of esophageal adenocarcinoma was only 14% in the mid 1990s [13]. Survival is stage dependent, and early spread of cancer prior to the onset of symptoms is an unfortunate characteristic of this tumor: lymph node metastases may be found in up to 5% of intramucosal carcinoma cases and in up to 24% of submucosal carcinoma cases due to the rich lymphatic supply of the esophagus that extends into the lamina propria [14] (Fig. 12.2 [15]). However, the 5-year survival for *in situ* tumors is in excess of 68% giving impetus to a strategy of early detection [16]. Thus, the only hope for improved survival of patients with esophageal adenocarcinoma is detection of cancer at an early and potentially curable stage.

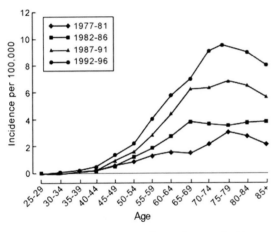

Fig. 12.1 The age distribution of cases diagnosed with esophageal adenocarcinoma in the USA between 1977 and 1996. Reprinted with permission from El-Serag *et al.* [5].

Endoscopic Surveillance

What is Surveillance?

Surveillance is a technique applied to individuals who warrant continued ongoing investigation until they either develop a target lesion while in a surveillance program or exit a surveillance program for some other reason, such as declining health [17]. Surveillance is applied to individuals thought to be at increased risk for a particular malignancy, in this case, esophageal adenocarcinoma.

Rationale for Endoscopic Surveillance

Given the dismal outcome of advanced esophageal adenocarcinoma, current practice guidelines recommend endoscopic surveillance of patients with Barrett's esophagus in an attempt to detect cancer at an early and potentially curable stage [18]. A number of observational studies suggest that patients with Barrett's esophagus in whom adenocarcinoma was detected in a surveillance program have their cancers detected at an earlier stage (Fig. 12.3), with markedly improved 5-year survival compared to similar patients not undergoing routine endoscopic surveillance [19–25] (Fig. 12.4). Furthermore, nodal involvement is far less likely in surveyed patients compared to non-surveyed patients [23]. Since esophageal cancer survival is stage-dependent, these studies suggest that survival may be enhanced by endoscopic surveillance. Several decision-analysis models support the concept of endoscopic surveillance as well (see below) [24–29].

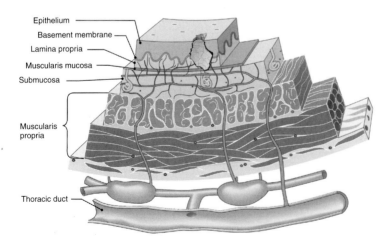

Fig. 12.2 Lymphatic anatomy of the esophagus. Lymphatics extend into the lamina propria, which explains why lymphatic spread is so common in esophageal cancer. Reprinted with permission from Falk [15].

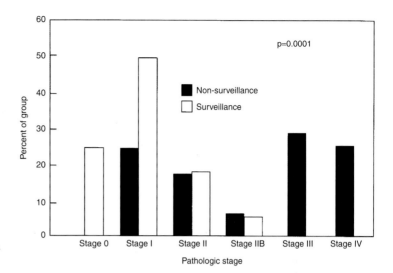

Fig. 12.3 Improved pathologic stage at diagnosis of esophageal adenocarcinoma for patients diagnosed during endoscopic surveillance compared to patients diagnosed without prior surveillance. Reproduced with permission from Corley *et al.* [19].

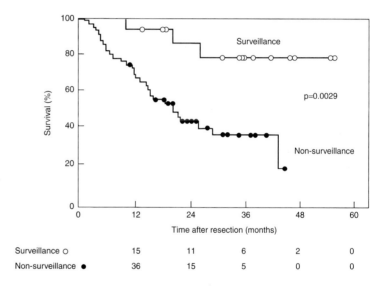

Fig. 12.4 Improved postoperative survival in esophageal adenocarcinoma for patients diagnosed during endoscopic surveillance compared to patients diagnosed without prior surveillance. Reproduced with permission from Corley *et al.* [19].

However, others argue that since most patients with Barrett's esophagus will not die from esophageal cancer, the benefit of surveillance remains uncertain and as such, endoscopic surveillance is not warranted until substantiated by prospective studies [30–32]. Recent work from Northern Ireland has again demonstrated this conundrum [33]. While the overall mortality rate among patients with Barrett's esophagus was no different than that of the general population, mortality from esophageal cancer was increased in Barrett's esophagus patients, but only 4.7% of these patients died of esophageal adenocarcinoma [33]. Others point out that since approximately 95% of esophageal adenocarcinomas are diagnosed in patients without a prior diagnosis of Barrett's esophagus, the entire premise of surveillance should be questioned [34].

Furthermore, all cancer surveillance strategies have a number of potential pitfalls [17]. Selection bias may result in patients accepting surveillance who are less likely to develop cancer or who would have presented with symptoms of cancer at an earlier stage regardless of surveillance. Lead time bias in a surveillance program may lead to cancer detection at an earlier stage, prior to the development of symptoms, resulting in a longer apparent survival. Finally, surveillance programs may simply detect slower growing, more indolent cancers that may never be fatal to the patient in contrast to faster growing aggressive tumors (length time bias).

The resources encumbered by vigorous endoscopic surveillance are considerable. Despite the concern regarding the esophageal cancer "epidemic" the overall burden of disease is rather limited in the Western world in comparison to other malignancies such as colon cancer. A randomized controlled trial of surveillance versus no surveillance in Barrett's esophagus has not been performed and probably never will be. While it is scientifically appealing to wait for evidence to support endoscopic surveillance, we still have the clinical dilemma of dealing with individual patients at increased risk for the development of esophageal cancer [35].

The Risk of Esophageal Adenocarcinoma in an Individual Patient

Despite the alarming increase in the incidence of esophageal adenocarcinoma, the precise incidence of adenocarcinoma in patients with Barrett's esophagus is uncertain, with rates varying from 1/52 to 1/297 years of follow-up [30,36–38]. Shaheen *et al.* found a strong inverse relationship between cancer risk and study size, with small studies reporting much higher cancer risks than large studies [38]. This finding suggests that there is a publication bias that has led to an overestimate of cancer risk in Barrett's esophagus: small studies were published or submitted for publication only if they indicated high cancer risk. Most recent studies suggest a much lower risk than what was previously thought, approximately 0.5% or less annually [30,38]. However, regional variations of cancer risk exist in the Western world, and the annual incidence rate in the UK is approximately twice that (1%) found in

the USA (0.5%) [39]. The evolving epidemiologic data suggest that despite the alarming increase in the incidence of esophageal adenocarcinoma, the vast majority of patients with Barrett's esophagus will never develop cancer. Furthermore, the survival of patients with Barrett's esophagus is similar to that of the general population, despite an increased risk of esophageal adenocarcinoma [33].

Development of Esophageal Adenocarcinoma from Barrett's Esophagus

Cancer risk in Barrett's esophagus appears to be limited to patients with specialized columnar epithelium, a finding that may be explained by the increased rate of cellular proliferation encountered in these cells compared to cardiac or fundic type epithelium [40,41]. Compelling evidence exists for a dysplasia–carcinoma sequence in Barrett's esophagus whereby specialized columnar epithelium progresses to low-grade dysplasia, high-grade dysplasia, and finally to carcinoma. Foci of carcinoma typically appear adjacent to dysplasia [42]. However, the time course for this progression is highly variable (Fig. 12.5), and most patients never progress to dysplasia.

It is hypothesized that cancer develops in a subset of patients who have acquired genomic instability in Barrett's epithelium [43]. This predisposes to the development of abnormal clones of cells that then accumulate progressively more genetic errors which include numerical and structural chromosomal rearrangements, gene mutations, loss of normal cell cycle control, and increased cell proliferation rates [44–46]. However, there is no clearly predictable sequence of genetic abnormalities that leads to the development of cancer. Upregulation of cyclooxygenase-2 (COX-2) expression also occurs in the metaplasia–dysplasia–carcinoma sequence [47]. Increased COX-2 expression is associated with increased cellular proliferation and decreased apoptosis *in vitro* [48].

Candidates for Endoscopic Surveillance

Only patients at increased risk for the development

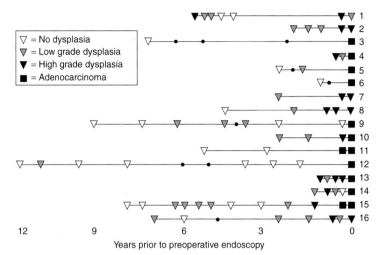

Fig. 12.5 The dysplasia–carcinoma sequence in Barrett's esophagus in 16 patients undergoing endoscopic surveillance of Barrett's esophagus. Note the variable time frame for the evolution of Barrett's esophagus without dysplasia to low-grade dysplasia, high-grade dysplasia, and adenocarcinoma. Reproduced with permission from Van Sandick *et al.* [23].

of carcinoma, that is those with intestinal metaplasia, should undergo endoscopic surveillance. It is generally agreed that all otherwise healthy patients with Barrett's esophagus should undergo surveillance, with an endpoint of either high-grade dysplasia or adenocarcinoma. Elderly patients or patients with comorbid illnesses who are not candidates for esophagectomy generally would not undergo surveillance or would be dropped from surveillance at a certain undetermined age. However, new ablation techniques may make more of these patients eligible for surveillance in the future. This area remains unsettled.

Surveillance Techniques

Current guidelines suggest obtaining systematic four quadrant biopsies at 2 cm intervals along the entire length of the Barrett's segment once inflammation related to GERD is controlled with antisecretory therapy [18] (Fig. 12.6). At the time of endoscopy, landmarks including the diaphragmatic hiatus, esophagogastric junction, and squamocolumnar junction should be carefully defined prior to commencing the biopsy protocol. Subtle mucosal abnormalities no matter how trivial, such as ulceration, erosion, plaque, nodule, stricture, or other luminal irregularity in the Barrett's segment, should also be biopsied, as there is an association of such lesions with underlying cancer [49]. A systematic biopsy protocol clearly detects more dysplasia and early

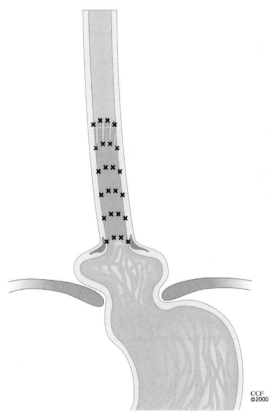

Fig. 12.6 Technique of endoscopic surveillance. Landmarks including the diaphragm, proximal margin of gastric folds, and squamocolumnar junction should be identified first. Four quadrant biopsies should then be obtained every 2 cm in the involved segment. Reproduced with permission from Falk [15].

cancer compared to ad hoc random biopsies [50]. The "turn and suction" technique (Fig. 12.7) allows acquisition of biopsies that are significantly larger than those obtained by the traditional techniques of advancing an open biopsy forceps into the lumen and then closing it to obtain the biopsy sample [51]. With this technique, the biopsy forceps is advanced out of the biopsy channel of the endoscope and opened. The forceps is then drawn back until it is flush with the tip of the endoscope and turned into the esophageal wall. Air is then suctioned from the lumen to collapse the mucosa into the forceps cup, which is then advanced slightly until resistance is appreciated. The forceps is then closed while maintaining suction and the endoscope tip is straightened followed by withdrawal of the biopsy forceps to avulse the mucosal sample. The safety of systematic endoscopic biopsy protocols has been demonstrated [52].

The rational for such a comprehensive biopsy program comes from observations that high-grade dysplasia and early carcinoma in Barrett's esophagus often occur in the absence of endoscopic abnormalities, and from the focal nature of dysplasia. Systematic esophagectomy mapping studies demonstrate just how focal dysplasia and superficial cancer may be [53]. In 30 esophagectomy specimens from patients undergoing surgery for either high-grade dysplasia or early invasive adenocarcinoma with no endoscopic evidence of cancer, the median surface area of total Barrett's esophagus was found to be $32\,cm^2$; low-grade dysplasia $13\,cm^2$; high-grade dysplasia $1.3\,cm^2$; and adenocarcinoma $1.1\,cm^2$ [53] (Fig. 12.8). The three smallest cancers had surface areas of 0.02, 0.30, and $0.40\,cm^2$.

Because of the focal nature of dysplasia and cancer, some experts recommend that endoscopic surveillance should utilize a large particle (jumbo) forceps to obtain biopsies [54]. Studies suggest that a systematic jumbo biopsy protocol at 1 cm intervals plus biopsy of any mucosal abnormalities can reliably distinguish patients with high-grade dysplasia alone from those with intramucosal or submucosal adenocarcinoma, thereby avoiding the risk of unnecessary surgery in these patients [49,54]. Reid *et al.* evaluated the utility of this technique in 45 high-grade dysplasia patients who eventually devel-

oped cancer [49]. Interestingly, 82% of patients had cancer in only a single 1 cm segment and 69% had cancer in a single biopsy. Furthermore, only 39% of patients with cancer by endoscopic biopsy had cancer found at surgery. Using this "Seattle protocol," 100% of cancers were detected. If biopsies were obtained at 2 cm intervals, only 50% of cancers would have been detected. Others have confirmed that jumbo biopsies performed at 2 cm intervals will miss cancer in patients with high-grade dysplasia [55]. However, this technique requires passage of a therapeutic endoscope and the generalizability of this technique to clinical practice is problematic. Survey data suggest that only 17% of gastroenterologists in the USA use the jumbo biopsy forceps [56].

The aim of surveillance is the detection of dysplasia and early cancer. The description of dysplasia should use a standard five tier system: (i) negative for dysplasia; (ii) indefinite for dysplasia; (iii) low-grade dysplasia; (iv) high-grade dysplasia; (v) carcinoma [57]. Dysplasia describes a change that is unequivocally neoplastic. It is characterized by nuclear pleomorphism, nuclear hyperchromatism, and an alteration in nuclear polarity. Low-grade dysplasia is characterized by abnormal nuclei in the basal half of the cell whereas high-grade dysplasia is characterized by nuclei in the upper half of the cell, nuclear crowding and stratification, and more marked nuclear pleomorphism and hyperchromasia. Intramucosal carcinoma is defined as carcinoma cells extending into the lamina propria or muscularis mucosa but not beyond whereas submucosal carcinoma is defined as infiltration of carcinoma cells beyond the muscularis mucosa into the submucosa. Active inflammation makes it more difficult to distinguish dysplasia from reparative changes. As such, surveillance endoscopy should not be done until any active inflammation related to GERD is controlled with antisecretory therapy.

Surveillance Intervals

Surveillance intervals, determined by the presence and grade of dysplasia, are based on our limited knowledge of the biology of esophageal adenocarcinoma (Table 12.1). However, these intervals are arbitrary, have never been subject to a clinical trial

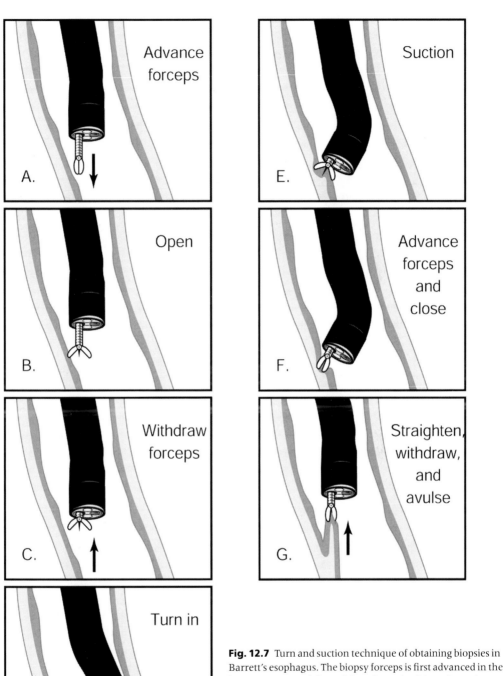

A. Advance forceps

B. Open

C. Withdraw forceps

D. Turn in

E. Suction

F. Advance forceps and close

G. Straighten, withdraw, and avulse

Fig. 12.7 Turn and suction technique of obtaining biopsies in Barrett's esophagus. The biopsy forceps is first advanced in the lumen (a), opened (b) and then drawn back into the endoscope until it is flush with the endoscope tip (c). The endoscope is then turned into the esophageal wall (d) after which suction is applied (e). The biopsy forceps is advanced slightly and closed (f), after which the endoscope is straightened followed by withdrawal of the forceps to avulse a mucosal sample. Reproduced with permission from Levine and Reid [51].

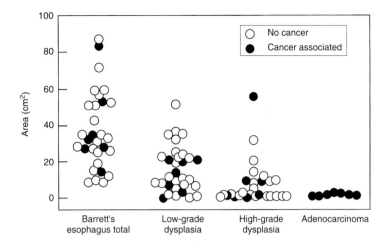

Fig. 12.8 Surface area involved with Barrett's esophagus, low-grade dysplasia, high-grade dysplasia, and adenocarcinoma in 30 patients without obvious carcinoma undergoing resection for high-grade dysplasia or superficial adenocarcinoma. Reproduced with permission from Cameron and Carpenter [53].

Table 12.1 2002 American College of Gastroenterology practice guidelines for endoscopic surveillance of Barrett's esophagus. Adapted with permission from Sampliner [18].

Dysplasia grade	Interval
None	Every 3 years after two are negative
Low-grade	Repeat endoscopy with intensive biopsy of area with dysplasia while on maximum acid suppression
	Every year until no dysplasia
High-grade	Repeat endoscopy with intensive biopsy protocol preferably with therapeutic endoscope and large capacity biopsy forceps to rule out cancer and document high-grade dysplasia. Special attention to mucosal irregularity
	Expert pathologist confirmation
	Focal high-grade dysplasia (< 5 crypts): continued surveillance every 3 months
	Multifocal (≥ 5 crypts): intervention
	Mucosal irregularity: endoscopic mucosal resection

and likely never will be. Surveillance every 3 years is now recommended as adequate in patients without dysplasia after two negative examinations [18]. In patients with low-grade dysplasia, biopsies should first be reviewed by an expert gastrointestinal pathologist to confirm the diagnosis. The patient should then undergo a repeat endoscopy within 3–6 months using a therapeutic endoscope with large capacity forceps to exclude the possibility of a higher grade lesion [58], Biopsy intervals of 1 cm make sense in this setting. If low-grade dysplasia is confirmed, then annual surveillance is now recommended until the lesion disappears [18]. These patients should receive aggressive antisecretory

therapy for reflux disease with a proton pump inhibitor to decrease the changes of regeneration that make pathologic interpretation of this category so difficult.

If high-grade dysplasia is found, the diagnosis should first be confirmed by an experienced gastrointestinal pathologist. The endoscopic biopsy protocol should then be repeated within 1 month to exclude an unsuspected carcinoma. However, biopsies should now be obtained at 1 cm intervals with large particle "jumbo" forceps to maximize the ability to detect unsuspected cancer [49,54]. If high-grade dysplasia is confirmed, there is no agreement on the most appropriate management of these patients. Esophagectomy is recommended by many authors to eliminate the risk of carcinoma or to detect and treat cancer at an early curable stage, because of the marked variability in the finding of unsuspected cancer in patients with high-grade dysplasia which ranges from 0% to 73% [59]. Surgical mortality in high volume centers is now less than 5%, but is still unacceptably high in centers with low surgical volume [55].

However, this approach has been criticized because of the potential risks associated with esophagectomy and the variable natural history of high-grade dysplasia [54]. Others recommend a continued program of rigorous endoscopic surveillance utilizing the systematic biopsy protocol described above, reserving esophagectomy for patients with a preoperative diagnosis of intramucosal or submucosal carcinoma [54]. Still others recommend endoscopic ablation therapy, and a recent cost-effectiveness model suggested that photodynamic therapy was the most effective strategy for patients with high-grade dysplasia, yielding the greatest gain in quality adjusted life years while also providing the greatest gain in incremental cost-effectiveness ratio when compared to continued surveillance or esophagectomy [60]. The optimal strategy for these patients remains to be defined but clearly must factor in local expertise in surgery, pathology and ablative techniques, availability of endoscopic intervention clinical trials, patient age, length of the Barrett's segment, and willingness of a patient and physician to adhere to rigorous surveillance.

Limitations of Surveillance

Endoscopic surveillance of Barrett's esophagus, as currently practiced, has numerous shortcomings. Dysplasia and early adenocarcinoma are endoscopically indistinguishable from intestinal metaplasia without dysplasia. The distribution of dysplasia and cancer is highly variable, and even the most thorough biopsy surveillance program has the potential for sampling error. There is considerable interobserver variability and quality control problems in the interpretation of dysplasia in both the community and academic settings [57,61]. Montgomery *et al.* found that interobserver agreement was moderate

to substantial for intestinal metaplasia without dysplasia (kappa score of 0.58), slight for indefinite for dysplasia (kappa score of 0.15), fair for low-grade dysplasia (kappa score of 0.32), but substantial for high-grade dysplasia or adenocarcinoma (kappa score of 0.65) [57]. However, there are even larger quality control problems in the community setting where a study of 20 pathologists found that only 35% correctly identified intestinal metaplasia without dysplasia and only 38% could identify gastric metaplasia without intestinal metaplasia [61]. Many pathologists continue to classify gastric metaplasia without intestinal metaplasia as Barrett's esophagus, thereby subjecting many individuals to unnecessary surveillance endoscopy. Problems with interobserver variability are even encountered with esophageal resection specimens among experienced gastrointestinal pathologists with a kappa score of 0.6 (moderate agreement) for high-grade dysplasia and 0.56 for high-grade dysplasia versus intramucosal carcinoma (moderate) [62]. It is precisely this type of problem that may explain the highly variable natural history of dysplasia.

Current surveillance programs are expensive and time consuming. Survey data indicate that while surveillance is widely practiced, there is considerable variability in the technique and interval of surveillance, and most do not even follow current practice guidelines [56,63,64]. Furthermore, there are no prospective clinical trials that have tested the efficacy of surveillance in the prevention of esophageal adenocarcinoma. Such a study would require patients to be randomized to surveillance versus no surveillance and followed prospectively over many years. Given the low incidence of cancer in individual patients, such a study is deemed by many to be impractical logistically and economically.

Modeling Strategies of Endoscopic Surveillance of Barrett's Esophagus

Despite the current practice guidelines, there are no data from randomized controlled trials that demonstrate the value of surveillance. Such a trial would take a long period of time to complete, considerable financial resources, and a large number of patients. A number of computer-generated modeling strategies have examined the cost-effectiveness of endoscopic surveillance of Barrett's esophagus. These generally demonstrate that endoscopic surveillance can be cost-effective in selected patients under certain conditions [28]. A decision-analysis study by Provenzale *et al.* of the optimal surveillance strategy for Barrett's esophagus with an endpoint of esophagectomy for high-grade dysplasia found that surveillance every 5 years was the most effective strategy to increase both length and quality of life [27]. A decision analysis model by Inadomi *et al.* examined screening of 50-year-old White men with chronic GERD symptoms for Barrett's esophagus, and found that one time screening was probably cost-effective only if subsequent surveillance was limited to patients with dysplasia on initial examination [26]. This strategy would result in a cost of $10 440 per quality adjusted life year saved compared to a strategy of no screening or surveillance. However, if surveillance was subsequently performed in patients without dysplasia on a screening examination, even at 5-year intervals, the strategy would cost approximately $596 000 per quality adjusted life year.

In contrast, a cost-effectiveness model by Gerson *et al.* found that screening of 50-year-old men with chronic GERD symptoms followed by surveillance of patients with both dysplastic and non-dysplastic Barrett's esophagus with either esophagectomy or endoscopic therapy for patients with high-grade dysplasia or adenocarcinoma was indeed cost-effective [29]. They found that such a strategy would result in a cost of $12 140 per life-year gained compared to a strategy of no screening or surveillance. What accounts for such disparate results? As is usually the case with modeling studies, the assumptions and methods used by Inadomi *et al.* and Gerson *et al.* are different, especially with respect to cancer epidemiology, treatment strategies, and cancer detection rates.

All modeling studies to date suggest that following parameters influence cost-effectiveness: (a) cost and frequency of surveillance; (b) sensitivity and specificity of endoscopy for detecting dysplasia; (c) incidence of neoplasia; and (d) impact of therapy be it surgical or non-surgical on length and quality of life [65]. Thus, when taken together, modeling studies suggest that endoscopic surveillance followed by efficacious intervention in selected patients can be cost-effective [65].

Potential Strategies to Enhance Surveillance

Currently, all Barrett's esophagus patients are handled in a similar fashion unless dysplasia is present. However, most patients do not have dysplasia and will never develop cancer. In order to make surveillance techniques more effective, new approaches are necessary. This can be accomplished conceptually by either sampling larger areas of Barrett's mucosa, targeting our biopsies to areas with a higher probability of harboring dysplasia, or developing risk stratification tools to allow us to concentrate our efforts on individuals at greatest risk of developing cancer while decreasing the frequency and intensity of surveillance for individuals at lower cancer risk.

Cytology   Brush cytology may be complementary to endoscopic biopsies and is recommended by some to be part of the routine endoscopic surveillance of Barrett's patients [66]. Cytology has a number of potential advantages compared to routine endoscopic biopsies: ability to sample a greater area of involved epithelium, preferential exfoliation of the less cohesive dysplastic cells, simplicity, and lower cost. There are clear cytologic criteria for dysplasia and biomarker studies can be performed on cytologic specimens [66–68]. Studies to date suggest that endoscopic cytology has excellent sensitivity and specificity for the extremes of Barrett's esophagus: no dysplasia or high-grade dysplasia/adenocarcinoma [66]. However, there are problems in the cytologic detection of low-grade dysplasia and it is imperfect for the detection of goblet cells alone. Survey data indicate that only 17% of gastroenterologists utilize brush cytology as part of endoscopic surveillance of Barrett's esophagus [56] and questions remain regarding the generalizability of cytology to the community setting [69].

Chromoendoscopy   Methylene blue is a vital stain that selectively diffuses into the cytoplasm of absorptive epithelium of the small intestine and colon. The presence of staining in the esophagus indicates the presence of intestinal metaplasia [70]. Some studies suggest that methylene blue chromoendoscopy increases the efficiency of detecting dysplasia: fewer biopsies are required and more patients are identified with dysplasia compared to four quadrant biopsies obtained at 2 cm intervals [71]. However, others are unable to detect any differences in dysplasia detection between methylene blue directed biopsies compared to a standard biopsy protocol [72]. Chromoendoscopy is appealing because it is simple and inexpensive. However, there is no agreement on application technique in terms of the concentration, volume and "dwell time" of various reagents, and interpretation of staining remains subjective. Methylene blue chromoendoscopy also adds additional procedure time and there are some concerns regarding carcinogenesis related to the dye itself [73].

Optical Biopsy Techniques   A variety of endoscopic optical techniques including fluorescence spectroscopy, light spectroscopy, optical coherence tomography, light scattering spectroscopy, light induced fluorescence endoscopy, confocal microscopy, and molecular imaging with injected probes have the potential to obtain "light" biopsies of Barrett's esophagus. All of these techniques are based on the principle that benign and malignant tissues have different optical qualities. In theory, this would permit optical sampling of larger areas of the columnar-lined esophagus and improve the efficiency of biopsies by targeting areas thought to harbor dysplasia or cancer.

Initial work with laser-induced fluorescence spectroscopy in a group of 36 patients had a sensitivity of 100% for high-grade dysplasia and a specificity of 70% for no dysplasia, but all six patients with low-grade dysplasia were classified as benign by laser-induced fluorescence spectroscopy [74]. A spectroscopic probe that combined the techniques of fluorescence, reflectance, and light scattering spectroscopy in 16 patients with Barrett's esophagus had a sensitivity and specificity of 100% for separating high-grade dysplasia from low-grade dysplasia and no dysplasia and a sensitivity of 93% with a specificity of 100% for separating any dysplasia from no dysplasia [75]. However, spectroscopic techniques,

as currently configured, require a "point and shoot" method of touching the mucosa with the probe followed by biopsy. To be clinically helpful, these techniques will need to image a larger field by "spraying light" followed by targeted biopsies of abnormal optical regions.

Optical coherence tomography uses infrared light to produce high-resolution images of mucosal tissue *in vivo*. Current technology again is limited to a "touch and image" technique and is not yet able to sample large areas rapidly.

Light induced fluorescence endoscopy is a technique that allows one to "spray" light on the entire esophagus. It is based on the principal that tissue excited by light of a specific wavelength will emit fluorescent light of a longer wavelength, and that normal, metaplastic, and dysplastic tissues have different autofluorescence colors visible to the naked eye. This will permit targeting biopsies to areas of abnormal light. In theory, this technique has the potential to rapidly assess large areas of epithelium prior to targeting biopsies. A preliminary report found that light induced fluorescence endoscopy identified 14 of 14 early cancers, seven of 11 "severe" dysplasias, but only four of 22 areas of low-grade dysplasia [76]. However, once an area is biopsied, the resulting blood can interfere with imaging. Endoscopic fluorescence detection may be enhanced further by using a sensitizer, such as 5-aminolevulinic acid, which accumulates selectively in tumors and dysplasia. Illumination by light of a specific wavelength allows one to see fluorescence from these lesions that is not visible at normal white light endoscopy.

However, validation, standardization, and comparison of all of these techniques are still lacking and as such, none are as yet ready for clinical use [77,78]. It is anticipated that a combination of techniques that permit efficient sampling of a wide surface area of involved mucosa accompanied by deep tissue penetration and high cellular resolution will be the most useful strategy in the future [78].

Risk Stratification   A number of clinical and biologic markers may define patients at increased risk for the development of adenocarcinoma. Clinical risk factors for the development of high-grade dysplasia or adenocarcinoma include male gender,

Caucasian ethnicity, increasing age, dysplasia at either index endoscopy or at any time during surveillance, hiatal hernia size, length of the Barrett's segment, BMI, use of lower esophageal sphincter relaxing medications, low selenium levels, and smoking [5,7,79–86]. A recent case control study found that 79% of the population attributable risk of esophageal adenocarcinoma, that is the proportion of disease attributable to a given risk factor or set of risk factors, was due to ever having smoked, BMI above the lowest quartile, history of gastroesophageal reflux, and low fruit and vegetable consumption [86]. That means that in theory, elimination of all of these factors could eliminate most cases of esophageal adenocarcinoma.

Dysplasia still remains the best available marker of cancer risk despite recognized problems with interobserver variability [57]. Dysplasia is recognized adjacent to and distant from Barrett's esophagus associated adenocarcinoma in resection specimens from patients with Barrett's esophagus [42,43]. Patients progress through a phenotypic sequence of no dysplasia, low-grade dysplasia, high-grade dysplasia, and adenocarcinoma although the time course is highly variable [23].

Indefinite for dysplasia is used to characterize lesions not wholly diagnostic of dysplasia but too atypical to dismiss as normal [87]. Work by Montgomery *et al.* found that the median progression-free interval to cancer was 62 months for indefinite for dysplasia, 60 months for low-grade dysplasia, and 8 months for high-grade dysplasia [87]. This finding supports the concept of grouping indefinite for dysplasia and low-grade dysplasia together for clinical decision making.

The natural history of low-grade dysplasia is poorly understood. In part, this may be due to the high degree of interobserver variability in establishing this diagnosis and the variable protocols by which these patients are followed [57]. Recent studies suggest that approximately 10–28% of low-grade dysplasia patients go on to develop high-grade dysplasia or adenocarcinoma, whereas regression is seen in approximately 60–75% [30,88,89]. The remainder will have persistent low-grade dysplasia. However, complete interobserver agreement among experienced gastrointestinal pathologists may im-

prove the prognostic value of the finding of low-grade dysplasia that progresses on to high-grade dysplasia or cancer [90].

Unsuspected carcinoma is detected at esophagectomy in approximately 40% of patients with high-grade dysplasia, with a range of 0–73% [59]. However, while high-grade dysplasia remains a worrisome lesion, progression to carcinoma may take many years and is not inevitable. Buttar *et al.* followed 100 patients with high-grade dysplasia with continued endoscopic surveillance and found cancer at 1 and 3 years in 38% and 56% of individuals with diffuse high-grade dysplasia and 7% and 14% of individuals with focal high-grade dysplasia [91]. Reid *et al.* followed 76 patients for 5 years and encountered cancer in 59% [92]. On the other hand, Schnell *et al.*, in a study of 79 patients, found cancer in 5% during the first year of surveillance and in 16% of the remaining patients followed for a mean of 7 years (20% of the total group developed cancer) [93]. Others have reported regression of high-grade dysplasia over time as well [93,94]. Extent of high-grade dysplasia is thought by some to be a risk factor for the subsequent development of adenocarcinoma [91]. However, there are currently no uniform criteria for defining the extent of high-grade dysplasia and there are conflicting data on the clinical significance of extent of high-grade dysplasia in biopsy specimens and risk for unsuspected carcinoma [91,95].

Unfortunately, dysplasia is not distinguishable endoscopically, and the focal nature of dysplasia makes targeting of biopsies problematic. Furthermore there is considerable interobserver variability in the grading of dysplasia in both the community and academic settings [57,61]. The ability of pathologists to distinguish between intramucosal carcinoma and high-grade dysplasia is problematic even in esophagectomy specimens, thus providing a potential explanation for the wide variation in behavior of high-grade dysplasia reported in the literature [62]. Therefore, a less subjective marker for cancer risk that could supplement or replace the current dysplasia grading system is needed.

Biomarkers of Increased Risk   A number of biologic markers may define patients at increased risk for the development of esophageal adenocarcinoma.

Among the most frequently described molecular changes that precede the development of adenocarcinoma in Barrett's esophagus are alterations in *p53* (mutation, deletion or loss of heterozygosity [LOH]), *p16* (mutation, deletion, promoter hypermethylation, or LOH) and aneuploidy by flow cytometry. Neoplastic progression in Barrett's esophagus is accompanied by flow cytometric abnormalities such as aneuploidy or increased G2/tetraploid DNA contents, and these abnormalities may precede the development of high-grade dysplasia or adenocarcinoma [45]. The potential importance of flow cytometry as a prognostic biomarker was illustrated in work by Reid *et al.*, who found that for patients with no flow cytometric abnormalities at baseline and with histology that showed no dysplasia, indefinite or low-grade dysplasia, the 5-year incidence of cancer was 0% [92]. In contrast, aneuploidy, increased 4N fractions or high-grade dysplasia was detected in each of the 35 patients who went on to develop cancer within 5 years.

Mutations of *p53* and *17p* LOH have been reported in up to 92% and 100%, respectively, of esophageal adencocarcinomas [96]. Furthermore, both abnormalities have been detected in Barrett's epithelium prior to the development of carcinoma [96,97]. For example, Reid *et al.* found that the prevalence of 17p (*p53*) LOH at baseline increased from 6% in patients negative for dysplasia to 20% in patients with low-grade dysplasia, and to 57% in patients with high-grade dysplasia [97]. More importantly, the 3-year incidence of cancer was 38% for individuals with 17p (*p53*) LOH compared to 3.3% for individuals with two 17p alleles. However, techniques to detect *p53* mutations and 17p LOH are labor intensive and have not achieved widespread acceptance in clinical practice to date. Immunohistochemistry, a much simpler technique, has been extensively studied in the dysplasia–carcinoma sequence of Barrett's esophagus, but is hampered by false positive and negative rates of approximately 25% [97]. Similarly, *p16* LOH and inactivation of the *p16* gene by promoter region hypermethylation have been reported frequently in esophageal adenocarcinoma [47,98]. Furthermore, 9p LOH is commonly encountered in premalignant Barrett's epithelium and can be detected over large regions of the Barrett's mucosa

[98]. It is hypothesized that clonal expansion occurs in conjunction with *p16* abnormalities creating a field in which other genetic lesions leading to esophageal adenocarcinoma can arise [98].

Unfortunately, none of these biomarkers has been validated in large-scale clinical trials. In the future, it is hoped that risk stratification may be accomplished by a panel of biomarkers obtained from genomic profiling of Barrett's esophagus patients using rapidly advancing genomic technology. If risk stratification is successful in the future, it is anticipated that endoscopic surveillance intervals will be lengthened for patients at low risk for developing adenocarcinoma and shortened for patients at increased risk of developing adenocarcinoma.

References

1. Wei JT, Shaheen NJ. The changing epidemiology of esophageal adenocarcinoma. *Sem Gastrointest Disease* 2003;**3**:112–27.
2. Bollschweiler E, Wolfgarten E, Gutschow C, Holscher AH. Demographic variations in the rising incidence of esophageal adenocarcinoma in White males. *Cancer* 2001;**92**:549–55.
3. Jemal A, Tiwari RC, Murray T *et al.* Cancer Statistics 2004. *CA Cancer J Clin* 2004;**54**:8–29.
4. Wong A, Fitzgerald RC. Epidemiologic risk factors for Barrett's esophagus and associated adenocarcinoma. *Clin Gastroenterol Hepatol* 2005;**3**:1–10
5. El-Serag HB, Mason AC, Petersen N, Key CR. Epidemiologic differences between adenocarcinoma of the oesophagus and adenocarcinoma of the gastric cardia in the USA. *Gut* 2002;**50**:368–72.
6. Lagergren J, Bergstrom R, Lindgren A, Nyren O. Symptomatic gastroesophageal reflux as a risk factor for esophageal adenocarcinoma. *N Engl J Med* 1999;**340**:825–31.
7. Lagergren J, Bergstrom R, Nyren O. Association between body mass and adenocarcinoma of the esophagus. *Ann Intern Med* 1999;**130**:883–90.
8. Chow WH, Blot WJ, Vaughan TL *et al.* Body mass index and risk of adenocarcinoma of the esophagus and gastric cardia. *J Natl Cancer Inst* 1998;**90**:150–5.
9. Brown LM, Swanson CA, Gridley G *et al.* Adenocarcinoma of the esophagus: role of obesity and diet. *J Natl Cancer Inst* 1995;**87**:104–9.
10. Gammon MD, Schoenberg JB, Ahsan H *et al.* Tobacco, alcohol, and socioeconomic status and adenocarcino-

mas of the esophagus and gastric cardia. *J Natl Cancer Inst* 1997;**89**:1277–84.

11. Chow WH, Blaser MJ, Blot WJ *et al.* An inverse relation between *cagA*⁺ strains of *Helicobacter pylori* infection and risk of esophageal and gastric cardia adenocarcinoma. *Cancer Research* 1998;**58**:588–90.

12. Enzinger PC, Mayer RJ. Esophageal cancer. *N Engl J Med* 2003;**349**:2241–52.

13. Brown LM, Devesa SS. Epidemiologic trends in esophageal and gastric cancer in the United States. *Surg Oncol Clin N Am* 2002;**11**:235–56.

14. Sabik JF, Rice TW, Goldblum JR *et al.* Superficial esophageal carcinoma. *Ann Thorac Surg* 1995;**60**:896–902.

15. Falk GW. Endoscopic surveillance of Barrett's esophagus. *Techniques in Gastrointestinal Endoscopy* 2000;**2**:186–93.

16. Farrow DC, Vaughan TL. Determinants of survival following the diagnosis of esophageal adenocarcinoma. *Cancer Causes Control* 1996;**7**:322–7.

17. Parsonnet J, Axon AT. Principles of screening and surveillance. *Am J Gastroenterol* 1996;**91**:847–9.

18. Sampliner RE. Updated guidelines for the diagnosis, surveillance, and therapy of Barrett's esophagus. *Am J Gastroenterol* 2002;**97**:1888–95.

19. Corley DA, Levin TR, Habel LA, Weiss NS, Buffler PA. Surveillance and survival in Barrett's adenocarcinomas: a population-based study. *Gastroenterology* 2002;**122**:633–40.

20. Incarbone R, Bonavina L, Saino G, Bona D, Peracchia A. Outcome of esophageal adenocarcinoma detected during endoscopic biopsy surveillance for Barrett's esophagus. *Surg Endosc* 2002;**16**:263–6.

21. Ferguson MK, Durkin A. Long-term survival after esophagectomy for Barrett's adenocarcinoma in endoscopically surveyed and nonsurveyed patients. *J Gastrointest Surg* 2002;**6**:29–36.

22. Streitz JM, Andrews CW, Ellis FH. Endoscopic surveillance of Barrett's esophagus. Does it help? *J Thorac Cardiovasc Surg* 1993;**105**:383–8.

23. Van Sandick JW, van Lanschot JJ, Kuiken BW *et al.* Impact of endoscopic biopsy surveillance of Barrett's esophagus on pathological stage and clinical outcome of Barrett's carcinoma. *Gut* 1998;**43**:216–22.

24. Peters JH, Clark GW, Ireland AP *et al.* Outcome of adenocarcinoma arising in Barrett's esophagus in endoscopically surveyed and nonsurveyed patients. *J Thorac Cardiovasc Surg* 1994;**108**:813–22.

25. Fountoulakis A, Zafirellis KD, Dolan K *et al.* Effect of surveillance of Barrett's esophagus on the clinical outcome of oesophageal cancer. *Br J Surg* 2004;**91**:997–1003.

26. Inadomi JM, Sampliner R, Lagergren J *et al.* Screening and surveillance for Barrett esophagus in high risk groups: a cost–utility analysis. *Ann Intern Med* 2003;**138**:176–86.

27. Provenzale D, Schmitt C, Wong JB. Barrett's esophagus: a new look at surveillance based on emerging estimates of cancer risk. *Am J Gastroenterol* 1999;**94**:2043–53.

28. Sonnenberg A, Soni A, Sampliner RE. Medical decision analysis of endoscopic surveillance of Barrett's oesophagus to prevent oesophageal adenocarcinoma. *Aliment Pharmacol Ther* 2002;**16**:41–50.

29. Gerson LB, Groeneveld PW, Triadafilopoulos G. Cost-effectiveness model of endoscopic screening and surveillance in patients with gastroesophageal reflux disease. *Clin Gastroenterol Hepatol* 2004;**2**:868–79.

30. Conio M, Blanchi S, Lapertosa G *et al.* Long-term endoscopic surveillance of patients with Barrett's esophagus: incidence of dysplasia and adenocarcinoma: a prospective study. *Am J Gastroenterol* 2003;**98**:1931–9.

31. Van der Burgh A, Dees J, Hop WC, van Blankenstein M. Oesophageal cancer is an uncommon cause of death in patients with Barrett's oesophagus. *Gut* 1996;**39**:5–8.

32. MacDonald CE, Wicks AC, Playford RJ. Final results from 10-year cohort of patients undergoing surveillance for Barrett's oesophagus: observational study. *Br Med J* 2000;**321**:1252–5.

33. Anderson LA, Murray LJ, Murphy SJ *et al.* Mortality in Barrett's oesophagus: results from a population based study. *Gut* 2003;**52**:1081–4.

34. Dulai GS, Guha S, Kahn KL, Gornbein J, Weinstein WM. Preoperative prevalence of Barrett's esophagus in esophageal adenocarcinoma: a systematic review. *Gastroenterology* 2002;**122**:26–33.

35. Sampliner RE. Adenocarcinoma of the esophagus and gastric cardia: is there progress in the face of increasing cancer incidence? *Ann Intern Med* 1999;**130**:67–9.

36. Drewitz DJ, Sampliner RE, Garewal HS. The incidence of adenocarcinoma in Barrett's esophagus: a prospective study of 170 patients followed 4.8 years. *Am J Gastroenterol* 1997;**92**:212–5.

37. O'Connor JB, Falk GW, Richter JE. The incidence of adenocarcinoma and dysplasia in Barrett's esophagus: report on the Cleveland Clinic Barrett's esophagus registry. *Am J Gastroenterol* 1999;**94**:2037–42.

38. Shaheen NJ, Crosby MA, Bozymski EM, Sandler RS. Is there a publication bias in the reporting of cancer risk in Barrett's esophagus? *Gastroenterology* 2000;**119**:333–8.

39. Jankowski JA, Provenzale D, Moayyedi P. Esophageal adenocarcinoma arising from Barrett's metaplasia has regional variations in the West [letter]. *Gastroenterology* 2002;**122**:588–90.

40. Reid BJ, Sanchez CA, Blount PL, Levine DS. Barrett's esophagus: cell cycle abnormalities in advancing stages of neoplastic progression. *Gastroenterology* 1993;**105**: 119–29.

41. Gray MR, Hall PJ, Nash J *et al*. Epithelial proliferation of Barrett's esophagus by proliferating cell nuclear antigen immunolocalization. *Gastroenterology* 1992;**103**:1769–76.

42. McArdle JE, Lewin KJ, Randall G, Weinstein W. Distribution of dysplasias and early invasive carcinoma in Barrett's esophagus. *Human Pathol* 1992;**23**: 479–82.

43. Reid BJ, Barrett MT, Galipeau PC *et al*. Barrett's esophagus: ordering the events that lead to cancer. *Eur J Cancer Prev* 1996;**5**(suppl 2):57–65.

44. Klump B, Hsieh CJ, Holzmann K, Gregor M, Porschen R. Hypermethylation of the CDKN2/p16 promoter during neoplastic progression in Barrett's esophagus. *Gastroenterology* 1998;**115**:1381–6.

45. Reid BJ, Blount PL, Rubin CE *et al*. Flow-cytometric and histological progression to malignancy in Barrett's esophagus: prospective endoscopic surveillance of a cohort. *Gastroenterology* 1992;**102**:1212–9.

46. Rabinovitch PS, Reid BJ, Haggitt RC, Norwood TH, Rubin CE. Progression to cancer in Barrett's esophagus is associated with genomic instability. *Lab Invest* 1988;**60**:65–71.

47. Shirvani VN, Ouatu-Lascar R, Kaur BS, Omary MB, Triadafilopoulos G. Cyclooxygenase 2 expression in Barrett's esophagus and adenocarcinoma: *ex vivo* induction by bile salts and acid exposure. *Gastroenterology* 2000;**118**:487–96.

48. Morris CD, Armstrong GR, Bigley G, Green H, Attwood SE. Cyclooxygenase expression in the Barrett's metaplasia–dysplasia–adenocarcinoma sequence. *Am J Gastroenterol* 2001;**96**:990–6.

49. Reid BJ, Blount PL, Feng Z, Levine DS. Optimizing endoscopic biopsy detection of early cancers in Barrett's high-grade dysplasia. *Am J Gastroenterol* 2000;**95**: 3089–96.

50. Fitzgerald RC, Saeed IT, Khoo D, Farthing MJ, Burnham WR. Rigorous surveillance protocol increases detection of curable cancers associated with Barrett's esophagus. *Dig Dis Sci* 2001;**46**:1892–8.

51. Levine DS, Reid BJ. Endoscopic biopsy technique for acquiring larger mucosal samples. *Gastrointest Endosc* 1991;**37**:332–7.

52. Levine DS, Blount PL, Rudolph RE, Reid BJ. Safety of a systematic endoscopic biopsy protocol in patients with Barrett's esophagus. *Am J Gastroenterol* 2000; **95**:1152–7.

53. Cameron AJ, Carpenter HA. Barrett's esophagus, high-grade dysplasia and early adenocarcinoma. *Am J Gastroenterol* 1997;**92**:586–91.

54. Levine DS, Haggitt RC, Blount PL *et al*. An endoscopic biopsy protocol can differentiate high-grade dysplasia from early adenocarcinoma in Barrett's esophagus. *Gastroenterology* 1993;**105**:40–50.

55. Falk GW, Rice TW, Goldblum JR, Richter JE. Jumbo biopsy forceps protocol still misses unsuspected cancer in Barrett's esophagus with high-grade dysplasia. *Gastrointestinal Endosc* 1999;**49**:170–6.

56. Falk GW, Ours TM, Richter JE. Practice patterns for surveillance of Barrett's esophagus in the United States. *Gastrointest Endosc* 2000;**52**:197–203.

57. Montgomery E, Bronner MP, Goldblum JR *et al*. Reproducibility of the diagnosis of dysplasia in Barrett's esophagus: a reaffirmation. *Hum Pathol* 2001;**32**: 368–78.

58. Sharma P. Low-grade dysplasia in Barrett's esophagus. *Gastroenterology* 2004;**127**:1233–8.

59. Pellegrini CA, Pohl D. High-grade dysplasia in Barrett's esophagus: surveillance or operation? *J Gastrointest Surg* 2000;**4**:131–4.

60. Shaheen NJ, Inadomi JM, Overholt BF, Sharma P. What is the best management strategy for high grade dysplasia in Barrett's esophagus? A cost effectiveness analysis. *Gut* 2004;**53**:1736–44.

61. Alikhan M, Rex D, Khan A *et al*. Variable pathologic interpretation of columnar lined esophagus by general pathologists in community practice. *Gastrointest Endosc* 1999;**50**:23–6.

62. Ormsby AH, Petras RE, Hendricks WH *et al*. Observer variation in the diagnosis of superficial oesophageal adenocarcinoma. *Gut* 2002;**51**:671–6.

63. Gross CP, Canto MI, Hixson J, Powe NR. Management of Barrett's esophagus: a national study of practice patterns and their cost implications. *Am J Gastroenterol* 1999;**94**:3440–7.

64. Moss A, Clarke E, Crowe J, Lennon J, Mathuna PM. Management of Barrett's oesophagus in 2001 in Ireland. *Ir J Med Sci* 2003;**172**:174–6.

65. Sharma P, McQuaid K, Dent, J *et al*. A critical review of the diagnosis and management of Barrett's esophagus: the AGA Chicago workshop. *Gastroenterology* 2004; **127**:310–30.

66. Falk GW. Cytology in Barrett's esophagus. *Gastrointest Endosc Clin N Am* 2003;**13**:335–8.

67. Falk GW, Skacel M, Gramlich TL *et al.* Fluorescence *in situ* hybridization of cytologic specimens from Barrett's esophagus: a pilot feasibility study. *Gastrointest Endosc* 2004;**60**:280–4.

68. Doak SH, Jenkins GJ, Parry EM *et al.* Chromosome 4 hyperploidy represents an early genetic aberration in premalignant Barrett's oesophagus. *Gut* 2003;**52**: 623–8.

69. Alexander JA, Jones SM, Smith CJ *et al.* Usefulness of cytopathology and histology in the evaluation of Barrett's esophagus in a community hospital. *Gastrointest Endosc* 1997;**46**:318–20.

70. Canto MI, Setrakian S, Petras RE *et al.* Methylene blue selectively stains intestinal metaplasia in Barrett's esophagus. *Gastrointest Endosc* 1996;**44**:1–7.

71. Canto MI, Setrakian S, Willis J *et al.* Methylene-blue directed biopsies improve detection of intestinal metaplasia and dysplasia in Barrett's esophagus. *Gastrointest Endosc* 2000;**51**:560–8.

72. Egger K, Werner M, Meining A *et al.* Biopsy surveillance is still necessary in patients with Barrett's oesophagus despite new imaging techniques. *Gut* 2003; **52**:18–23.

73. Oliver JR, Wild CP, Sahay P, Dexter S, Hardie LJ. Chromoendoscopy with methylene blue and associated DNA damage in Barrett's oesophagus. *Lancet* 2003; **362**:373–4.

74. Panjehpour M, Overholt BF, Vo-Dinh T *et al.* Endoscopic fluorescence detection of high-grade dysplasia in Barrett's esophagus. *Gastroenterology* 1996;**111**:93–101.

75. Georgakoudi I, Jacobson BC, Van Dam J *et al.* Fluorescence, reflectance, and light-scattering spectroscopy for evaluating dysplasia in patients with Barrett's esophagus. *Gastroenterology* 2001;**120**:1620–9.

76. Haringsma J, Prawirodirdjo W, Tytgat GN. Accuracy of fluorescence imaging of dysplasia in Barrett's esophagus. *Gastroenterology* 1999;**116**:A418.

77. Wang T, Triadafilopoulos G. S, M, L, XL methods of surveillance for Barrett's oesophagus. *Gut* 2003;**52**: 5–6.

78. Wang TD, Van Dam J. Optical biopsy: a new frontier in endoscopic detection and diagnosis. *Clin Gastroenterol Hepatol* 2004;**2**:744–53.

79. Rudolph RE, Vaughan TL, Storer BE *et al.* Effect of segment length on risk for neoplastic progression in patients with Barrett's esophagus. *Ann Intern Med* 2000;**132**:612–20.

80. Weston AP, Badr AS, Hassanein RS. Prospective multivariate analysis of clinical, endoscopic, and histological factors predictive of the development of Barrett's multifocal high-grade dysplasia or adenocarcinoma. *Am J Gastroenterol* 1999;**94**:3413–9.

81. Menke-Pluymers MB, Hop WC, Dees J, van Blankenstein M, Tilanus HW. Risk factors for the development of an adenocarcinoma in the columnar-lined esophagus. *Cancer* 1993;**72**:1155–8.

82. Weston AP, Sharma P, Mathur S *et al.* Risk stratification of Barrett's esophagus: updated prospective multivariate analysis. *Am J Gastroenterol* 2004;**99**:1657–66.

83. Avidan B, Sonnenberg A, Schnell TG *et al.* Hiatal hernia size, Barrett's length, and severity of acid reflux are all risk factors for esophageal adenocarcinoma. *Am J Gastroenterol* 2002;**97**:1930–6.

84. Gopal D, Lieberman DA, Margaret N *et al.* Risk factors for dysplasia in patients with Barrett's esophagus (BE). Results from a multicenter consortium. *Dig Dis Sci* 2003;**48**:1537–41.

85. Lagergren, J, Bergstrom R, Adami HO, Nyren O. Association between medication that relax the lower esophageal sphincter and risk for esophageal adenocarcinoma. *Ann Intern Med* 2000;**133**:165–75.

86. Engel LS, Chow WH, Vaughan TL *et al.* Population attributable risks of esophageal and gastric cardia cancers. *J Natl Cancer Inst* 2003;**95**:1404–13.

87. Montgomery E, Goldblum JR, Greenson JK *et al.* Dysplasia as a predictive marker for invasive carcinoma in Barrett esophagus: a follow-up study based on 138 cases from a diagnostic variability study. *Hum Pathol* 2001;**32**:379–88.

88. Skacel M, Petras RE, Gramlich TL *et al.* The diagnosis of low-grade dysplasia in Barrett's esophagus and its implications for disease progression. *Am J Gastroenterol* 2000;**95**:3383–7.

89. Weston AP, Banerjee SK, Sharma P *et al.* p53 protein overexpression in low grade dysplasia (LGD) in Barrett's esophagus: immunohistochemical marker predictive of progression. *Am J Gastroenterol* 2001;**96**: 1355–62.

90. Skacel M, Petras RE, Rybicki LA *et al.* p53 expression in low grade dysplasia in Barrett's esophagus: correlation with interobserver agreement and disease progression. *Am J Gastroenterol* 2002;**97**:2508–13.

91. Buttar NS, Wang KK, Sebo TJ *et al.* Extent of high-grade dysplasia in Barrett's esophagus correlates with risk of adenocarcinoma. *Gastroenterology* 2001;**120**: 1630–9.

92. Reid BJ, Levine DS, Longton G, Blount PL, Rabinovitch PS. Predictors of progression to cancer in Barrett's esophagus: baseline histology and flow cytometry identify low- and high-risk patient subsets. *Am J Gastroenterol* 2000;**95**:1669–76.

93. Schnell TG, Sontag SJ, Chejfec G *et al.* Long-term nonsurgical management of Barrett's esophagus with high-grade dysplasia. *Gastroenterology* 2001;**120**: 1607–19.

94. Weston AP, Sharma P, Topalovski M *et al.* Long-term follow-up of Barrett's high-grade dysplasia. *Am J Gastroenterol* 2000;**95**:1888–93.

95. Dar M, Goldblum JR, Rice TW, Falk GW. Can extent of high-grade dysplasia predict the presence of adenocarcinoma at esophagectomy? *Gut* 2003;**52**:486–9.

96. Reid BJ. *p53* and neoplastic progression in Barrett's esophagus [editorial]. *Am J Gastroenterol* 2001;**96**: 1321–3.

97. Reid BJ, Prevo LJ, Galipeau PC *et al.* Predictors of progression in Barrett's esophagus II: baseline 17p (*p53*) loss of heterozygosity identifies a patient subset at increased risk for neoplastic progression. *Am J Gastroenterol* 2001;**96**:2839–48.

98. Wong DJ, Paulson TG, Prevo LJ *et al.* $p16^{INK4a}$ lesions are common, early abnormalities that undergo clonal expansion in Barrett's metaplastic epithelium. *Cancer Res* 2001;**61**:8284–9.

CHAPTER 13

The Cost-Effectiveness of Screening and Surveillance to Decrease Mortality from Esophageal Adenocarcinoma

John M. Inadomi and Joel H. Rubenstein

Introduction

Medical decision analysis relies on a set of mathematical tools based on probability theory to quantitatively compare the expected outcomes of two or more competing medical management strategies. Cost-effectiveness analysis (CEA) includes costs in the comparisons of competing strategies to identify the optimal medical strategy in an environment with limited economic resources. Previous guidelines for the conduct and interpretation of economic analyses in medicine have been published [1–3]. This chapter examines the cost-effectiveness of screening and surveillance for Barrett's esophagus to decrease mortality from esophageal adenocarcinoma using evidence-based medicine principles. We will first present the results of our systematic review of the literature to identify studies of the economic impact of screening and/or surveillance to decrease mortality from esophageal adenocarcinoma. We will then introduce the criteria by which economic analysis of health care interventions should be conducted. Finally, we will critically examine the retrieved studies to determine whether consensus is achieved regarding the implementation of screening and surveillance strategies, and identify key areas to which the models are sensitive in order to provide potential hypotheses to guide future clinical research.

This chapter will follow the format recommended by the Panel on Cost-Effectiveness in Health and Medicine [1,2,4]. We will examine retrieved studies to determine whether the methods are valid, discuss the results, and determine whether the results will help in caring for patients.

Systematic Review of the Literature

We performed a systematic review of the literature to identify articles that examined the economic impact of screening or surveillance to decrease mortality from esophageal adenocarcinoma. Search terms included: (Barrett esophagus OR Barrett oesophagus OR adenocarcinoma) AND (economic analysis OR cost-effectiveness OR decision support techniques). Databases searched included Medline and Embase; studies were limited to full publications (abstracts excluded) in the English language that included a calculation of the cost-effectiveness of screening or surveillance to decrease cancer mortality, and excluded reviews without new data. Two reviewers independently confirmed the inclusion of articles for inclusion and data abstraction; discrepancy was resolved through consensus. Methods for constructing formal meta-analysis of economic studies have not been devised, thus thorough discussion to compare and contrast results are provided.

Results of Systematic Review

Computerized literature searches yielded 14 original cost-effectiveness studies of strategies to decrease mortality from esophageal adenocarcinoma (Table 13.1). Three examined screening and surveillance among patients with symptoms of gastroesophageal reflux disease (GERD) [5–7], one examined screen-

Table 13.1 Studies included in systematic review.

Author	Journal	Year	Population
Screening with surveillance			
Nietert et al. [5]	*Gastrointest Endosc*	2003	GERD
Inadomi et al. [6]	*Ann Intern Med*	2003	GERD
Gerson et al. [7]	*Clin Gastroenterol Hepatol*	2004	GERD
Screening alone			
Soni et al. [8]	*Am J Gastroenterol*	2000	GERD
Surveillance alone			
Provenzale et al. [9]	*Am J Gastroenterol*	1994	BE
Sonnenberg & El-Serag [10]	*Gastrointest Endosc Clin N Am*	1997	BE
Streitz et al. [11]	*Am J Gastroenterol*	1998	BE
Provenzale et al. [12]	*Am J Gastroenterol*	1999	BE
Sonnenberg et al. [13]	*Aliment Pharmacol Therapeut*	2002	BE
PDT for dysplasia			
Hur et al. [14]	*Dig Dis Sci*	2003	BE with HGD
Vij et al. [15]	*Gastrointest Endosc*	2004	BE with HGD
Shaheen et al. [16]	*Gut*	2004	BE with HGD
Chemoprevention			
Sonnenberg & Fennerty [17]	*Gastroenterology*	2003	BE
Hur et al. [18]	*J Nat Canc Inst*	2004	BE

BE, Barret's esophagus; GERD, gastroesophageal reflux disease symptoms; HGD, high-grade dysplasia; PDT, photodynamic therapy.

ing of this population without surveillance [8], and five focused on surveillance among patients already diagnosed with Barrett's esophagus [9–13]. Recall that screening is the use of a test in order to identify a group of patients who possess an elevated risk of disease, while surveillance is the repeated application of tests or interventions in an already identified high-risk group. Three other studies evaluated management of patients with Barrett's esophagus and high-grade dysplasia (HGD) [14–16], and two compared cancer chemoprevention using aspirin or other non-steroidal anti-inflammatory drugs (NSAIDs) with traditional surveillance methods [17,18].

Of the three analyses that examined screening patients with reflux symptoms to identify patients at high-risk for progression to esophageal adenocarcinoma (EAC), one focused on the potential for reduced cost using unsedated ultrathin endoscopy as a screening tool [5]. This study found that while standard sedated endoscopy would likely result in the greatest number of life-years saved, unsedated ultrathin endoscopy could save almost as many lives at a much reduced cost.

Two other analyses estimated the relative yield of screening for prevalent cancers compared to surveillance for incident cancers. Those analyses examined screening patients with reflux symptoms using different surveillance strategies (Table 13.2). Although one study found that continued surveillance of patients with Barrett's esophagus in the absence of dysplasia required resources beyond those customarily appropriated for health care interventions [6], the other reported that surveillance for all Barrett's esophagus patients was cost-effective [7]. Additionally, while the former found that heightened surveillance among Barrett's esophagus patients with HGD was most cost-effective, the latter advocated the use

Table 13.2 Screening with surveillance.

Author	Nietert *et al.* [5]	Inadomi *et al.* [6]	Gerson and Groeneveld [7]
Lowest cost	No screening	No screening	No screening
Cost	$11 785	$104	$655
Benefit	19.327 dQALYs	16.47 dQALYs	18.16 life years
Lowest ICER	Ultrathin endoscopy screening	Screen; surveillance for BE with dysplasia	N/A
Cost	$12 119	$1748	N/A
Benefit	19.333 dQALYs	16.624 dQALYs	N/A
Most effective	Standard EGD screening; BE surveillance every 2 years; surgery for HGD or cancer	Screen; BE surveillance every 2 years; surgery for cancer	Screen; BE surveillance every 3 years; surgery for HGD and cancer
Cost	$12 332	$2 587	$1 920
Benefit	19.333 dQALYs	16.626 dQALYs	18.27 life-years
ICER	$709 260	$414 233	$12 140

BE, Barrett's esophagus; dQALYs, discounted quality-adjusted life-years; EGD, esophagogastroduodenoscopy; HGD, high-grade dysplasia; ICER, incremental cost-effectiveness ratio, compared to next least expensive intervention; N/A, not applicable.

of prophylactic esophagectomy for patients with HGD in Barrett's esophagus. The divergent results between these two studies will be examined in the following section (Evidence-Based Criteria to Assess Validity of an Economic Analysis).

One analysis restricted its focus to screening patients with GERD symptoms to detect Barrett's esophagus with dysplasia or cancer [8]. This study illustrated that prevalence rates may allow the initial screening endoscopy to be a cost-effective intervention (i.e. <$100 000 per life-year gained). It was noted, however, that relatively small changes in assumptions regarding the prevalence of Barrett's esophagus and EAC, the rate of cancer development among Barrett's esophagus patients, and the impact of esophagectomy on health-related quality of life caused the incremental cost-effectiveness ratio (ICER) to rise above the threshold usually allotted for health care interventions.

Among the five studies that focused on surveillance among patients already diagnosed with Bar-

rett's esophagus, it appeared that performing surveillance at almost any interval was cost-effective, if compared to no surveillance. However, surveillance intervals of 1–2 years required substantial increases in resource allocation with little benefit compared to longer intervals (Table 13.3). Note that one study did not use techniques standard to most economic analyses, thus the costs and outcomes reported vary widely from other estimates [11]. The ICER between longer and shorter intervals could be as great as $276 000 per quality-adjusted life-year (QALY) saved, exceeding the standard $50 000–100 000 per QALY benchmark commonly used in economic analysis. Revised national guidelines published subsequent to release of these data reflect recommendations to lengthen the surveillance interval [19]. As could be expected, sensitivity analysis noted several variables to which the models were sensitive, including the *incidence of cancer* among patients with Barrett's esophagus, the *efficacy of surveillance* to decrease cancer mortality, and the *utility of the*

Table 13.3 Screening or surveillance alone.

Strategy	Lowest cost	Cost ($)	Benefit (dQALYs)	Most effective	Cost ($)	Benefit	ICER	ICER comparator
Screening alone								
Soni et al. 2000 [8]	No screening	258	15.30	Screen; surgery for HGD and cancer	1 036	15.33 dQALYs	$24 718/dQALY gained	No screening
Surveillance alone								
Provenzale et al. 1994 [9]	No surveillance	5 750	11.81	Surveillance every 4 years	N/S	N/S	$276 700/dQALY gained	Surveillance every 5 years
Sonnenberg & El-Serag 1997 [10]	No surveillance	N/S	N/S	Surveillance every year	N/S	N/S	$59 514/life-year gained	No surveillance
Streitz et al. 1998 [11]	No surveillance	N/S	N/S	Surveillance (variable interval)	59 529	8.96 life-years gained	$4 151/life-year gained	No surveillance
Provenzale et al. 1999 [12]	No surveillance	4 100	12.64	Surveillance every 5 years	13 900	12.74 dQALYs	$98 000/dQALY gained	No surveillance
Sonnenberg et al. 2002 [13]	No surveillance	2 061	N/S	Surveillance every 2 years	6 262	N/S	$16 965/dQALY gained	No surveillance

dQALYs, discounted quality-adjusted life-years; HGD, high-grade dysplasia; ICER, incremental cost-effectiveness ratio; N/S, not stated.

postesophagectomy state. These three topics are thus identified as critical areas in which to perform research to more fully define the economic impact of surveillance to decrease mortality from EAC.

Utilities reduce the value of certain states of disease in order to reflect patient preferences. Since it may be assumed that a year living in health is valued more highly than an equal amount of time living with cancer, or in the case of Barrett's esophagus with the morbidity of having undergone an esophagectomy for cancer or HGD, utilities allows weighting of various states of health to be incorporated in an economic analysis. In most studies perfect health is valued as 1.0 while death is 0. It is standard to include utilities in CEA in order to allow comparison of interventions across diseases [1–3].

Three studies examined endoscopic therapy for patients with Barrett's esophagus and HGD (Table 13.4). All compared photodynamic therapy (PDT) to esophagectomy or continued surveillance. While there was discrepancy among the studies with regards to the least expensive strategy, there was consensus that the most effective strategy was to employ ablative therapy. Compared to the least expensive strategy, PDT provided an ICER of $12 400–47 410 per QALY gained. Although the models were sensitive to assumptions of effectiveness of PDT to decrease the risk of cancer, and the relative utilities associated with Barrett's esophagus and after esophagectomy, the conclusions regarding the economic viability of PDT remained despite extensive sensitivity analysis. Non-surgical interventions that decreased the incidence of cancer were more likely to be cost-effective than strategies to detect early cancer development. In short, it is cheaper to prevent cancer than to treat cancer after it develops.

Similarly, the two studies that examined chemoprevention of cancer among patients with Barrett's esophagus found that aspirin and/or non-aspirin NSAIDs need only to be marginally effective in reducing cancer incidence in order to achieve superior cost-effectiveness compared to current surveillance strategies (see Table 13.4). In one study, aspirin use was found to be both less expensive and more beneficial than providing no intervention, and surveillance with or without aspirin was prohibitively expensive in comparison to aspirin alone

(>$200 000 per QALY gained) [18]. The other study reported that no intervention was still cheapest, but NSAIDS increased life-years at low cost [17]. In that analysis, combining surveillance with NSAIDs improved outcomes and cost less than $30 000 per QALY gained. As with PDT, the strategy that decreased cancer incidence was superior to strategies that relied entirely on detection and treatment of early cancers.

Evidence-Based Criteria to Assess Validity of an Economic Analysis

Criteria governing the conduct and critique of economic analysis in health care management have been previously published [1–4]. In this section we will review these criteria to assist the reader in interpretation of CEA, and to understand the reasons why the results of seemingly similar studies vary so greatly. As an example, we will highlight the differences between studies that examined screening patients with reflux symptoms to identify patients with Barrett's esophagus and/or surveillance of patients with Barrett's esophagus for the purposes of detecting dysplasia or cancer. The structure of this section is to first examine the methods of analysis, interpret the results, and finally determine whether the conclusions may be applied to one's own population.

Are the Methods Sound?
Did the Analysis Provide a Full Economic Comparison of Health Care Strategies?
The answer to this question requires identifying the perspective of the analysis and determining whether all relevant strategies were compared.

What Was the Perspective of the Analysis?
Construction of a CEA requires establishment of the perspective of the analysis, or the viewpoint from which costs and effects are observed. A societal perspective is preferred in which direct health care costs, direct non-health care costs and indirect costs are included [1–3]. Determination of direct non-health care costs, such as the cost of transportation to and from office visits, or indirect costs, such as the cost of lost time from work, are difficult to define. For this

Table 13.4 Therapeutic interventions.

	Lowest cost	Cost ($)	Benefit (dQALYs)	Most effective	Cost ($)	Benefit (dQALYs)	ICER ($)
PDT for dysplasia							
Hur et al. [14]	Surveillance*	27 800	9.96	PDT with surgery for cancer and residual HGD	48 200	11.61	12 400
Vij et al. [15]	Esophagectomy*	24 045	11.82	PDT with surveillance for residual HGD; surgery for cancer	47 300	12.31	47 410
Shaheen et al. [16]	No intervention	748	13.90	PDT with surveillance for residual HGD; surgery for cancer	41 998	15.51	25 621
Chemoprevention							
Sonnenberg & Fennerty [17]	No intervention	N/S	N/S	NSAID with surveillance very 2 years (annually for HGD); surgery for cancer	N/S	N/S	27 000
Hur et al. [18]	Aspirin	4 200	13.11	Aspirin with surveillance every 3 years; surgery for HGD or cancer	20 500	13.19	203 800

dQALYs, discounted quality-adjusted life-years; HGD, high-grade dysplasia; ICER, incremental cost-effectiveness ratio; PDT, photodynamic therapy.
* A strategy without intervention was not considered.

reason, other perspectives may be utilized that involve a subset of the societal perspective. These include a third-party payer (insurer), hospital or clinic, or the patient perspective. Depending on the perspective applied, costs will include different components. All studies included in our systematic review used a third-party payer perspective.

For a CEA, the outcomes of interest include costs and effects, such as life-years saved, or number of cancer cases prevented. Cost–utility analysis, a subtype of CEA, accounts for patient preferences for differing health states so that time spent in less desirable states such as cancer or chemotherapy is valued less than time spent in perfect health. Cost–utility analysis is particularly useful when alternative treatments produce outcomes of different types, or if increased survival is associated with a reduction in the quality of life. The outcome of a cost–utility analysis is a ratio of costs to QALYs. Note that it is preferable to base a CEA on an outcome common to other diseases, such as QALYs, in order to provide global comparison of resources required to achieve health outcomes.

Of the two CEAs examining the relative contributions of screening and surveillance, there exist differences in preferred strategies, especially with regards to the use of prophylactic esophagectomy among patients with HGD. One study incorporated patient preferences for health states, or utilities, to address the potential negative impact of therapeutic interventions in patients who are otherwise asymptomatic [6]. Performance of esophagectomy for patients who do not yet have a diagnosis of cancer, and who may never have developed cancer, was of particular concern, so data from previous studies examining patient preferences were utilized to estimate the decrement in the quality of one's life due to performance of esophagectomy. The other study did not incorporate utilities, and this in part explains their differing conclusions [7]. It is difficult to compare the results of the latter study with other CEAs, since this was only one of two studies included in our systematic review that did not incorporate patient preferences [7,11].

Were All Relevant Strategies Compared?
All reasonable clinical management strategies should be considered in a CEA. Authors generally provide a figure summarizing their proposed model in order that readers may critique the structure. This may be in the form of a decision tree, or perhaps a Markov model. Decision trees are designed to model the temporal flow from one initial decision point to multiple subsequent chance points in a tree-like fashion. Markov models, in contrast, are recursive, in that they allow for movement of hypothetical patients back and forth between a set of recurrent health states. Because of this feature, Markov models take into account the effect of time spent in each health state more easily than simple trees.

The majority of studies retrieved in our systematic review modeled management based on published guidelines for screening and surveillance [19]. Several studies included alternative strategies not included in guidelines, such as the use of PDT, chemoprevention or other novel interventions [7,14–18]. It is unlikely that the base-case scenarios were significantly affected by these additions, and differences in conclusions were likely the result of other parameter and structural assumptions made by the investigators.

Were Costs and Outcomes Properly Measured?
Was Clinical Effectiveness Established?
The clinical effectiveness of competing strategies of management must be established prior to comparing the cost-effectiveness of these strategies. Assumptions of efficacy may be based on the results of individual trials, a range of values from several trials, or meta-analyses of published studies. Published results from randomized clinical trials is considered the best evidence for answering questions of *efficacy* of therapy, although economic studies may be more valid if *effectiveness* data that reflect normal clinical practice are available.

The efficacy of screening and surveillance strategies has been discussed thoroughly in previous chapters and will not be further examined. The studies included in the systematic review utilized extensive literature searches upon which the values for each of the variables within the models were derived. Within the limitations of published data, the studies used appropriate values for their parameter estimates.

Were Costs Measured Accurately?

The components of cost used in the model as well as the numerical value assigned to each component should be stated and referenced. Depending on the perspective of the analysis, different direct and indirect cost components should be included. Direct costs are composed of direct health care costs and direct non-health care costs. Direct health care costs include the costs to provide medical care including tests, drugs, supplies, health care personnel, and medical facilities. Direct non-health care costs include additional costs incurred by patients as a result of health care encounters, such as child- or eldercare costs, transportation costs, and other time costs resulting from clinic visits or procedures. Indirect, or productivity costs are those associated with lost or impaired ability to work or engage in leisure activities due to morbidity, and lost economic productivity due to death.

Importantly, there is a difference between costs and charges. Costs represent the resources foregone by society to provide medical services, while charges may deviate from this value depending on the accuracy of accounting systems, relative bargaining power of payers and providers, and inclusion of profit margins.

The majority of studies in our systematic review used costs based on reimbursements by Medicare to health care providers and facilities, thus representing the actual costs incurred by the Center for Medicare and Medicaid Services (CMS) for care of patients. This is an acceptable cost subgroup to consider, especially since the value of direct non-health care and indirect (productivity) costs have not been determined for GERD or Barrett's esophagus patients.

Were Costs and Outcomes Data Appropriately Integrated?

The costs and outcomes (such as life-years or QALYs) associated with each of the modeled strategies in a CEA should be reported; however, it is more important to compare the ICER between strategies. The ICER describes the additional cost incurred by providing an alternative strategy in order to achieve increased effectiveness. Similarly, identification of dominant strategies, or those strategies associated

with both greater effectiveness and lower costs, is warranted.

CEAs commonly employ discounting and time preference for outcomes. Discounting reflects people's preference for having money and material goods in the present rather than in the future. This concept accounts for the opportunity cost incurred by spending money now in order to derive benefit at some later time, and is generally based on the marginal return that would otherwise be gained had the money to implement an intervention been instead invested. In a similar manner, health benefits must also be adjusted to reflect time preferences of patients; if not, delaying implementation of an intervention would always appear more cost-effective. For example, patients with a given symptomatic disorder will generally prefer to obtain a year of health without this disorder immediately as opposed to delaying this benefit to a later time. This is because the benefit may otherwise never be realized (due to death from alternative cause) or may be associated with additional comorbid conditions that counteract improved quality of life achieved from the disorder in question.

The studies under review reported ICERs between competing strategies, in addition to incorporating time preferences through the use of discounting.

Was Appropriate Allowance Made for Uncertainties in the Analysis?

In the opinion of the authors, this is the most important question to answer when critiquing a decision analytic study. Appropriate testing of the assumptions of the model may cause the conclusions of the analysis to change. Uncertainty may be present in the parameter estimates (numerical values of variables) as well as structural assumptions (how the model was constructed). The conventional manner in which to examine uncertainty is through a sensitivity analysis. Parameter estimates may be tested to determine whether variation of variable values within reasonable clinical bounds will significantly alter the results; if so, the model is said to be sensitive to these variables. The model structural assumptions may be tested by changing the relationship between various parts of the model and determining whether these changes result in different conclusions.

Uncertainty may be evaluated through one-way sensitivity analyses, which examine changes in outcome following variation of a single variable at a time. In two- and three-way analyses, two or three variables are varied simultaneously to assess their joint influence on the outcome of the model. Multiple (*n*-way) sensitivity analysis is performed through specialized modeling techniques such as Monte Carlo simulations, in which multiple variables in the model are varied simultaneously. In this type of analysis, variables are represented by probability distributions around an expected value. The model is run multiple times; however, instead of using fixed values for variables, the computer randomly selects a new set of input values from the probability distributions. The outcome of such an analysis will be in the form of an expected value with a statistical distribution defining its boundaries, for example, a mean value and standard deviation.

It is difficult to assess the structural assumptions of models because only an outline of the model is presented in the manuscript. Without the actual model available for scrutiny, many of the structural assumptions of decision analytic models remain hidden to even astute reviewers. It is possible to indirectly assess differences in structural assumptions between models by using a common set of values for each of the variables contained in the models. It may be assumed that any residual variance between model results arises from differences in structural assumptions.

Are Estimates of Costs and Outcomes Related to the Baseline Risk in the Treatment Population?

It is important to note the population modeled in a CEA. The generalizability of an analysis depend heavily on whether the hypothetical subjects examined in the model are representative of the population as a whole, or represent a subpopulation at high- or low-risk for the outcomes evaluated. All studies of screening in the systematic review examined a subpopulation of the USA consisting of people with long-standing symptoms of GERD [5–7]. Studies of surveillance focused on the subgroup of patients already diagnosed with Barrett's esophagus [9–13], as did studies examining the potential use of chemo-

prevention to decrease the incidence of CEA [17,18]. Studies involving endoscopic therapy selected an even more restrictive population to model, thus PDT was examined only among patients with Barrett's esophagus and HGD [14–16], or for non-surgical candidates with EAC [7].

What Are the Results?

Only if the methods by which a study is conducted are sound is it appropriate to examine the results. There are several criteria governing the presentation of the results of health economic studies.

What Were the Incremental Costs and Outcomes of Each Strategy?

The main outcomes of a CEA compare the costs and health outcomes of competing strategies. Once stated, the next step is to identify dominated strategies (strategies costing more despite providing less benefit than other strategies), and calculate the ICER between non-dominated strategies. A table containing the average cost per patient, remaining life expectancy or QALYs, ICER (cost per life-year or QALY gained), and reduction in the cancer incidence and cancer-associated mortality associated with each strategy should be presented.

The results of a CEA may also be graphically presented, with the effect or benefit on the abscissa and the cost on the ordinate. The results of each strategy are plotted, starting with the least expensive strategy and progressing through increasingly more expensive ones. Dominated strategies, or those that cost more despite achieving less benefit, are eliminated, and lines connecting non-dominated strategies are drawn. The slope of the line represents the ICER between strategies, which is defined as the difference in costs divided by the difference in effectiveness between two strategies.

It should be noted that among the published studies there were deviations from accepted practice with regards to reporting of strategies dominated either by simple or extended dominance. Thus, conclusions presented by authors regarding optimal strategies of management were not supported by data presented within the manuscripts. Future publications of CEA should adhere to published criteria when reporting results of economic analysis.

Do Incremental Costs and Outcomes Differ Between Subgroups?

Barrett's esophagus provides an opportunity to discuss identification of subgroups within an examined population to determine whether differing costs and health outcomes may be expected. Patients with Barrett's esophagus and HGD may be used as an example of a subgroup in which interventions not otherwise cost-effective in a general population might prove to be economically reasonable. Multiple studies identified patients with dysplasia to possess higher rates of cancer development that allowed continued surveillance to become cost-effective [9–13]; in addition, one study revealed that patients with Barrett's esophagus in the absence of dysplasia were an expensive group in which to intervene [6]. Another study provided a different conclusion, stating that continued surveillance in the entire Barrett's esophagus population was also cost-effective compared to limiting surveillance to patients with Barrett's esophagus and dysplasia alone [7]. Although heterogeneity between the studies in the parameter assumptions exists, it is the structural assumptions that likely form the basis for these differences.

One major structural difference was that the latter study did not incorporate patient utilities in the analysis [7]. As a result, the outcome of the study was limited to the difference in life-years between competing strategies. This study found that prophylactic esophagectomy for patients with Barrett's esophagus and HGD was a dominant strategy compared to continued surveillance. In the absence of utilities, the decision to perform esophagectomy is limited to weighing the risk of death from EAC with the mortality rate with esophagectomy. Other studies opposed this result, finding that incorporation of patient preferences for avoiding esophagectomy caused the equation to shift in favor of continued surveillance [6,11,17] or endoscopic therapy [14–16]. More importantly, these studies highlighted the importance of performing clinical research on this topic, since small variations in patient preferences causes large differences in the cost-effectiveness of screening and surveillance among Barrett's esophagus patients.

How Much Does Allowance for Uncertainty Change the Results?

A sensitivity analysis is performed to assess whether variations in baseline assumptions of the model significantly alter the results. As uncertainty exists in the estimates of the variables of all models, use of a range of clinically reasonable values obtained through literature searches or expert opinion will allow the reader to determine whether existing data are sufficient to answer the question posed.

Model structural assumptions may be addressed by varying the various interventions applied (i.e. prophylactic esophagectomy versus continued surveillance in Barrett's esophagus patients with HGD), or by varying the interaction between variables within the model (i.e. restricting cancer to arise from Barrett's esophagus with HGD, or allow its development from Barrett's esophagus with low-grade dysplasia or without dysplasia).

Although all studies included in the systematic review used some form of sensitivity analysis, it should be noted that no standard set of parameter estimates or structural assumptions were applied to each model. Thus, it remains unknown whether the differences in conclusions between models arises from variation in the values of the variables, or from variation in the interactions between variables modeled by the investigators.

Will the Results Help in Caring for My Patients?

All CEAs should address a clinical question that has the potential to improve the management of patients. A critical assessment of the risks, benefits and costs associated with implementation of tested strategies should be provided.

Are the Treatment Benefits Worth the Costs?

When comparing competing strategies in terms of their costs and benefits, three outcomes are possible. A strategy may be both less costly and associated with greater benefit than an alternative strategy, in which case it is said to be a dominant strategy. Conversely the strategy may itself be dominated by being both more costly and associated with less benefit than the alternative. Lastly one strategy may be

		Difference in Effectiveness	
		A > B	A ≤ B
Difference	A > B	ICER A vs B	B Dominant
in Costs	A ≤ B	A Dominant	ICER B vs A*

Fig. 13.1 Possible economic outcomes between competing strategies of management. ICER, incremental cost-effectiveness ratio. *If costs and effects are equal, strategies are equivalent.

more costly, but achieve greater benefit than the alternative; in this case the ICER may be calculated in order to determine whether the "bang is worth the buck." Figure 13.1 illustrates these possibilities graphically. The potential difference in costs between strategies is aligned in rows, while the difference in effectiveness is listed in columns. The lower left quadrant depicts the case where strategy A is less expensive (or the same cost) than strategy B, while achieving a larger effect. Assuming that the outcome is desirable, strategy A is dominant compared to strategy B. The upper right quadrant examines the converse where strategy A is both more expensive and associated with less (or equal) effect compared to strategy B; in this case strategy B dominates strategy A. The remaining two quadrants, upper left and lower right, depict examples where one strategy is associated with greater costs, but also greater benefit. In these cases, the ICER can be calculated, representing the additional resources required to improve outcome by using one strategy instead of another.

Although no true gold standard for acceptable ICERs exists, previous studies have presented the value of $50 000–100 000 per life-year saved as an amount society has shown a willingness to pay [3,20]. This standard, however, is based more on tradition than on science and represented the cost per life-year saved when performing hemodialysis in patients with renal failure. Estimates of the cost per life-year gained when screening for other malignancies are as low as $22 000 (breast cancer screening), and as high as $250 000 (cervical cancer screening) [21]. It is likely that the amount society is willing to pay to

achieve improved health outcomes depends on the available resources, the perceived impact of the specific disease in that society, and social issues not directly addressable through quantitative analysis. One of the insights gained through economic analysis is an estimation of the quantity of resources that will be foregone in order to implement health care programs. It is then a matter of prioritizing the allocation of resources to determine whether these programs should be embraced.

Could My Patients Expect Similar Health Outcomes?

Outcomes achieved in clinical trials may not be realized in clinical practice. One must consider the difference between the *efficacy* of an intervention in a clinical trial compared to the *effectiveness* of that intervention in a general practice setting. As clinical trials are usually performed in highly selected patient populations at specialized research institutions, it must be questioned whether patients in one's own healthcare population are similar enough to those in clinical trials to expect similar results. Additionally, the infrastructure to successfully implement the intervention must be demonstrated to function as effectively as that possessed in the clinical trial.

Could I Expect Similar Costs?

Depending on the perspective of the analysis, different categories of costs are included in a CEA. Even when limiting an economic analysis to direct health care costs, considerable differences may exist between costs reported in a study and one's own health system. This is because prices for resources may differ geographically, and more importantly, clinical practice variations may induce cost differences that do not translate from the study to one's own practice environment.

Problems With Screening and Surveillance in Barrett's Esophagus

Prevalence Versus Incidence

Current methods of screening are inadequate. Guidelines recommend screening patients with long-standing symptoms of GERD to detect Barrett's esophagus [19,22,23]. The use of GERD symptoms as the marker for the presence of Barrett's of esophagus is hindered by two facts. The first is that a substantial proportion of the population who develop adenocarcinoma of the esophagus do not reliably report a history of significant GERD symptoms. Lagergren *et al.* reported that 40% of patients with EAC did not state the presence of significant heartburn 5-years prior to the diagnosis of cancer [24]. Gerson *et al.* found 25% of the population of veterans who did not complain of heartburn had intestinal metaplasia confirmed on biopsy within the tubular esophagus [25]. It is evident that a substantial proportion of patients with Barrett's esophagus are not identified as screening candidates. Although heartburn is definitely a significant predictor for cancer occurrence, its absence does not rule out the possibility of cancer development.

The second is the fact that prevalent cancers outnumber incident cancers [26]. This means that by the time we diagnose Barrett's esophagus in a patient destined to develop cancer it is already present. It should be noted that most studies identifying this dilemma do not separate true screening cases from those detected due to the presence of symptoms, thus this may reflect the propensity of case-finding of esophageal cancer and overestimate the rate of cancer detection through "screening." However, the issue remains that current methods to identify patients at high-risk for cancer development are insufficient. Heartburn is a poor marker for the presence of Barrett's esophagus.

Lack of Reliable Markers of Progression to Cancer

Only a minority of patients with Barrett's esophagus develop EAC. The overall risk, previously overestimated, is approximately 0.5 % annually [27]. Currently dysplasia is the biomarker used to identify patients with Barrett's esophagus at highest risk for development of cancer [19,22,28–37]; however, the interobserver variability for interpreting dysplasia is high, and dysplasia itself appears to be a transient state [38–41]. Dysplasia is inconsistently diagnosed among patients with Barrett's esophagus undergoing surveillance examinations, which may be a result of sampling error, but may alternatively indicate

the evanescent nature of this biomarker. Moreover, studies examining the natural history of HGD note that the competing risk of mortality from other disease result in cancer mortality to be rare [26]. As a result, dysplasia is an inadequate marker for identifying patients with Barrett's esophagus at high-risk for development of cancer.

The majority of costs incurred in current strategies to decrease mortality from EAC are derived from the multiple surveillance examinations required among the population of Barrett's esophagus patients. Several analyses illustrate that the greatest benefit from any strategy occurs with the first screening endoscopy [6,8]. The yield and cost-effectiveness of surveillance would be greatly improved if a better marker to identify patients destined to develop EAC were developed, that could be used independently of the presence or absence of GERD symptoms, and could recognize the high-risk group more reliably than dysplasia. An ideal biomarker would be able to identify these patients prior to the development of cancer (thus shifting prevalent cancers to incident cancers), where interventions to decrease the risk of cancer could be implemented. A biomarker possessing these characteristics does not exist; however, promising results have been reported using *p16* [42,43], cyclin-D1 overexpression [44], 17p (*p53*) loss of heterozygosity [45,46], and aneuploidy or abnormal tetraploidy [47,48].

Inadequate Therapy

Current surveillance strategies in Barrett's esophagus focus on detection of early cancer that may be curable with surgical therapy. Compare this to colorectal cancer, for which polypectomy has been shown to decrease both the incidence of, and mortality from cancer [49]. The theoretical models identified in this systematic review illustrate the tenet that interventions that decrease the incidence of EAC, despite high cost and low efficacy, are more efficient than surveillance to detect EAC after it has developed [14–18]. In truth, the models using aspirin, non-aspirin NSAIDs, and PDT are interchangeable; all incorporate an intervention that is characterized by a certain cost, benefit, and side-effect profile. These models should not be cited to promulgate the widespread use of NSAIDs and PDT among all

Barrett's esophagus patients, but rather to point out that these strategies may be viable in comparison to surveillance using current technology. Truly, almost anything that has the potential to decrease the incidence of EAC is more cost-effective than our current practice of surveillance.

Conclusions

Although there is discussion regarding the current impact of EAC associated with Barrett's esophagus, there is little doubt that strategies to decrease mortality from EAC must be defined for use in the future, since the prevalence of Barrett's esophagus and EAC are predicted to increase. CEA is not designed to dictate how providers treat individual patients, but rather highlight the key elements of the management process that influence effectiveness for patients on average, and elements that must be considered from a societal perspective in order to appropriately allocate resources. To this end, economic analysis has revealed the following points: GERD symptoms are insensitive and non-specific for the presence of Barrett's esophagus; Barrett's esophagus is an inadequate marker for the development of EAC; interventions that reduce the incidence of cancer will be more cost-effective than strategies that rely on detection of cancer; and proposed treatment for Barrett's esophagus should not negatively affect patients' quality of life.

References

1. Siegel JE, Weinstein MC, Russell LB, Gold MR. Recommendations for reporting cost-effectiveness analyses. Panel on Cost-Effectiveness in Health and Medicine. *JAMA* 1996;**276**(16):1339–41.
2. Russell LB, Gold MR, Siegel JE, Daniels N, Weinstein MC. The role of cost-effectiveness analysis in health and medicine. Panel on Cost-Effectiveness in Health and Medicine. *JAMA* 1996;**276**(14):1172–7.
3. Gold MR, Siegel JE, Russell LB, Weinstein MC. *Cost-effectiveness in Health and Medicine*. New York: Oxford University Press, 1996.
4. Weinstein MC, Siegel JE, Gold MR, Kamlet MS, Russell LB. Recommendations of the Panel on Cost-Effectiveness in Health and Medicine. *JAMA* 1996;**276**(15):1253–8.
5. Nietert PJ, Silverstein MD, Mokhashi MS *et al*. Cost-effectiveness of screening a population with chronic gastroesophageal reflux. *Gastrointest Endosc* 2003;**57**(3):311–8.
6. Inadomi JM, Sampliner R, Lagergren J *et al*. Screening and surveillance for Barrett esophagus in high-risk groups: a cost–utility analysis. *Ann Intern Med* 2003;**138**(3):176–86.
7. Gerson LB, Groeneveld PW, Triadafilopoulos G. Cost-effectiveness model of endoscopic screening and surveillance in patients with gastroesophageal reflux disease. *Clin Gastroenterol Hepatol* 2004;**2**(10):868–79.
8. Soni A, Sampliner RE, Sonnenberg A. Screening for high-grade dysplasia in gastroesophageal reflux disease: is it cost-effective? *Am J Gastroenterol* 2000;**95**(8):2086–93.
9. Provenzale D, Kemp JA, Arora S, Wong JB. A guide for surveillance of patients with Barrett's esophagus. *Am J Gastroenterol* 1994;**89**(5):670–80.
10. Sonnenberg A, El-Serag HB. Economic aspects of endoscopic screening for intestinal precancerous conditions. *Gastrointest Endosc Clin N Am* 1997;**7**(1):165–84.
11. Streitz JM, Jr, Ellis FH, Jr, Tilden RL, Erickson RV. Endoscopic surveillance of Barrett's esophagus: a cost-effectiveness comparison with mammographic surveillance for breast cancer. *Am J Gastroenterol* 1998;**93**(6):911–5.
12. Provenzale D, Schmitt C, Wong JB. Barrett's esophagus: a new look at surveillance based on emerging estimates of cancer risk. *Am J Gastroenterol* 1999;**94**(8):2043–53.
13. Sonnenberg A, Soni A, Sampliner RE. Medical decision analysis of endoscopic surveillance of Barrett's oesophagus to prevent oesophageal adenocarcinoma. *Aliment Pharmacol Ther* 2002;**16**(1):41–50.
14. Hur C, Nishioka NS, Gazelle GS. Cost-effectiveness of photodynamic therapy for treatment of Barrett's esophagus with high grade dysplasia. *Dig Dis Sci* 2003;**48**(7):1273–83.
15. Vij R, Triadafilopoulos G, Owens DK, Kunz P, Sanders GD. Cost-effectiveness of photodynamic therapy for high-grade dysplasia in Barrett's esophagus. *Gastrointest Endosc* 2004;**60**(5):739–56.
16. Shaheen NJ, Inadomi JM, Overholt BF, Sharma P. What is the best management strategy for high grade dysplasia in Barrett's oesophagus? A cost effectiveness analysis. *Gut* 2004;**53**(12):1736–44.
17. Sonnenberg A, Fennerty MB. Medical decision analysis of chemoprevention against esophageal adenocarcinoma. *Gastroenterology* 2003;**124**(7):1758–66.

18. Hur C, Nishioka NS, Gazelle GS. Cost-effectiveness of aspirin chemoprevention for Barrett's esophagus. *J Natl Cancer Inst* 2004;**96**(4):316–25.

19. Sampliner RE. Updated guidelines for the diagnosis, surveillance, and therapy of Barrett's esophagus. *Am J Gastroenterol* 2002;**97**(8):1888–95.

20. Petitti DB. *Meta-Analysis, Decision Analysis and Cost-Effectiveness Analysis*. New York: Oxford University Press, 1994.

21. Weinstein MC, Siegel JE, Gold MR, Kamlet MS, Russell LB. Recommendations of the Panel on Cost-Effectiveness in Health and Medicine. *JAMA* 1996; **276**(15):1253–8.

22. Morales TG, Sampliner RE. Barrett's esophagus: update on screening, surveillance, and treatment. *Arch Intern Med* 1999;**159**(13):1411–6.

23. van Sandick JW, Bartelsman JF, van Lanschot JJ, Tytgat GN, Obertop H. Surveillance of Barrett's oesophagus: physicians' practices and review of current guidelines. *Eur J Gastroenterol Hepatol* 2000;**12**(1):111–7.

24. Lagergren J, Bergstrom R, Lindgren A, Nyren O. Symptomatic gastroesophageal reflux as a risk factor for esophageal adenocarcinoma. *N Engl J Med* 1999; **340**(11):825–31.

25. Gerson LB, Shetler K, Triadafilopoulos G. Prevalence of Barrett's esophagus in asymptomatic individuals. *Gastroenterology* 2002;**123**(2):461–7.

26. Schnell TG, Sontag SJ, Chejfec G *et al.* Long-term nonsurgical management of Barrett's esophagus with high-grade dysplasia. *Gastroenterology* 2001;**120**(7): 1607–19.

27. Shaheen NJ, Crosby MA, Bozymski EM, Sandler RS. Is there publication bias in the reporting of cancer risk in Barrett's esophagus? *Gastroenterology* 2000;**119**(2): 333–8.

28. O'Connor JB, Falk GW, Richter JE. The incidence of adenocarcinoma and dysplasia in Barrett's esophagus: report on the Cleveland Clinic Barrett's Esophagus Registry. *Am J Gastroenterol* 1999;**94**(8): 2037–42.

29. Katz D, Rothstein R, Schned A *et al.* The development of dysplasia and adenocarcinoma during endoscopic surveillance of Barrett's esophagus. *Am J Gastroenterol* 1998;**93**(4):536–41.

30. Sharma P, Morales TG, Bhattacharyya A, Garewal HS, Sampliner RE. Dysplasia in short-segment Barrett's esophagus: a prospective 3-year follow-up. *Am J Gastroenterol* 1997;**92**(11):2012–6.

31. Clark GW, Ireland AP, DeMeester TR. Dysplasia in Barrett's esophagus: diagnosis, surveillance and treatment. *Dig Dis* 1996;**14**(4):213–27.

32. Weston AP, Sharma P, Topalovski M *et al.* Long-term follow-up of Barrett's high-grade dysplasia. *Am J Gastroenterol* 2000;**95**(8):1888–93.

33. Weston AP, Krmpotich PT, Cherian R, Dixon A, Topalosvki M. Prospective long-term endoscopic and histological follow-up of short segment Barrett's esophagus: comparison with traditional long segment Barrett's esophagus. *Am J Gastroenterol* 1997;**92**(3): 407–13.

34. Hirota WK, Loughney TM, Lazas DJ *et al.* Specialized intestinal metaplasia, dysplasia, and cancer of the esophagus and esophagogastric junction: prevalence and clinical data. *Gastroenterology* 1999;**116**(2):277–85.

35. Weston AP, Badr AS, Hassanein RS. Prospective multivariate analysis of clinical, endoscopic, and histological factors predictive of the development of Barrett's multifocal high-grade dysplasia or adenocarcinoma. *Am J Gastroenterol* 1999;**94**(12):3413–9.

36. Hameeteman W, Tytgat GN, Houthoff HJ, van den Tweel JG. Barrett's esophagus: development of dysplasia and adenocarcinoma. *Gastroenterology* 1989;**96**(5 Pt 1):1249–56.

37. Sharma P, Reker D, Falk G *et al.* Progression of Barrett's esophagus to high grade dysplasia and cancer: preliminary results of the BEST (Barrett's Esophagus Study) trial. *Gastroenterology* 2001;**120**(5, suppl 1):A16.

38. Reid BJ, Haggitt RC, Rubin CE *et al.* Observer variation in the diagnosis of dysplasia in Barrett's esophagus. *Hum Pathol* 1988;**19**(2):166–78.

39. Alikhan M, Rex D, Khan A *et al.* Variable pathologic interpretation of columnar lined esophagus by general pathologists in community practice. *Gastrointest Endosc* 1999;**50**(1):23–6.

40. Montgomery E, Bronner MP, Goldblum JR *et al.* Reproducibility of the diagnosis of dysplasia in Barrett esophagus: a reaffirmation. *Hum Pathol* 2001;**32**(4):368–78.

41. Sagan C, Flejou JF, Diebold MD, Potet F, Le Bodic MF. Reproducibility of histological criteria of dysplasia in Barrett mucosa. *Gastroenterol Clin Biol* 1994;**18**(1 Pt 2):D31–4.

42. Wong DJ, Paulson TG, Prevo LJ *et al.* p16^{INK4a} lesions are common, early abnormalities that undergo clonal expansion in Barrett's metaplastic epithelium. *Cancer Res* 2001;**61**(22):8284–9.

43. Reid BJ, Blount PL, Rabinovitch PS. Biomarkers in Barrett's esophagus. *Gastrointest Endosc Clin N Am* 2003;**13**(2):369–97.

44. Bani-Hani K, Martin IG, Hardie LJ *et al.* Prospective study of cyclin D1 overexpression in Barrett's esophagus: association with increased risk of adenocarcinoma. *J Natl Cancer Inst* 2000;**92**(16):1316–21.

45. Weston AP, Banerjee SK, Sharma P *et al.* p53 protein overexpression in low grade dysplasia (LGD) in Barrett's esophagus: immunohistochemical marker predictive of progression. *Am J Gastroenterol* 2001;**96**(5): 1355–62.

46. Reid BJ, Prevo LJ, Galipeau PC *et al.* Predictors of progression in Barrett's esophagus II: baseline 17p (*p53*) loss of heterozygosity identifies a patient subset at increased risk for neoplastic progression. *Am J Gastroenterol* 2001;**96**(10):2839–48.

47. Rabinovitch PS, Longton G, Blount PL, Levine DS, Reid BJ. Predictors of progression in Barrett's esophagus III: baseline flow cytometric variables. *Am J Gastroenterol* 2001;**96**(11):3071–83.

48. Reid BJ, Levine DS, Longton G, Blount PL, Rabinovitch PS. Predictors of progression to cancer in Barrett's esophagus: baseline histology and flow cytometry identify low- and high-risk patient subsets. *Am J Gastroenterol* 2000;**95**(7):1669–76.

49. Winawer SJ, Zauber AG, Ho MN *et al.* Prevention of colorectal cancer by colonoscopic polypectomy. The National Polyp Study Workgroup. *N Engl J Med* 1993;**329**(27):1977–81.

CHAPTER 14

Chromoendoscopy in Barrett's Esophagus

M. Brian Fennerty

Introduction

Tissue staining, more often referred to as chromoscopy, is widely used throughout the world as an adjunct to endoscopy to improve the yield and/or accuracy of the endoscopic examination in identifying abnormal gastrointestinal mucosa [1–5]. Chromoscopy, as it is used endoscopically, is an imaging technique used to identify either specific epithelia or enhance the surface characteristics of the mucosa allowing for the recognition of epithelial changes such as neoplastic change (dysplasia). Used in this fashion, chromoendoscopy has been proven to improve the utility of the endoscopic examination when examining the esophagus, stomach, small intestine, and colon for various mucosal pathologies and disease states. Chromoscopy has evolved from a specific term describing "contrast enhancement of surface topography" into a more generic term referring to a variety of these techniques for tissue staining during endoscopy. Despite this generic term, chromoendoscopy, or endoscopic tissue staining, has generally been divided into the following categories: (i) traditional mucosal contrast staining (or true "chromoendoscopy") that specifically refers to the use of stains which accentuate the surface topography of the gastrointestinal epithelium allowing for recognition of abnormal mucosa that could otherwise go unrecognized during routine inspection of mucosa with standard video endoscopy; (ii) vital staining, which refers to the use of dyes which when applied to the gastrointestinal epithelial surface are subsequently absorbed into mucosal lining cells allowing visual identification of epithelia with specific characteristics, e.g. metaplastic absorptive epithelium or a lack of absorption capability where it would normally be expected from an epithelial surface; (iii) reactive tissue staining refers to use of agents during endoscopy that identify specific epithelia related to their ability to catalyze a chemical reaction (e.g. effect of acid on a reagent causing a color reaction); and (iv) mucosal tattooing with either a temporary "stain" or the implantation of a permanent mucosal mark (e.g. India Ink) to allow repeat inspection of a specific gastrointestinal mucosal site that otherwise could not be accurately relocated.

Contrast stains used endoscopically include cresyl violet and indigo carmine, vital stains include Lugol's solution, indocyanine green, methylene blue and toluidine blue, reactive stains include Congo red and phenol red, and finally tattooing has been done with both India Ink and indocyanine green.

Cresyl violet, a contrast stain, is useful as it pools in the margins of the mucosal pits and crevices highlighting the surface topography of the mucosa. It has been used most often in chromoendoscopy of the colon. The other mucosal contrast stain, indigo carmine, consists of a non-toxic blue dye (indigo) obtained from plants along with carmine (a compound composed of cochineal and alum) that forms a red coloring agent, that then collects in the sulci and grooves of the surface epithelium also highlighting and accentuating the surface topography of the mucosa.

Of the vital stains used during chromoendoscopy, Lugol's solution, named after the 19th century Paris physician, Jean Auguste Lugol, is a non-toxic mixture of iodine and potassium iodide that forms a compound iodine solution. Lugol's stains the non-keratinized epithelia of the esophagus green–brown related to the affinity of glycogen found in the normal esophageal epithelium for iodinated agents. This uptake of stain is rapid and immediate but short-lived lasting usually for 30–60 min at the most. Indocyanine green, composed of small dimmers and polymers of carbon, nitrogen and sulfur compounds in a solution has been used to stain normally functioning hepatocytes. As a chromoendoscopy agent though, its use has largely been relegated to that of a temporary tattooing agent. Methylene blue (methylthionine chloride) has been the most popular vital stain used endoscopically. It is considered a non-toxic vital stain used to reversibly stain "absorptive" epithelial blue. Stain uptake with this compound occurs within minutes and this coloration of absorptive epithelia is resistant to washing once the compound is absorbed into the mucosal cells. Staining with methylene blue persists long enough for recognition to occur endoscopically following rinsing of extraneous contrast. Toluidine blue is a vital stain largely used to stain neoplastic nuclei blue. Its use endoscopically has been relatively limited. All of the vital stains mentioned above (except for Lugol's solution), when used as chromoendoscopy agents within the luminal gastrointestinal tract, are only effective when the surface mucus has been first removed with a mucolytic agent. This "pretreatment" allows the vital (absorptive) stain to come into direct contact with the epithelium so absorption can then take place. Mucolytic compounds used during chromoendoscopy include pronase (a proteolytic agent not available for human use in the USA), mucomyst (N-acetylcysteine, most recognized as a protective agent used to mitigate the hepatic toxicity following acetaminophen overdose) or acetic acid. Mucomyst's free sulfhydryl groups disrupt the disulfide bridges of the glycoprotein gel structure of the mucus layer thereby destroying the component integral to maintaining the mucus cap normally adherent to the gastrointestinal mucosa.

Reactive stains include Congo red that changes color from red to blue–black at a pH of less than 3 and phenol red that is a yellow stain that turns red in the presence of an alkaline pH.

Finally tattooing of the gastrointestinal mucosa at the time of endoscopy can be accomplished with either India Ink, which is a colloidal suspension of carbon particles or indocyanine green (see above).

It has been my experience that the performance of chromoendoscopy and the application of these compounds to the surface of the gastrointestinal mucosa are best facilitated during an endoscopic examination by the use of a spraying catheter. The use of these type catheters ensures a uniform application of the agent as well as avoidance of spraying excessive material that will later have to be removed. Following application, endoscopic examination is continued with targeted biopsy of abnormally staining areas, but in the case of vital staining, washing off the extra contrast from the mucosa has to first be performed in order to clearly identify and target stained tissue.

Chromoscopy, used as the generic term for all types of tissue staining, has been used for decades as an adjunct to endoscopic examination of the gastrointestinal mucosa. Use of chromoscopy in this fashion has been demonstrated to improve the accuracy of determination of a colon polyp's histology (adenoma vs. hyperplasia), identify small bowel epithelium affected by celiac disease, highlight intestinal metaplasia in the stomach (including the cardia), and identify neoplastic squamous epithelium in the esophagus, among many other uses. In regards to the esophagus, traditional application of chromoscopy has focused on use of Lugol's solution to identify dysplasia and carcinoma in patients at risk for squamous cell cancer of the esophagus.

Another clinically important premalignant lesion of the esophagus is Barrett's esophagus [6]. Barrett's esophagus refers to a premalignant esophageal epithelium that is thought to occur as a consequence of a genetically determined inappropriate repair of esophageal mucosal injury (esophagitis/esophageal ulcer) with a metaplastic epithelium in the setting of an abnormal milieu, e.g. acid reflux, found in patients with chronic gastroesophageal reflux disease (GERD). For reasons as yet unknown, only some patients (predominantly White men) will repair their esophageal injury by forming this metaplastic premalignant columnar epithelium (Barrett's). GERD affects at least 20% of adult Americans with 10–15% of these GERD patients having Barrett's esophagus [7,8]. Extrapolation of these data indicate that as many as 1–2% of the adult population in the USA may therefore have Barrett's esophagus. This likely represents a conservative estimate as more recently screening of "asymptomatic" individuals undergoing screening for colorectal neoplasia suggests the prevalence of Barrett's in the US population may be as high as 5–15% [9,10]. This large at-risk pool of patients with Barrett's esophagus is the probable explanation for the rapidly rising incidence of the Barrett's associated cancer, esophageal adenocarcinoma, seen over the last 30 years in the USA and other Western countries [11].

Current clinical recommendations call for screening patients with chronic GERD for Barrett's esophagus, and enrolling those found to have the premalignant Barrett's lesion into an endoscopic surveillance programs [12]. The intent of both endoscopic screening and subsequent surveillance of patients for Barrett's esophagus is to detect neoplasia at an early, treatable and, in the case of malignancy, curable stage. Hampering current screening and surveillance practice is the inability to endoscopically recognize all and especially smaller zones of Barrett's, the high-risk subtype, intestinal metaplasia, as well early neoplastic lesions (dysplasia or cancer) in a field of Barrett's, as these areas are not usually recognizable with current widely used video endoscopic systems. Whether magnification or other methods of endoscopic imaging can obviate this lack of recognition of Barrett's and its neoplastic elements has not yet been determined, but clearly some sort of adjunctive endoscopic method(s) (e.g. chromoendoscopy) will be necessary to improve recognition of neoplastic Barrett's as well as smaller areas of Barrett's versus that obtained with current endoscopic imaging technology. Additionally, current endoscopic surveillance practice is to perform random biopsies throughout the entire field of Barrett's esophagus in order to maximize detection of dysplasia or early stage cancer [12]. This "random-biopsy" approach to surveillance is an effective technique for detecting early stages of neoplasia if saturation biopsies are taken from all four quadrants of the involved esophagus every 1–2 cm. However, this approach is difficult, tedious, expensive, and rarely applied in clinical practice. Technique(s)

that would increase the yield of an endoscopic surveillance examination's detection of Barrett's metaplasia or neoplasia, while limiting the number of biopsies necessary to accomplish this task would be of intuitive clinical benefit.

One potential means of improving the yield of detection of Barrett's metaplasia would be to accentuate the squamocolumnar junction. Similarly, another method to increase the ability to detect neoplasia while limiting the needed number of biopsies in a patient with Barrett's esophagus undergoing surveillance endoscopy would be to target only higher-risk tissue. Chromoendoscopy could be of benefit in both of these regards if it could either more accurately define the presence and extent of the metaplastic Barrett's epithelium to insure recognition and sampling of the full extent of the disease, or if tissue staining accurately identified areas of intestinal metaplasia/dysplasia. Intestinal metaplasia is now considered to be a prerequisite for the diagnosis of Barrett's esophagus as it represents the premalignant epithelium from which neoplasia arises [12]. However, within the length of Barrett's esophagus, there may be areas of columnar mucosa lacking intestinal metaplasia. As there is little or no risk of malignancy in these other regions of columnar epithelia, tissue sampling from these locations is unnecessary and wasteful. Thus targeting only the "at-risk" tissue (intestinal metaplasia) could also be of benefit and improve cost and/or yield of surveillance endoscopy in these patients.

This chapter will focus on the use of chromoscopy as an adjunct to endoscopy during screening and/or surveillance of Barrett's esophagus (see Tables 14.1 and 14.2). Unfortunately, there are little data available at this time on which to base strong clinical recommendations regarding use of chromoendoscopy in patients with Barrett's esophagus [1,3–5]. But where there are data it is quite compelling and it has identified areas where further research may be rewarding.

Use of Chromoendoscopy in Screening (Detecting) for Barrett's Esophagus

Lugol's solution, as mentioned previously, is an

Table 14.1 Tissue stains.

Stain	Type	Use
Methylene blue	Vital stain	Surveillance: identifies intestinal metaplasia and possibly dysplasia
Toluidine blue	Vital stain	Surveillance: identifies columnar mucosa
Lugol's solution	Vital stain	Screening: accentuates squamocolumnar border and highlights small islands and tongues of columnar mucosa
Acetic acid	Contrast stain	Screening: accentuates squamocolumnar border and highlights small islands and tongues of columnar mucosa
Indigo carmine	Contrast stain	Surveillance: identifies intestinal metaplasia and dysplasia when used with magnification endoscopy

Table 14.2 Tissue stain techniques.

Stain	Concentration	Volume	Application
Methylene blue	0.5–1.0% solution	10–50 cc	Spraying catheter (Olympus PW-5V) over surface of Barrett's following mucolytic (mucomyst or acetic acid) application
Toluidine blue	0.5–1.0% solution	10–50 cc	Same as for methylene blue
Lugol's solution	1–10% solution	20–50 cc	Spraying catheter at squamocolumnar junction
Acetic acid	1.0–1.5% solution	5–30 cc	Same as for Lugol's solution
Indigo carmine	0.1–2.0% solution	20–50 cc	Same as for methylene blue (mucolytic not needed)

iodine-based solution containing iodine and potassium iodide, that has an avidity for glycogen containing mucosa such as is found in the normal non-keratinized squamous epithelium of the esophagus [1]. The normal squamous mucosa of the native esophagus stains a distinctive green–brown following application of Lugol's solution. Lugol's solution has been extensively studied as a contrast agent to identify dysplasia and malignant areas within the squamous lined esophagus as it clearly demarcates normal squamous mucosa from abnormal neoplastic mucosa.

Based on the affinity of Lugol's solution to stain squamous mucosa, this chromoendoscopic agent has also been used as a vital stain to accentuate the border between normal esophageal squamous mucosa and metaplastic Barrett's esophagus columnar epithelium (Plate 14.1; color plate section falls between pp. 148–9.). In doing so, it may also be useful in identifying otherwise unrecognized areas of Barrett's mucosa, such as small islands or tongues of Barrett's mucosa adjacent to or distant from the squamocolumnar junction, that otherwise would have gone undetected. Woolf et al. demonstrated that use of Lugol's in this fashion allowed for more precise localization of the squamocolumnar border with a sensitivity and specificity of approximately 90% and 95% respectively [13]. My own personal experience with the use of Lugol's solution as a chromoendoscopic agent has been that is has also allowed for improved recognition of small residual tongues and islands of Barrett's mucosa following endoscopic reversal therapies. While the clinical relevance of such precise determination of the extent of the involvement of the esophagus by Barrett's metaplasia following staining with Lugol's solution is uncertain, this chromoendoscopic technique clearly allows for more complete sampling of the entirety of the metaplastic premalignant epithelium. Additionally in research of endoscopic ablation/reversal techniques for Barrett's esophagus, use of Lugol's allowed more precise determination of whether all of the endoscopically apparent Barrett's has been eradicated (personal observation).

Acetic acid has also been used as a contrast agent to accentuate the squamocolumnar junction. A dilute solution of acetic acid produces protein denaturation within the normal esophageal-squamous mucosa resulting in a "whitening" of the tissue. Thus like Lugol's solution, acetic acid (but used here as a contrast stain vs. a vital stain) can be used to accentuate the border between the squamous and metaplastic epithelia present within the esophagus. Guelrud was able to clearly demonstrate the utility of acetic acid when used for this type of application [14]. Whether Lugol's solution or an acetic acid solution is the superior chromoendoscopic agent in this regard, remains to be determined.

Use of Chromoendoscopy for Surveillance of Barrett's Esophagus

As noted previously, vital staining refers to the use of contrast agents during endoscopy that are taken up by an absorptive epithelium and thereby can be used to identify specific epithelia that are present but could otherwise go unrecognized. As originally described, Barrett's esophagus consisted of a non-absorptive gastric-type of epithelium. In actuality, three distinct metaplastic columnar epithelia have been identified within the tubular esophagus and may co-exist within a segment of Barrett's esophagus: (i) a gastric-type columnar epithelium; (ii) a junctional-type columnar epithelium; and (iii) an intestinal metaplasia (absorptive) columnar epithelium. The cancer risk in Barrett's esophagus is almost exclusively related to the intestinal metaplasia subtype, and thus it is this specific epithelial change that is regarded as the precursor lesion for adenocarcinoma of the esophagus [6,12]. Moreover, Barrett's esophagus is now defined by the presence of this type metaplastic epithelium within the esophagus, and Barrett's esophagus should only be diagnosed when

intestinal metaplasia is documented within the tubular esophagus as this is the at-risk lesion [12]. Importantly, Barrett's related intestinal metaplasia is similar to gastric intestinal metaplasia in that it has absorptive characteristics. This absorptive ability can be used to differentiate and detect intestinal metaplasia within a field of Barrett's esophagus by employing chromoendoscopy (Plate 14.3; color plate falls between pp. 148–9.). Tissue stains used to identify absorptive epithelia within Barrett's esophagus have included methylene blue and toluidine blue, agents shown to identify intestinal metaplasia elsewhere in the gut previously [15].

In 1987, Chobanian *et al.* were the first to use a vital stain as a chromoendoscopic technique to detect Barrett's epithelium [16]. In 58 patients undergoing endoscopy, they used acetic acid as a prestain wash to remove the surface mucus layer followed by application of a toluidine blue solution. Biopsies were obtained from both darkly stained versus lightly stained or unstained areas following the application of this vital stain. The use of this tissue staining technique improved the yield of detection of Barrett's esophagus from 86% to 98% in 110 biopsies, but this improvement in sensitivity was also associated with a decrease in a specificity of the diagnosis of Barrett's from 88% to 80%. Six patients had Barrett's esophagus diagnosed based on detection by toluidine blue staining alone. Somewhat surprisingly, vital staining with this agent did not correlate with the presence of intestinal metaplasia, but identified junctional and gastric-type epithelia as well. Similar data using toluidine blue was later reported by Katzka *et al.* [17].

However, it took 9 years from the seminal observation of Chobanian's for chromoendoscopy of Barrett's to really capture investigators' attention. At that time Canto *et al.* reported the results correlating chromoendoscopy with methylene blue staining to the presence of intestinal metaplasia and dysplasia [18]. In this prospective trial of 31 patients with known Barrett's esophagus, routine four-quadrant biopsy with jumbo forceps versus methylene blue directed biopsies were performed in a randomized order. In patients with short segment Barrett's esophagus, the yield of intestinal metaplasia in each biopsy increased from 54% to 94%, and in long segment Barrett's esophagus from 72% to 92% ($P = 0.0006$) when targeting of methylene blue stained mucosa was used. Additionally, neoplasia was detected significantly more frequently, with 8% of samples and 40% of patients in randomly obtained specimens having either dysplasia or cancer versus 11% of samples and 52% of patients ($P = 0.03$) in those biopsies directed by staining with methylene blue. Canto *et al.* also subsequently reported the utility of chromoendoscopy using methylene blue in a controlled trial of patients with and without Barrett's esophagus undergoing endoscopic examination [19]. They first removed the mucus from the esophageal epithelial surface with *N*-acetylcysteine and following this procedure methylene blue was applied with subsequent stain positive and stain negative directed biopsies in both the 14 patients with Barrett's esophagus and the 12 control patients thought not to have Barrett's esophagus undergoing routine endoscopy. In this study they were able to demonstrate accuracy in detecting specialized intestinal metaplasia in methylene blue staining directed biopsies of 95%. Only 3.5% of biopsies from stained areas contained no intestinal metaplasia, and only 5% of biopsies from unstained areas contained intestinal metaplasia. Somewhat surprising, chromoendoscopy using methylene blue directed biopsy also resulted in the detection of low-grade or indefinite dysplasia in six patients, high-grade dysplasia in one patient, and an unrecognized intramucosal cancer in one patient. The odds ratio for detection of neoplasia in a biopsy from a positive "stained" area versus a biopsy obtained from an unstained area was 17.7 ($P = 0.0004$). Interestingly, methylene blue staining detected intestinal metaplasia in the esophagus of 42% of the "control" patients, thought to have been normal. Staining with methylene blue was reproducible when reapplied later in the same patients, and the estimated cost of applying chromoendoscopy in this fashion was less than $9 per patient.

Canto *et al.* has also evaluated the accuracy and correlation of the staining intensity with methylene blue in detecting dysplasia in an *ex vivo* study [20]. In this study the intensity of staining inversely correlated with the dysplasia grade. More recently, Gangarosa *et al.* also correlated the presence of dysplasia to staining intensity with methylene blue

[21]. In those with prominent staining, intestinal metaplasia was more frequently detected. Areas of low-grade dysplasia showed blue staining less frequently than non-dysplastic Barrett's (52% vs. 74%, $P < 0.05$) but the positive predictive value for poor staining indicating the presence of dysplasia was still 41%. Thus the intensity of staining with methylene blue at the time of chromoendoscopy may be an important determinate of the presence of both intestinal metaplasia (strong staining) and dysplasia (light staining). Finally, Canto *et al.* also demonstrated in a randomized trial that the utilization of chromoendoscopy during routine surveillance endoscopy in patients with Barrett's esophagus increased the percentage of biopsies and patients found to have dysplasia [22]. In this study the yield of neoplasia from methylene blue directed biopsies was 12% of specimens and 44% of patients versus random biopsies detecting neoplasia in 6% of samples and 28% of patients. Moreover, this increased yield of neoplasia with methylene blue directed biopsy was seen in both short and long segment Barrett's patients. Other investigators have also confirmed the utility of chromoendoscopy using methylene blue for surveillance in patients with Barrett's esophagus. Sharma *et al.* confirmed that use of methylene blue directed biopsies in short segment Barrett's yielded intestinal metaplasia in 61% of biopsies versus 42% of the randomly obtained biopsies ($P = 0.024$) [23]. In those with 1–2 cm lengths of Barrett's the yield of intestinal metaplasia in a biopsy rose from 45% to 77% when directed by methylene blue staining, and in those with 2–3 cm of Barrett's it increased from 58% of samples containing intestinal metaplasia to 90%. Both of these differences in yield were statistically significant. More data are still needed in order to determine the exact clinical relevance of these findings, but these above findings strongly suggest that if the goal of surveillance endoscopy in patients with Barrett's esophagus is to detect patients with neoplasia, then the use of methylene blue chromoendoscopy is superior to that of the current standard of random biopsies in targeting at-risk tissue and finding the lesion. One conundrum that still needs to be resolved is the relevance of an unstained segment. As Barrett's frequently has segments of columnar mucosa that is not intestinalized (cardia or junctional mu-

cosa), these areas will not take up staining and could potentially be classified as being more likely neoplastic and targeted unnecessarily. This issue has not been specifically addressed but remains a potential problem with chromoendoscopy using a vital stain such as methylene blue. In a similar demonstration of the utility of chromoendoscopy with methylene blue staining to detect intestinal metaplasia in the region of the esophagogastric junction, Morales *et al.* also reported an increase in the detection of intestinal metaplasia in the cardia from 38% with random biopsies to 67% with methylene blue targeted biopsies from this anatomic location [24]. Finally, Sharma *et al.* has also used magnification endoscopy combined with vital staining with indigo carmine in attempting to improve the detection of neoplastic Barrett's [25]. They found this technique to be reliable for detecting intestinal metaplasia as well as high-grade dysplasia but not in differentiating low-grade dysplasia from surrounding intestinal metaplasia.

It should be noted that not all investigators have been able to reproduce this high degree of accuracy with methylene blue staining of Barrett's. Wo *et al.* preformed a crossover study of chromoendoscopy with methylene blue staining in patients with Barrett's esophagus [26]. These investigators found a low sensitivity and specificity for the diagnosis of intestinal metaplasia using methylene blue directed biopsies and no statistical significant improvement in the detection of either metaplasia or dysplasia with this technique. Meining *et al.* using a combination of chromoendoscopy with and without methylene blue staining, demonstrated a high level of interobserver variability in its accuracy (all kappa <0.4) [27]. Others have also found less impressive results with use of methylene blue staining chromoendoscopy [28,29]. The reasons for the discordance results reported with methylene blue chromoendoscopy in Barrett's is unclear but, as mentioned above, I suspect it is likely related to differences in the skill and experience with chromoendoscopy between investigators, as this technique appears to be very operator dependent, or to differences in chromoendoscopy technique (amount of stain, washing technique, time observed, etc.) employed in these studies. One final note, although

methylene blue staining has been found to be exceedingly safe and there are no reports of toxicity in the literature when used in this fashion, a recent report suggests that we must remain vigilant in assessing safety of this chromoendoscopic technique. Olliver *et al.* reported oxidative damage in tissues exposed to methylene blue, and this observation is thought to possibly be related to the photosensitization of the compound in the presence of white light used endoscopically [30]. While this hypothesis and observation is in itself not sufficient for recommending caution in using methylene blue chromoendoscopy, it does suggest that further work regarding the safety of this and other chromoendoscopy agents is still needed.

However, when the data regarding use of methylene blue chromoendoscopy in the screening and surveillance of Barrett's esophagus are viewed in their entirety, targeted biopsy of methylene blue stained areas increases the recognition and diagnostic accuracy not only for the presence of Barrett's esophagus and intestinal metaplasia but also increases the ability to diagnose dysplasia within Barrett's esophagus. These data strongly suggest that this simple and relatively inexpensive technique has been and remains underutilized in the screening for and subsequent surveillance of patients with Barrett's esophagus.

As noted previously, contrast staining refers to the use of agents to accentuate topography of the epithelium. As mentioned above, Barrett's esophagus is not a single epithelium, but may be a mixture of different types of columnar epithelia (intestinal metaplasia, cardia or junctional-type and fundic-type columnar mucosa). Dysplasia and/or early cancer arises exclusively from the intestinal metaplasia subtype and can exist unrecognized within otherwise normal appearing Barrett's esophagus when using currently available video-endoscopy. Theoretically, subtle unrecognized epithelium abnormalities, such as are found in neoplastic tissues, could be detected by using a contrast staining technique. Additionally, the recognition of areas of intestinal metaplasia, allowing targeted biopsy of these zones and an increased yield in detecting otherwise unrecognizable neoplasia within the tissue, could also conceivably be accomplished with such a chromoendoscopy technique.

Indigo carmine is a contrast stain that has been used to accentuate topographical variations in the surface epithelium related to pooling within crevices and depressions allowing recognition of subtle differences in topography [1]. Stevens *et al.* studied the utility of chromoendoscopy using contrast staining with indigo carmine combined with high-resolution magnification endoscopy to detect areas of intestinal metaplasia within Barrett's esophagus [31]. Accentuation of the squamocolumnar junction was first achieved by application of Lugol's solution (see above) then indigo carmine was sprayed on the surface of the Barrett's epithelium. Specialized intestinal metaplasia had a characteristic villiform pattern and additionally dysplasia was associated with a raised irregular surface within this tissue. Unfortunately, I am not aware of any follow-up studies validating the use of contrast chromoendoscopy to identify intestinal metaplasia or dysplasia during endoscopic surveillance of Barrett's esophagus and thus the value of this procedure remains unknown.

The final chromoendoscopic technique I would like to briefly discuss is the ability to relocate lesions or mucosal areas accurately by means of a tissue "tattoo." (Plate 14.2; color plate section falls between pp. 148–9.) Tattooing of the esophagus has been demonstrated to be both safe and effective at ensuring precision of measurement, relocalization, and rebiopsy of the same site [32]. Moreover, the tattoo has persisted with 95% of tattoos still being present at 36 months. Its use in Barrett's esophagus seems to be most applicable in tattooing sites undergoing endoscopic mucosal resection (EMR) to be able to later rebiopsy from that site to ensure complete removal of all neoplastic tissue.

Conclusions

Chromoendoscopy has a number of possible applications in the management of Barrett's esophagus. Both vital staining and contrast staining appear to be potentially useful both in screening for Barrett's esophagus and in the surveillance of the lesion for the development of neoplasia. The use of Lugol's solution as a vital stain and acetic acid as a contrast stain for squamous mucosa appear to be useful in highlighting the squamocolumnar border and thus increasing the ability to identify an otherwise unrecognized existence of columnar mucosa within the esophagus, thus confirming the presence and the diagnosis of Barrett's esophagus. As such this technique may be a valuable adjunct to endoscopic screening for Barrett's esophagus. Similarly the use of methylene blue during endoscopy (following removal of surface mucus) as a vital stain for intestinal metaplasia and/or dysplasia increases the detection of the at-risk tissue (intestinal metaplasia) as well as the yield of dysplasia during surveillance endoscopy of Barrett's patients. Combination of these two chromoendoscopic staining techniques and/or contrast staining with indigo carmine combined with high resolution magnifying endoscopy may improve the utility of endoscopic screening and surveillance of Barrett's esophagus and increasing use of the these techniques must be encouraged.

The ideal tissue stain to use for endoscopic screening and surveillance of Barrett's esophagus is probably as yet undiscovered. A contrast agent accurately identifying neoplastic epithelium would be of obvious clinical benefit and perhaps immunohistochemical stains that target neoplastic tissue and be readily recognizable during routine video endoscopy could be developed. Putative targets for such "molecular beacons" include *p53* or similar mutations associated with genomic instability and cancer risk in Barrett's esophagus.

There are ample opportunities that remain for clinical research in the field of chromoendoscopy and Barrett's esophagus. More importantly, development and validation of these techniques may provide an opportunity to improve patient outcomes. Areas needing to be addressed include those such as: Why does dysplastic epithelium absorb methylene blue, if it does at all? Does staining really identify dysplasia in this setting, or is it identifying a field of intestinal metaplasia from which dysplasia is arising? Can we decrease the number of biopsies needed and thus time and cost when surveying these patients by using chromoendoscopy? Are these techniques cost-effective? Further research employing well-designed, controlled clinical studies may be able to answer these and other important questions related to chromoendoscopy in Barrett's esophagus.

References

1. Fennerty MB. Tissue staining. *Gastroenterol Clin North Am* 1997;**4**:297–311.

2. Shim CS. Staining in gastrointestinal endoscopy. *Endoscopy* 1999;**31**:487–96.

3. Fennerty MB. Tissue staining (chromoscopy) of the gastrointestinal tract. *Can J Gastroenterol* 1999;**13**: 423–9.

4. Canto MI. Vital staining and Barrett's esophagus. *Gastrointest Endosc* 1999;**49**:S12–6.

5. Fennerty MB. Should chromoscopy be part of the proficient endoscopist's armamentarium? *Gastrointest Endosc* 1998;**47**:313–5.

6. Fennerty MB, Sampliner RE, Garewal HS. Barrett's esophagus–cancer risk, biology and therapeutic management. *Aliment Pharmacol Ther* 1993;**7**:339–45.

7. Locke GR, Talley NJ, Zinsmeister AR *et al*. Prevalence and clinical spectrum of gastroesophageal reflux: a population-based study in Olmstead County, Minnesota. *Gastroenterology* 1997;**112**:1448–56.

8. Winters C, Spurling TJ, Chobanian SJ *et al*. Barrett's esophagus. A prevalent, occult complication of gastroesophageal reflux disease. *Gastroenterology* 1987; **92**:118–24.

9. Rex DK, Cummings OW, Shaw M *et al*. Screening for Barrett's esophagus in colonoscopy patients with and without heartburn. *Gastroenterology* 2003;**125**:1670–7.

10. Gerson LB, Shetler K, Triadafilopoulos G. Prevalence of Barrett's esophagus in asymptomatic individuals. *Gastroenterology* 2002;**123**:461–7.

11. Blot WJ, Devesa SS, Kneller RW, Fraumeni JF. Rising incidence of adenocarcinoma of the esophagus and gastric cardia. *JAMA* 1991;**265**:1287–9.

12. Sampliner RE, The Practice Parameters Committee of the American College of Gastroenterology. Updated guidelines on the diagnosis, surveillance and therapy of Barrett's esophagus. *Am J Gastroenterol* 2002;**97**: 1888–95.

13. Woolf GM, Riddle RH, Irvine EJ *et al*. A study to examine agreement between endoscopy and histology for the diagnosis of columnar-lined (Barrett's) esophagus. *Gastrointest Endosc* 1989;**35**:541–5.

14. Guelrud M, Herrera I. Acetic acid improves identification of remnant islands of Barrett's epithelium after endoscopic therapy. *Gastrointest Endosc* 1998;**47**: 512–5.

15. Fennerty MB, Sampliner RE, McGee DL *et al*. Intestinal metaplasia of the stomach: identification by a selective mucosal staining technique. *Gastrointest Endosc* 1992; **38**:696–8.

16. Chobanian SJ, Cattau EL, Winters C *et al*. *In vivo* staining with toluidine blue as an adjunct to the endoscopic detection of Barrett's esophagus. *Gastrointest Endosc* 1987;**33**:99–101.

17. Katzka D, Plotkin A, Saul S *et al*. A controlled study of toluidine blue staining in patients with metaplasia of the esophagus. *Gastroenterol* 1986;**90**: 1485.

18. Canto MI, Setrakian S, Willis J *et al*. Methylene blue directed biopsy for improved detection of intestinal metaplasia and dysplasia in Barrett's esophagus: a controlled sequential trial [abstract]. *Gastrointest Endosc* 1996;**43**:331.

19. Canto MI, Setrakian S, Petras RE *et al*. Methylene blue selectively stains intestinal metaplasia in Barrett's esophagus. *Gastrointest Endosc* 1996;**44**: 1–7.

20. Canto MI, Setrakian S, Petras RE *et al*. Methylene blue staining of dysplastic and non-dysplastic Barrett's esophagus: an *in vivo* and *ex vivo* study [abstract]. *Gastrointest Endosc* 1996;**43**:332.

21. Gangarosa LM, Halter S, Mertz H. Methylene blue staining and endoscopic ultrasound evaluation of Barrett's esophagus with low-grade dysplasia. *Dig Dis Sci* 2000;**45**:225–9.

22. Canto MI, Setrakian S, Willis J *et al*. Methylene blue directed biopsies improve detection of intestinal metaplasia and dysplasia in Barrett's esophagus. *Gastrointest Endosc* 2000;**51**:560–8.

23. Sharma P, Topalovski M, Mayo MS, Weston AP. Methylene blue chromoendoscopy for detection of short segment Barrett's esophagus. *Gastrointest Endosc* 2001;**54**:289–93.

24. Morales T, Bhattacharyya A, Camargo E *et al*. Methylene blue staining for intestinal metaplasia of the gastric cardia with follow-up for dysplasia. *Gastrointest Endosc* 1998;**48**:26–31.

25. Sharma P, Weston AP, Topalovski M *et al*. Magnification chromoendoscopy for the detection of intestinal metaplasia and dysplasia in Barrett's oesophagus. *Gut* 2003;**52**:24–7.

26. Wo J, Ray M, Mayfield-Stokes S *et al*. Comparison of methylene blue directed biopsies and conventional biopsies in the detection of intestinal metaplasia and dysplasia in Barrett's esophagus: a preliminary study. *Gastrointest Endosc* 2001;**54**:294–301.

27. Meining A, Rosch T, Kiesslich R *et al*. Inter- and Intra-observer variability of magnification chromoendoscopy for detecting specialized intestinal metaplasia at the gastroesophageal junction. *Endoscopy* 2004;**36**: 160–4.

28. Dave U, Shousha AS, Westaby D. Methylene blue staining: is it really useful in Barrett's esophagus? *Gastrointest Endosc* 2001;**53**:333–5.

29. Breyer HP, Silva De Barros SG, Maguilnik I, Edelweiss MI. Does methylene blue detect intestinal metaplasia in Barrett's esophagus? *Gastrointest Endosc* 2003;**57**: 505–9.

30. Olliver JR, Wild CP, Sahay P, Dexter S, Hardie LJ. Chromoendoscopy with methylene blue and associated DNA damage in Barrett's esophagus. *Lancet* 2002;**362**: 373–4.

31. Stevens PD, Lightdale CJ, Green PHR *et al.* Combined magnification endoscopy with chromoendoscopy for the evaluation of Barrett's esophagus. *Gastrointest Endosc* 1994;**40**:747–9.

32. Schaffner RT, Francis JM, Carrougher JG *et al.* India Ink tattooing in the esophagus. *Gastrointest Endosc* 1998;**47**:257–60.

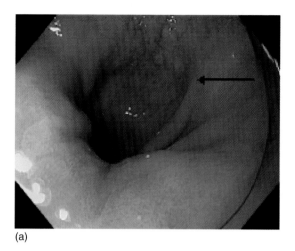

(a)

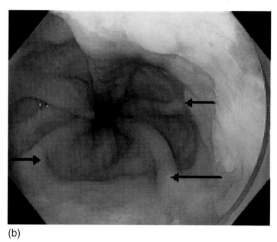

(b)

Plate 1.1 (a) Endoscopic picture of the gastroesophageal junction. During minimal insufflation, the gastroesophageal junction is seen as the point at which the proximal ends of the gastric folds appear and coincide with the pinch at the end of the tubular esophagus (arrow). Reproduced by permission from P. Sharma. (b) Endoscopic picture of Barrett's esophagus. The arrows identify the gastroesophageal junction. The columnar lined esophagus above the gastroesophageal junction is endoscopic or suspected Barrett's esophagus. If histology shows intestinal metaplasia, then this can be considered as confirmed Barrett's esophagus. Reproduced with permission from P. Sharma.

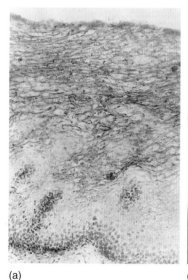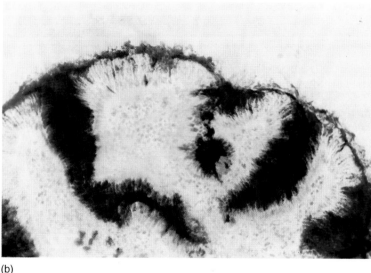

(a)   (b)

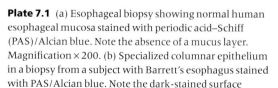

Plate 7.1 (a) Esophageal biopsy showing normal human esophageal mucosa stained with periodic acid–Schiff (PAS)/Alcian blue. Note the absence of a mucus layer. Magnification × 200. (b) Specialized columnar epithelium in a biopsy from a subject with Barrett's esophagus stained with PAS/Alcian blue. Note the dark-stained surface mucus gel layer. Magnification × 200. Modified and reproduced with permission from Dixon J, Strugala V, Griffin SM *et al.* Esophageal mucin: an adherent mucus gel barrier is absent in the normal esophagus but present in columnar-lined Barrett's esophagus. *Am J Gastroenterol* 2001;**96**:2575–83.

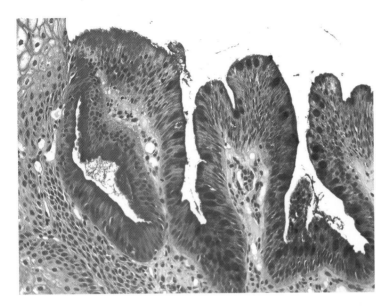

Plate 10.1 Periodic acid–Schiff (PAS)/Alcian blue at pH 2.5 demonstrates incomplete intestinal metaplasia. Goblet cells containing acid mucin stain intensely blue with Alcian blue (right), while the adjacent columnar cells containing neutral mucin stain with PAS (left).

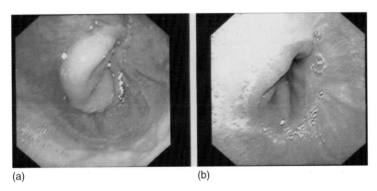

(a)   (b)

Plate 14.1 (a) This reveals the squamocolumnar junction as viewed with an endoscope before chromoendoscopy with Lugol's staining. (b) Reveals the same view of the junction after chromoendoscopic application of 1% Lugol's solution demonstrating a clear accentuation of the border between the squamous and columnar mucosa.

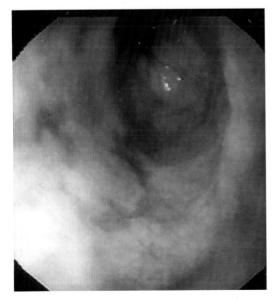

Plate 14.2 India Ink "tattoo" of the esophagus. This tattoo allows relocalization of a specific mucosal area for further study.

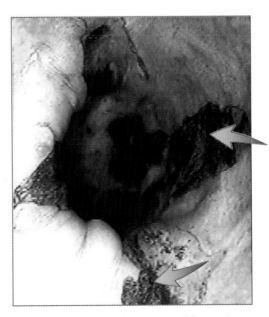

Plate 14.3 Methylene blue staining of the esophagus identifying areas of intestinal metaplasia within a Barrett's segment for targeted biopsy when screening for the lesion or surveillance for neoplasia.

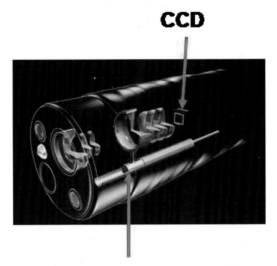

CCD

The focal distance can be adjusted by moving the lens

Plate 15.1 The proximal end of a high-resolution/magnification endoscope. CCD, charge-coupled device.

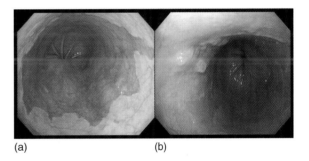

(a)   (b)

Plate 15.2 Overview images of Barrett's esophagus in two different patients examined with a high-resolution endoscope; (a) no visible lesions; (b) a nodular lesion is visible at the 10 o'clock position. This lesion was removed by endoscopic mucosal resection and was found to contain intramucosal carcinoma.

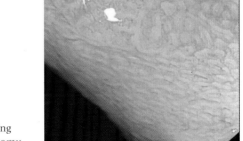

Plate 15.3 A minute superficial mucosal lesion detected by magnifying endoscopy in a Barrett's esophagus patient. The lesion shows irregular mucosal/vascular patterns and abnormal blood vessels (~80× magnification).

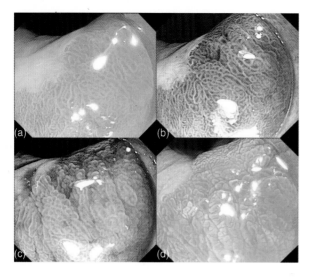

Plate 15.4 Magnified images of the same Barrett's esophagus area taken with (a) high-resolution endoscopy; (b) narrow band imaging (NBI); (c) indigo carmine chromoendoscopy (ICC); and (d) acetic acid chromoendoscopy (AAC). This area contains regular villous/gyrous-forming mucosal patterns corresponding to intestinal metaplasia without dysplasia (~80× magnification).

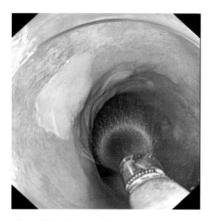

Plate 15.5 Spraying the esophagus of a Barrett's esophagus patient with acetic acid using a spraying catheter inserted through the working channel of an endoscope.

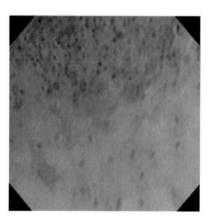

Plate 17.1 An endocytoscopic image esophagus at 450× magnification with methylene blue staining is shown of the region of mucosa at the border between esophageal cancer (top half) and normal squamous mucosa (bottom half). The region of cancer stains darker overall, and has a much higher density of nuclei than that of normal.

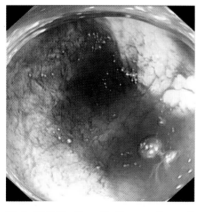

Plate 15.6 Pooling of indigo carmine at the left lateral position (6–7 o'clock) obscuring the mucosal surface.

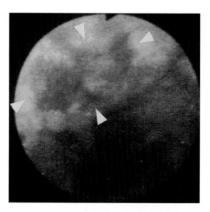

Plate 17.2 An autofluorescence image of the distal esophagus collected *in vivo* is shown. A region of red enhancement (arrowheads) reveals high-grade dysplasia in the setting of Barrett's.

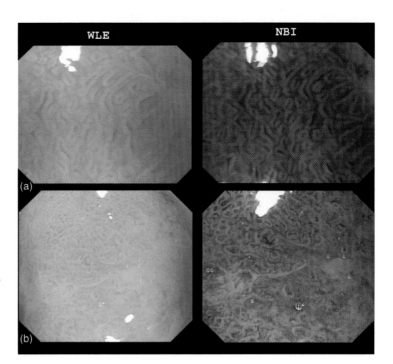

WLE   NBI

Plate 15.7 Magnified images of two Barrett's esophagus areas imaged with high-resolution white light endoscopy (WLE) and narrow band imaging (NBI). (a) An area with intestinal metaplasia showing regular mucosal and vascular patterns. (b) An area with high-grade dysplasia showing irregular/disrupted mucosal and vascular patterns (~ 115× magnification).

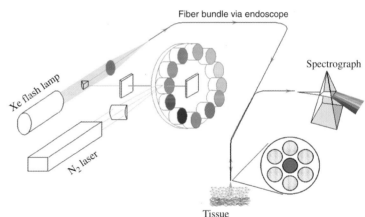

Plate 16.1 Apparatus for collecting trimodal spectroscopy. On the left are two light sources. A Xenon lamp that produces white light for reflectance and light scattering, and a nitrogen laser (output 337 nm) that is passed through a series of rotating die wells to produce 11 different wavelengths of light for laser-induced fluorescence spectroscopy. Both sources of light are focused on the back end of a fiber bundle, which is passed through the endoscope to the tissue. Light from the tissue is collected through the same bundle and split into separate colors and analyzed by a spectrometer.

Fiber bundle via endoscope

Xe flash lamp

N₂ laser

Spectrograph

Tissue

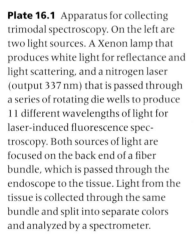

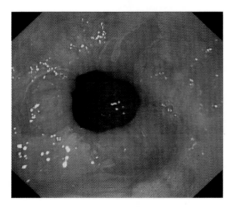

Plate 18.1 A patient with a diaphragmatic hernia, Barrett's epithelium, and erosive esophagitis.

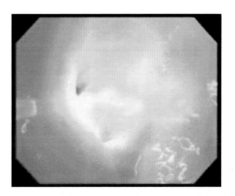

Plate 20.1 Photodynamic therapy (PDT) light delivery using a bare fiber. The fiber can be positioned through the biopsy port of a standard endoscope. During photoradiation, views of the mucosa are limited due to the intensity of light. The fiber can be difficult to center as shown.

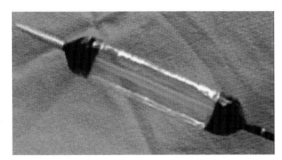

Plate 20.2 This is an over-the-wire photodynamic therapy (PDT) balloon, which is termed an Excel balloon. It comes in three sizes, with a 3, 5, or 7 cm diffusing window. This is designed to help center the lumen of Barrett's esophagus.

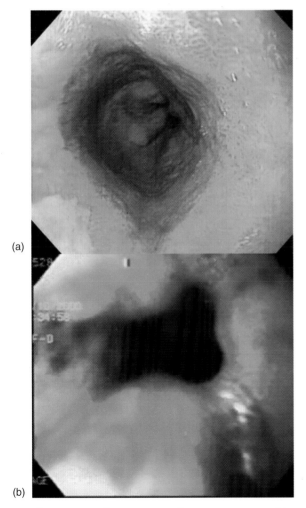

(a)

(b)

Plate 20.3 (a) The appearance of a Barrett's segment. (b) Twenty-four hours after photoradiation, the degree of tissue damage can be appreciated.

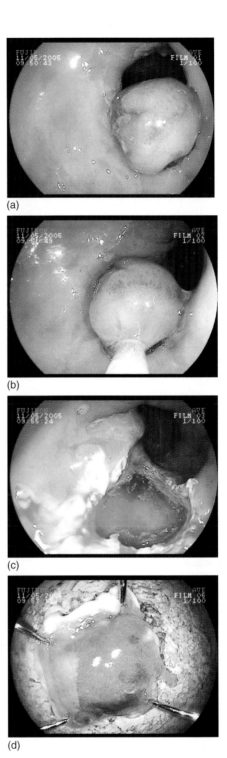

(a)

(b)

(c)

(d)

Plate 21.1 (a–d) Endoscopic resection of mucosal Barrett's adenocarcinoma with cap technique.

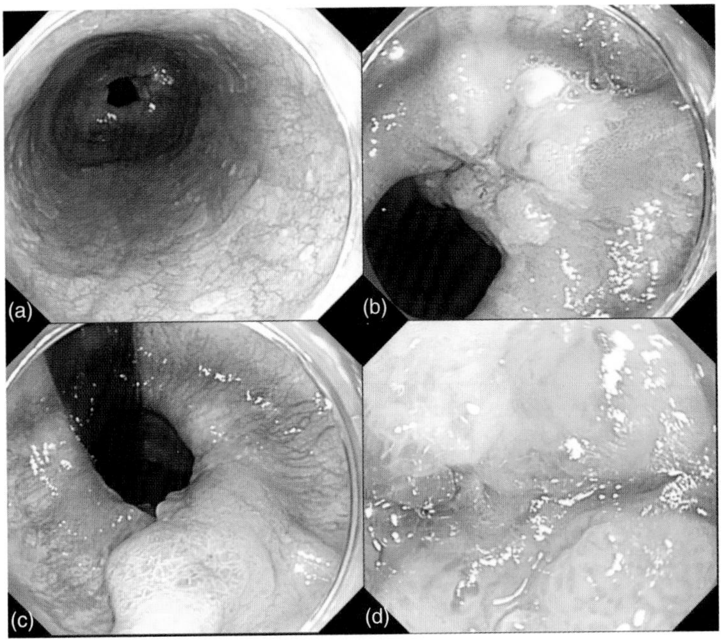

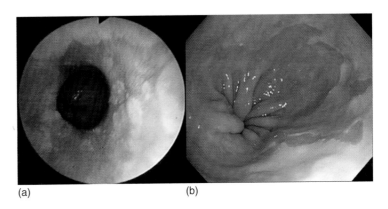

Plate 25.1 Endoscopic image of an esophageal cancer that developed in a Barrett's segment. (a) Shows a long segment Barrett's esophagus with a lesion distally at the right-hand side. (b) Shows a closer view of the lesion which shows retraction and stenosis of the esophagus. (c) Shows the lesion in the retroflexed position. (d) Shows the lesion using the zoom-mode of the endoscope.

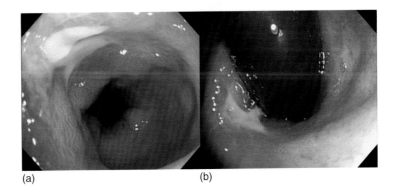

Plate 25.2 (a,b) Endoscopic image of an ulcerating lesion in a Barrett's esophagus. Any ulceration in a Barrett's segment should raise the suspicion of a malignancy but in this case the ulceration was secondary to active reflux esophagitis.

Plate 25.3 Endoscopic images obtained with a fiber-optical endoscope (a) and a high-resolution endoscope (b) showing a clear difference in image quality.

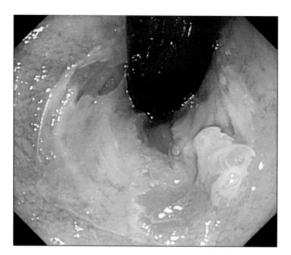

Plate 25.4 Endoscopic image of an early cancer in a Barrett's esophagus detected in the retroflexed position. Subtle lesions at the transition between the lower end of the Barrett's segment and the hiatal hernia are easily overlooked when inspected with the endoscope in the antegrade position only.

CHAPTER 15

Surface Imaging in Barrett's Esophagus: The Role of High-Resolution Endoscopy, Magnifying Endoscopy, and Related Techniques

Mohammed A. Kara, Prateek Sharma, and Jacques J. G. H. M. Bergman

Introduction

The rising incidence of Barrett's esophagus and associated adenocarcinoma has led to the establishment of endoscopic surveillance programs for Barrett's esophagus patients. Since malignancy develops through a metaplasia–dysplasia–cancer sequence, the goal of surveillance is to diagnose and treat dysplasia or early cancer and thus prevent the development of advanced cancer, which is associated with a poor prognosis. One of the challenges facing surveillance programs is the difficulty in detecting dysplasia/early cancer with standard endoscopy. In this chapter, we will discuss the use of high-resolution/magnifying endoscopy in routine endoscopic surveillance for detecting early neoplastic lesions in Barrett's esophagus patients.

What are High-Resolution Endoscopy and Magnifying Endoscopy?

In the last two decades, endoscopes with charge-coupled devices (CCDs), i.e. electronic endoscopes, have largely replaced fiberoptic endoscopes. A CCD is an integrated electrical circuit made of semiconductive material, usually silicon, which is inherently photosensitive. The surface of the CCD is divided into numerous photosensitive elements, better known as pixels. Light photons incident on the semi-conductive device alter the electrical charge in a directly proportionate relationship; i.e. the higher the light intensity (more photons), the higher the generated charge. Each pixel generates and stores electrons in proportion to the number of incident photons on the pixel. The charge stored in all of the pixels is transferred to an amplifier that measures the charge in each pixel. Various methods can be applied for the transfer and read-out of the electrical charge. Description of these methods can be found elsewhere [1]. Different pixels in the same CCD generate variable electrical charges depending on the number of photons received and therefore the information from a CCD is an analog signal. This signal is converted into a binary (i.e. digital) signal by using a computer processor that also converts the received information into a color image for display on a television screen.

Image resolution is the ability to discriminate between two closely adjacent points. For CCD-based instruments, the resolution depends, among other geometrical and electromechanical factors, on the total number of pixels on the CCD surface and on the total number of pixels used to generate the image. The CCDs in standard video endoscopes have 100 000–300 000 pixels [2]. Recently, endoscopes containing CCDs with larger numbers of pixels (600 000–1 000 000) have been introduced and these are called *high-resolution endoscopes*.

Gastrointestinal endoscopes (standard or high resolution) usually have a focal distance with a fixed range (e.g. 1–9 cm). This means that to be in focus, the target area should be within this range from the endoscope and bringing the tip of the endoscope closer to the mucosa results in blurring of the image. This limits the possibility of close detailed inspection of the mucosa, which may be necessary during endoscopy. This limitation can be overcome by two means. First, some endoscopes are equipped with a mechanical system that can be used to move the lens along the longitudinal axis of the endoscope, thus allowing the operator to adjust the focal length of the device (Plate 15.1; color plate section falls between pp. 148–9). When the endoscope is brought in close proximity to the tissue, the operator may manually adjust the focal length using a lever on the head of the endoscope or a food pedal. This maneuver results in *"optical magnification"* (or optical zoom) of the target area, thus allowing inspection of the fine details of a small area. Because of manual adjustment of the focal length, optical magnification allows the use of the total number of pixels and image resolution is preserved. Endoscopes with this feature are called *magnifying endoscopes* or zoom endoscopes. Second, magnification can also be achieved electronically by the video processor. When using this function, the area at the center of the view field is electronically magnified without changing the focal distance, i.e. *"electronic magnification"* or electronic zoom. Only the pixels originally involved in imaging the target area are used to generate the magnified view and therefore, image resolution is not preserved if electronic magnification is used. Higher levels of electronic magnification will thus result in loss of image details.

What can be Achieved by High-Resolution/Magnification Endoscopy?

The main purpose of using high-resolution endoscopy and magnifying endoscopy in the gastrointestinal tract is to detect early neoplastic lesions. Early mucosal lesions may be too small to be discriminated from the surrounding normal tissue by standard instruments. Small mucosal lesions such as diminutive colonic polyps and early lesions in Bar-

rett's esophagus may present in the form of a nodule or erosion of only a few millimeters in diameter. Such small macroscopic alterations in the mucosal topography may be detected by high-resolution endoscopy (Plate 15.2a,b; color plate section falls between pp. 148–9). Early neoplasia may not be readily visible macroscopically. Rather, it may be in the form of irregularities in the microscopic superficial structures that are only visible with optical magnification. With magnification endoscopy, therefore, detailed close-up inspection may aid in detecting abnormalities confined to the mucosal and vascular (micro) structures (Plate 15.3; color plate section falls between pp. 148–9).

Using magnifying endoscopy to investigate large surface areas may be laborious and not optimally effective because it entails investigating the entire area using the magnifying mode and overview of the segment may be lost. Magnification may, however, also be used for detailed inspection of an already suspected lesion. It is known that, in the colon, the type of mucosal pattern is a useful diagnostic tool for identification of precancerous polyps by means of magnifying endoscopy with or without dye-staining [3]. More recently, similar approaches have been evaluated in Barrett's esophagus. However, while there is a widely accepted mucosal pattern classification in the colon, there is no consensus yet in the classification and clinical relevance of mucosal patterns in Barrett's esophagus.

Generally, if used for mucosal and vascular pattern diagnosis, magnifying endoscopy may be a useful adjunct to high-resolution endoscopy and other techniques, such as autofluorescence endoscopy, that are associated with high sensitivity for early lesions but suffer from low specificity. Using magnifying endoscopy for a close-up detailed inspection of areas deemed to be suspicious with such techniques may raise the specificity of endoscopic detection of early lesions by excluding false positive lesions [4]. Magnifying endoscopy can also be useful for the detailed inspection of lesions including accurate delineation of lesion margins prior to endoscopic mucosal resection [5].

What Techniques can Enhance High-Resolution/Magnifying Endoscopy?

High-resolution/magnifying endoscopy can be combined with staining techniques (i.e. chromoendoscopy) in order to achieve a better visualization of the surface details. In the setting of Barrett's esophagus, acetic acid and indigo carmine are the most used staining agents for contrast enhancement. Plate 15.4a–d (color plate section falls between pp. 148–9) shows examples of magnified images of the same area taken by different techniques in Barrett's esophagus. Methylene blue has also been used in Barrett's esophagus but mainly in combination with standard endoscopes and less so with high-resolution/magnifying endoscopy. Recently, an optical contrast-enhancement imaging technique known as narrow band imaging has been developed as a potential alternative to using staining agents [6].

Acetic Acid Chromoendoscopy

Acetic acid, the shortest-chain fatty acid, is a weak acid with a pK_a of 4.8. When sprayed on the mucosal surface, acetic acid interacts with the superficial glycoproteins of the mucosa, predominantly cytokeratins. Due to a change in the pH, the disulfide bonds of these molecules undergo reversible breakdown with subsequent alteration in the tertiary (spatial) structure of these proteins [7]. This configuration change leads to a whitish discoloration of the epithelium (i.e. acetowhite reaction). The acetowhite reaction enhances visualization of mucosal patterns (pits, grooves and epithelial folds) but it also increases the opacity of the surface and thus masks the vascular network. In addition, the mucolytic action of acetic acid further improves visualization of the mucosal details.

Acetic acid has been used since decades for neoplasia detection in the genitourinary tract (cervical intraepithelial neoplasia) [8]. This approach has only recently been introduced in gastrointestinal endoscopy. A small amount (~10 mL) of a dilute solution of acetic acid (1–2%) is applied on the mucosal surface by means of a spray catheter (Plate 15.5; color plate section falls between pp. 148–9). The acetowhite effect can immediately be observed (Plate 15.4d; color plate section falls between pp. 148–9).

Excessive acid application may lead to localized bleeding that may hamper further inspection.

So far, two studies have reported on the use of acetic acid chromoendoscopy (AAC) in combination with magnifying endoscopy in Barrett's esophagus. Both studies concentrated on the detection of the mucosal patterns that may correlate with intestinal metaplasia and did not evaluate areas with dysplasia. Guelrud *et al.* used high-resolution endoscopy (GIF-200Z, Olympus America Inc., Melville, NY; maximum magnification 35-fold) with acetic acid enhancement in 49 patients with short segment Barrett's esophagus (<3 cm) without dysplasia [9]. After review of the mucosal patterns in 129 areas they identified four different patterns: (i) round pits; (ii) circular or oval reticular pits; (iii) fine villous appearance without pits; and (iv) ridged convoluted pattern. High-resolution endoscopy alone identified mucosal patterns in 38% of the examined areas. Contrast enhancement with acetic acid revealed a mucosal pattern in all 129 areas. In this study, intestinal metaplasia could be detected in 0%, 11%, 87%, and 100% in patterns one to four, respectively, suggesting that intestinal metaplasia is mainly characterized by a fine villous or ridged mucosal pattern.

Toyoda *et al.* assessed the value of magnifying endoscopy with AAC (1.5%) for the detection of intestinal metaplasia in the distal esophagus and esophagogastric junction in patients undergoing routine upper endoscopy [10]. The mucosal patterns were classified into three types: (i) normal pits corresponding to gastric-body type mucosa; (ii) slit-reticular pattern, corresponding to gastric cardia mucosa; and (iii) gyrus-villous pattern associated with intestinal metaplasia. The diagnostic value of the type three pattern for intestinal metaplasia in targeted biopsy specimens was as follows: sensitivity 89%, specificity 90%, positive predictive value 85%, negative predictive value 92%, and an overall accuracy of 90% [10].

Indigo Carmine Chromoendoscopy

Indigo carmine is a non-vital staining agent, i.e. it is not absorbed by the mucosal cells, but accumulates in the pits and grooves along the epithelial surface, thus highlighting the superficial mucosal architecture (Plate 15.4c; color plate section falls between pp.

148–9). Its application is relatively simple and can be combined with high-resolution/magnifying endoscopy. Typically, a solution of 0.4% is sprayed on the mucosal surface using a spray catheter. The distribution of the dye is affected by gravity and may therefore be uneven, making the left lateral side of the esophagus (i.e. 6 o'clock in the field of view) difficult to evaluate (Plate 15.6; color plate section falls between pp. 148–9). Excess dye can be immediately aspirated and multiple sprayings and aspirations may be necessary for optimal results.

Sharma *et al.* have demonstrated the feasibility of mucosal pattern detection in Barrett's esophagus by using indigo carmine chromoendoscopy (ICC) in combination with high-resolution/magnifying endoscopy [11]. They found three types of mucosal patterns within the columnar mucosa: (i) ridged/villous; (ii) circular; and (iii) an irregular/distorted pattern. Intestinal metaplasia was found in regular ridged/villous (89%, 24 of 27) and circular patterns (33%, three of nine). Six patients had an irregular/distorted pattern and all had high-grade dysplasia on the corresponding biopsies leading to a 100% identification of high-grade dysplasia based on the distorted irregular mucosal pattern. Eight patients had low-grade dysplasia on target biopsy; all had the ridged/villous pattern, hence identifying low-grade dysplasia was not possible since areas with low-grade dysplasia appeared similar to those with non-dysplastic intestinal metaplasia. These results suggest that magnifying endoscopy with ICC may be used for the detection and follow-up of high-grade dysplasia, but not for low-grade dysplasia.

Methylene Blue Chromoendoscopy

Methylene blue is a vital stain, i.e. it is taken up into the cytoplasm of actively absorbing epithelia and not by non-absorbing epithelia. Methylene blue is therefore absorbed by intestinal epithelia but not by squamous or gastric tissue. For Barrett's esophagus, areas with intestinal metaplasia show a homogenous dark staining pattern, while dysplasia/cancer may reveal irregular (heterogeneous) staining pattern or remain unstained. In expert hands, however, methylene blue chromoendoscopy (MBC) has been conducted successfully with a reported average procedure time prolongation of 6–7 min in randomized studies conducted by expert endoscopists [12,13].

In Barrett's esophagus, MBC has mainly been used with standard endoscopy for topographical detection of staining patterns [12–15]. Details can be found in a previous chapter. In one study, however, this technique was combined with high-resolution endoscopy/magnifying endoscopy for the detection of the mucosal patterns that correspond to intestinal metaplasia. In this study, Endo *et al.* reported the use of high-resolution endoscopy (GIF Q240Z, Olympus Optical Co., Ltd., Tokyo, Japan; maximum magnification 80-fold) followed by methylene blue staining in 30 Barrett's esophagus patients [16]. They identified five different mucosal patterns: (i) small round pits; (ii) straight lines; (iii) long oval pits; (iv) tubular (gyrus-like) pattern; and (v) villous projections. All tubular or villous areas contained intestinal metaplasia. Round pits and straight lines corresponded to gastric fundic type epithelium. In addition, the tubular and villous areas showed absorption of methylene blue, whereas this was lacking in areas with small round pits and/or straight lines.

Narrow Band Imaging

Narrow band imaging (NBI) is a novel endoscopic technique that combines high-resolution/magnifying endoscopy and mucosal contrast enhancement without the use of dye spraying. NBI is based on the phenomenon that the depth of light penetration depends on its wavelength: the longer the wavelength the deeper the penetration. Blue light penetrates only superficially, whereas red light penetrates into deeper layers. The prototype NBI-system (Olympus, Tokyo, Japan) uses a red, green, blue (RGB) sequential endoscopy system containing special NBI RGB-filters with narrowed RGB band-pass ranges, increased relative contribution of blue light, and diminished contribution of red light. NBI in combination with high-resolution/magnifying endoscopy has the ability to reveal the superficial details of the luminal esophageal surface without the need for dye spraying. Plate 15.7a,b (color plate section falls between pp. 148–9) shows a comparison between images of Barrett's mucosa taken with white light endoscopy and those taken with NBI.

Recently, preliminary reports have suggested that NBI improves the recognition of mucosal and vascular patterns in Barrett's esophagus. Kara *et al.* have found that magnified images taken by high-resolution endoscopy-NBI are superior to those taken by high-resolution endoscopy alone in revealing details of the mucosal patterns [17]. In this ongoing study, the preliminary observation was that the mucosal and vascular patterns in Barrett's esophagus obtained by NBI could be classified into two main groups: regular and irregular patterns (Plate 15.7a,b; color plate section falls between pp. 148–9). High-grade dysplasia and early cancer are predominantly found in the irregular patterns [17]. Sharma *et al.* have reported preliminary results of NBI in 24 patients with Barrett's esophagus [18]. They found that all patients with intestinal metaplasia had a fine capillary pattern and a ridge/villous pattern (sensitivity 100%, specificity 80%) whereas all high-grade dysplasia patients had an abnormal capillary pattern (increased number, tortuous, dilated, corkscrew type). Low-grade dysplasia patients had a similar pattern as intestinal metaplasia. All patients with long segment Barrett's esophagus had areas with intestinal metaplasia identified, whereas 10 of 12 (83%) patients with short segment Barrett's esophagus were identified with NBI as having intestinal metaplasia. Another study from Japan has confirmed some of these findings in a limited number of patients [19]. From these preliminary reports it can be concluded that NBI has the ability of surface mucosal and vascular pattern recognition without the need for chromoendoscopy. It provides a detailed image of the capillary and mucosal patterns in Barrett's esophagus and may be a useful clinical tool for the detection of intestinal metaplasia and high-grade dysplasia.

What Dye or Technique to Use?

With the wide range of techniques available for detailed endoscopic inspection of Barrett's esophagus and a relative lack of well-conducted studies in this field, it is not possible to give an evidence-based advice as to which technique is superior. ICC is easy to use but it may be hampered by unequal distribution of the dye over the mucosal surface necessitating multiple sprayings and aspirations. AAC is easier to apply and to interpret since pooling of "the dye" does not obscure visualizing the underlying mucosa as with indigo carmine. The opacity caused by acetic

acid, however, masks the superficial blood vessels making a comprehensive and accurate diagnosis of the vascular morphology difficult. MBC is also operator-dependant and associated with conflicting results when used in an overview mode with standard endoscopes [12–15,20–22]. Methylene blue application has also been recently reported to increase the genetic damage in Barrett's esophagus when followed by tissue exposure to endoscopic light [23]. Based on these practical and safety considerations, we prefer and recommend the use of indigo carmine for performing chromoendoscopy for contras-enhancement in Barrett's esophagus.

NBI has the advantage of high magnification imaging of the surface details without the need for dye staining. Using NBI is operator-friendly and may save time. Instant switching between standard white light endoscopy and NBI requires only a touch of a button. NBI also has the advantage of showing the superficial vascular bed lining the esophageal mucosa since blue light achieves a higher contrast for blood vessels than white light owing to absorption of blue light by hemoglobin. As shown by recent preliminary reports, these vascular patterns can be different in different histological states. The combination of mucosal and vascular pattern diagnosis may eventually prove to be an accurate endoscopic tool that may help target biopsies to areas with suspicious superficial morphology. However, NBI is still in the form of a proto-type available only to a few academic centers around the world. Meanwhile, magnification chromoendoscopy with indigo carmine may be the best alternative.

Remarks and Future Perspective

Visualization of the fine surface structure of the mucosa is an attractive approach to enhance endoscopic diagnosis. Particularly in Barrett's esophagus, which harbors various histopathological subtypes, endoscopists are struggling to distinguish these subtypes using standard techniques. The mucosal patterns in Barrett's esophagus can be seen by chromoendoscopy and high magnification. Studies have already shown that there are different mucosal patterns present in Barrett's esophagus as there is a mosaic of histological subtypes. There is already evidence that certain patterns as detected by magnifying chromoendoscopy are associated with intestinal metaplasia or high-grade dysplasia.

Studies using magnifying chromoendoscopy for mucosal pattern diagnosis in Barrett's esophagus have suffered from three major limitations. First, these studies concentrated on the distinction between normal gastric-type mucosal patterns and those corresponding with intestinal metaplasia. Less attention was given to the mucosal pattern appearance of dysplasia especially high-grade dysplasia, which may be more relevant from a clinical perspective. Second, there is as yet no consensus on the terminology and classification of mucosal patterns. Third, the proposed classifications are difficult to reproduce and interpret because they depend on detecting minute differences in the sizes and shapes of the mucosal pits and ridges. This may reduce inter-observer agreement as suggested in a recent study conducted in Germany [24].

Future studies should focus on developing and testing objective criteria for interpretation of these surface features. For clinical relevance, the primary focus should be on finding and validating criteria that differentiate between dysplastic and non-dysplastic tissues. Since NBI is an optical technique that appears less operator dependant than staining techniques, it may offer a better platform for objective interpretation and interobserver studies.

Prospective clinical studies comparing the various chromoendoscopic techniques with each other and with NBI may shed a light on the real clinically relevant strengths and weaknesses of each technique. In a recent randomized crossover study, high-resolution endoscopy was shown to have a relatively high sensitivity (~80%) for high-grade dysplasia and early cancer in high-risk patients attending a tertiary referral center. The lesions were detected using the overview mode of the high-resolution endoscope without the use of ICC or NBI (unpublished data). ICC and NBI were found to be useful in detecting a limited number of additional lesions with high-grade dysplasia or early cancer that were occult to high-resolution endoscopy alone. ICC and NBI were also found to improve the detailed inspection and delineation of lesions. This suggests that these techniques in combination with magnifying endoscopy may be more suitable for targeted inspection of areas of interest with the Barrett's segment. A more appropriate indication is maybe to combine these techniques with magnifying endoscopy for detailed examination of the mucosal and vascular patterns of suspicious areas that has been detected by high-resolution endoscopy. This may confirm the suspicion for dysplasia and help in precise targeting of biopsies to the most suspicious areas. These techniques can also be used prior to endoscopic mucosal resection for more accurate delineation of lesion margins.

Summary

High-resolution endoscopes that contain CCDs with a high number of pixels are currently available. These endoscopes may be used for the early detection of minute mucosal lesions in Barrett's esophagus. Magnifying endoscopy may further enhance the efficacy of high-resolution endoscopy. Magnifying endoscopy enables the detection of abnormalities of the surface mucosal and vascular pattern, thus enabling the distinction of early abnormalities that may accompany neoplastic transformation. Chromoendoscopy with various staining agents may enhance the surface structures and can be used with magnifying endoscopy. As yet, these techniques have only been used in a limited number of studies that focused mainly on the classification of "benign" mucosal patterns, i.e. the distinction between gastric-body, gastric cardia, and intestinal metaplasia. Chromoendoscopic techniques suffer from being labor-intensive and operator-dependant for optimal results. NBI is a new optical technique that enhances the mucosal and vascular patterns without dye spraying. This technique seems to be promising and preliminary studies have demonstrated that areas with high-grade dysplasia have distinct mucosal and vascular patterns. Future studies should focus on creating a clinically relevant classification of the mucosal and vascular patterns in Barrett's esophagus in order to distinguish between dysplastic and non-dysplastic patterns. Prospective studies should be conducted to compare the various techniques in order to determine the optimal setting for each technique.

References

1. Sivak MV, Jr. Video endoscopy, the electronic endoscopy unit and integrated imaging. *Baillieres Clin Gastroenterol* 1991;**5**(1):1–18.

2. Bruno MJ. Magnification endoscopy, high resolution endoscopy, and chromoscopy; towards a better optical diagnosis. *Gut* 2003;**52**(suppl 4):7–11.

3. Kudo S, Tamura S, Nakajima T *et al.* Diagnosis of colorectal tumorous lesions by magnifying endoscopy. *Gastrointest Endosc* 1996;**44**(1):8–14.

4. Kara M, Peters F, Fockens P *et al.* Video autofluorescence imaging (AFI) followed by narrow band imaging (NBI) for detection of high grade dysplasia (HGD) and early cancer (EC) in Barrett's esophagus (BE) [abstract]. *Endoscopy* 2004;**36**(suppl I):A7.

5. Ishiyama A, Fujisaki J, Hosaka H *et al.* NBI enables accurate enodoscopic diagnosis of early gastric cancer [abstract]. *Gut* 2004;**53**(suppl VI):A7.

6. Gono K, Obi T, Yamaguchi M *et al.* Appearance of enhanced tissue features in narrow-band endoscopic imaging. *J Biomed Opt* 2004;**9**(3):568–77.

7. Lambert R, Rey JF, Sankaranarayanan R. Magnification and chromoscopy with the acetic acid test. *Endoscopy* 2003;**35**(5):437–45.

8. Gaffikin L, Lauterbach M, Blumenthal PD. Performance of visual inspection with acetic acid for cervical cancer screening: a qualitative summary of evidence to date. *Obstet Gynecol Surv* 2003;**58**(8):543–50.

9. Guelrud M, Herrera I, Essenfeld H *et al.* Enhanced magnification endoscopy: a new technique to identify specialized intestinal metaplasia in Barrett's esophagus. *Gastrointest Endosc* 2001;**53**(6):559–65.

10. Toyoda H, Rubio C, Befrits R *et al.* Detection of intestinal metaplasia in distal esophagus and esophagogastric junction by enhanced-magnification endoscopy. *Gastrointest Endosc* 2004;**59**(1):15–21.

11. Sharma P, Weston AP, Topalovski M *et al.* Magnification chromoendoscopy for the detection of intestinal metaplasia and dysplasia in Barrett's oesophagus. *Gut* 2003;**52**(1):24–7.

12. Canto MI, Setrakian S, Willis J *et al.* Methylene blue-directed biopsies improve detection of intestinal metaplasia and dysplasia in Barrett's esophagus. *Gastrointest Endosc* 2000;**51**(5):560–8.

13. Ragunath K, Krasner N, Raman VS *et al.* A randomized, prospective cross-over trial comparing methylene blue-directed biopsy and conventional random biopsy for detecting intestinal metaplasia and dysplasia in Barrett's esophagus. *Endoscopy* 2003;**35**(12):998–1003.

14. Sharma P, Topalovski M, Mayo MS *et al.* Methylene blue chromoendoscopy for detection of short-segment Barrett's esophagus. *Gastrointest Endosc* 2001;**54**(3):289–93.

15. Kiesslich R, Hahn M, Herrmann G *et al.* Screening for specialized columnar epithelium with methylene blue: chromoendoscopy in patients with Barrett's esophagus and a normal control group. *Gastrointest Endosc* 2001;**53**(1):47–52.

16. Endo T, Awakawa T, Takahashi H *et al.* Classification of Barrett's epithelium by magnifying endoscopy. *Gastrointest Endosc* 2002;**55**(6):641–7.

17. Kara M, Ennahachi M, Fockens P *et al.* Narrow-band imaging (NBI) in Barrett's esophagus (BE): what features are relevant for the detection of high-grade dysplasia (HGD) and early cancer (EC)? *Gastroenterology* 2004;**126**(4):A50.

18. Sharma P, McGregor D, Cherian R, Weston A. Use of narrow band imaging, a novel imaging technique, to detect intestinal metaplasia and high-grade dysplasia in patients with Barrett's esophagus [abstract]. *Gastrointest Endosc* 2003;**57**(5):AB77.

19. Hamamoto Y, Endo T, Nosho K *et al.* Usefulness of narrow-band imaging endoscopy for diagnosis of Barrett's esophagus. *J Gastroenterol* 2004;**39**(1):14–20.

20. Dave U, Shousha S, Westaby D. Methylene blue staining: is it really useful in Barrett's esophagus? *Gastrointest Endosc* 2001;**53**(3):333–5.

21. Egger K, Werner M, Meining A *et al.* Biopsy surveillance is still necessary in patients with Barrett's oesophagus despite new endoscopic imaging techniques. *Gut* 2003;**52**(1):18–23.

22. Wo JM, Ray MB, Mayfield-Stokes S *et al.* Comparison of methylene blue-directed biopsies and conventional biopsies in the detection of intestinal metaplasia and dysplasia in Barrett's esophagus: a preliminary study. *Gastrointest Endosc* 2001;**54**(3):294–301.

23. Olliver JR, Wild CP, Sahay P *et al.* Chromoendoscopy with methylene blue and associated DNA damage in Barrett's oesophagus. *Lancet* 2003;**362**(9381):373–4.

24. Meining A, Rosch T, Kiesslich R *et al.* Inter- and intraobserver variability of magnification chromoendoscopy for detecting specialized intestinal metaplasia at the gastroesophageal junction. *Endoscopy* 2004;**36**(2):160–4.

CHAPTER 16

Emerging Techniques: Spectroscopy

Stephan M. Wildi and Michael B. Wallace

Abstract

Screening and surveillance of Barrett's esophagus may prevent esophageal adenocarcinoma by detecting precursor lesions. In most cases, however, dysplasia is invisible to the eye of the endoscopist. Therefore, surveillance requires extensive random biopsies and histologic examination of the excised tissue for dysplasia. This biopsy strategy has several limitations including sampling errors, increased time and cost of endoscopy, and limited reliability of histological interpretation of dysplasia. Spectroscopic methods have the potential to overcome many of these limitations by rapidly and safely evaluating wide regions of tissue for dysplasia without required excision of the tissue and providing a way to quantify cellular and molecular changes associated with neoplasia.

The basis of spectroscopy is to objectively quantify the color and brightness of light and use this information to detect changes within the mucosa that are too subtle to be appreciated by the naked eye. In addition, spectroscopic analysis can extract information that is outside the visible range including measurement of nuclear size, morphology, and density. Most spectroscopic techniques are initially developed and tested using optical fiber-probes. These probes have several advantages including ease of passage through the accessory channel of standard diagnostic endoscopes and highly predictable geometry between fibers, which provide the source of light, and those that deliver collected light to the detector. These factors make point-probes highly suitable for research and technology development; however, they are limited by the small surface area they examine at the tip of the probe. Methods developed with fiber-probe technology can usually be translated into broad-area imaging systems compatible with current video-endoscopes.

Although many types of spectroscopy have been applied for examining gastrointestinal disease, the four that have been used for examining dysplasia are fluorescence spectroscopy, reflectance spectroscopy, Raman spectroscopy and light-scattering spectroscopy (LSS). Fluorescence spectroscopy is based on the principle that certain molecules of gastrointestinal cells called fluorophores emit light of one wavelength (color) when stimulated by light of another wavelength. The term autofluorescence refers to the detection of endogenous molecules (fluorophores) that have the ability to fluorescence when stimulated with a certain wavelength of light. Fluorescence can also be stimulated by giving exogenous fluorophores; typically porphyrin compounds or their precursors. Dysplasia can be distinguished from normal or inflamed tissue based on differential concentrations (and thus spectra) of fluorphores such as porphyrins, collagen, nicotinamide adenine denucleotide (NADH) and flavine adenine dinucleotide (FADH), which are either increased or decreased in concentration in the setting of dysplasia.

Reflectance spectroscopy quantifies the color (wavelength) and intensity of reflected light. Unlike fluorescence spectroscopy, the reflected light always maintains the same wavelength although it differs in the degree of absorption and reflection. The spectrum of reflected light is altered by the tissue through absorption of certain wavelengths, most notably hemoglobin; thus providing information of vascularity and oxygenation status.

LSS measures the extent to which photons of light are scattered by structures they encounter. Dense objects in the cell scatter light to different degrees depending on the size, density, and number of the object (such as a nucleus) and the wavelength of light used. Based on mathematical modeling, LSS is capable of determining the size, density, and number of objects (such as nuclei) in epithelium and classifying dysplasia based on standard histological patterns of nuclear morphology and crowding. The ability to characterize dysplastic and non-dysplastic tissue is further improved by combining these three spectroscopic techniques (called trimodal spectroscopy).

Raman spectroscopy is one of the most recent techniques for evaluating dysplasia. Raman is based on detecting characteristic spectral "fingerprints" of molecules in the tissue based on how the molecules vibrate in response to light energy. The technique is very powerful in that almost all molecules give off some Raman spectra. Unfortunately, the Raman signal is very weak and can only be detected with very sensitive and precise instrumentation but offers significant promise for future development.

Promising clinical results demonstrate the ability of spectroscopic techniques to provide useful information for disease classification in a non-invasive manner. Although spectroscopic techniques have advanced substantially from their initial *in vitro* and animal studies, there remains much work to be done before these systems can be integrated into routine endoscopy. Point-probe technology continues to be a highly useful system for understanding the interaction of light and tissue, and developing algorithms for detecting disease. As these methods are developed, they can be adapted to more clinically suitable techniques such as broad area spectroscopy and imaging.

Introduction

The incidence of esophageal adenocarcinomas in the USA has been rising since the 1970s. Barrett's esophagus as a premalignant lesion is recognized in the majority of cases of adenocarcinomas of the esophagus and esophagogastric junction. A common phenotype of esophageal adenocarcinomas and all epithelial cancers is the progression from normal mucosa, through a stage of dysplasia, to cancer. In the last three decades, diagnostic gastrointestinal endoscopy has undoubtedly altered the approach to

precancerous and cancerous lesions of the gastrointestinal tract. There is strong evidence that endoscopic screening and surveillance can prevent gastrointestinal cancer by detecting precursor lesions of cancer. Three difficulties arise in the clinical diagnosis of dysplasia. Firstly, in many cases dysplasia is invisible to the eye of the endoscopist and endoscopic detection is largely dependent on the recognition of gross architectural changes like nodular lesions. Abnormalities of a microscopic nature, such as dysplasia in Barrett's esophagus, are usually unrecognizable by macroscopic inspection. Therefore, surveillance in these situations requires extensive random biopsies and histologic examination of the excised tissue for dysplasia. This biopsy strategy may overlook areas of dysplasia and is limited by sampling errors. Secondly, dysplastic changes within visible lesions can usually not be distinguished endoscopically from the surrounding non-dysplastic tissue. Histologic evaluation of biopsy specimens is required for accurate diagnosis of these lesions as well. Reliance on histology imposes a time delay between endoscopy and diagnosis, severely limiting the diagnostic accuracy of the endoscopic procedure since suspicious sites cannot be oversampled or treated at the time of endoscopy. Thirdly, there is also significant interobserver disagreement between pathologists in diagnosing dysplasia [1,2].

New optical methods have the potential to overcome many of these limitations by rapidly and safely evaluating wide regions for dysplasia without requiring excision of the tissue. Spectroscopy, the analysis of the wavelength (color) and intensity (brightness) of light, is one of these new emerging techniques. It can objectively quantify the color and brightness of light and uses this information to detect changes within the mucosa that are too subtle to be appreciated by the naked eye as well as evaluate wavelengths of light outside the visible range (infrared and ultraviolet). A great advantage of spectroscopic measurements is that they can be implemented *in vivo*, thus providing information about tissue in its native state, free of distortion introduced by tissue excision and processing. Therefore, spectroscopic techniques can be used to provide information about tissue morphology and biochemistry.

There are primarily two methods for measuring tissue fluorescence during endoscopy. Most spectroscopic techniques are initially developed and tested using optical fiber-probes. These probes have several advantages including ease of passage through the accessory channel of standard diagnostic endoscopes and highly predictable geometry between fibers, which provide the source of light, and those that deliver collected light to the detector. These factors make point-probes highly suitable for research and technology development; however, they are limited by the small surface area they examine at the tip of the probe. To overcome these limitations, fluorescence imaging systems were developed with the advantage of the visualization of a much larger surface area of the mucosa.

Technology

Limitations of Standard Endoscopy and Histopathology

Endoscopic detection of dysplasia relies on the recognition of visible lesions or random sampling of tissue (biopsy), as in the case of Barrett's esophagus. Endoscopy alone can neither reliably detect regions of invisible or flat dysplasia nor distinguish dysplasia from non-dysplastic changes within visible lesions. Histological examination of the excised material is required to diagnose and locate dysplasia. Random biopsy techniques are subject to sampling errors and increased risk because of long procedure time and multiple biopsy sites.

Although the microscopic examination of tissue remains the gold standard for pathologic assessment, it is not without its limitations. Histopathologic diagnosis of dysplasia often relies on the observation of particular features of the overall tissue morphology and of the morphometry of specific cellular organelles, such as the nucleus. The nuclei become enlarged, crowded and hyperchromatic. Normal nuclei have spheroid shape with a characteristic size in the range 4–7 μm. In precancerous and cancerous tissues, the cells proliferate and their nuclei can become as large as 20 μm, occupying almost the entire cell volume. Although the gross and microscopic appearance of dysplasia in different organs and different types of epithelium can vary significantly, these nuclear morphological features are common to all types of epithelial dysplasia. Based on these features, lesions are categorized as non-dysplastic, indefinite for dysplasia, or low-grade dysplasia (LGD) or high-grade dysplasia (HGD) [3]. The histopathologic diagnosis of dysplasia is problematic because there is poor interobserver agreement on the classification of a particular specimen, even among expert gastrointestinal pathologists [1,2]. One reason for such variation may be the subjective nature of determining increased nuclear size, nuclear crowding, or architectural disorganization [3].

The biochemical changes that take place during the development of neoplastic lesions are not typically considered during histopathologic diagnosis, since the cutting and processing of tissue before examination likely alters its biochemical state. As a result, potentially significant information is lost in this type of analysis.

New Techniques for Detecting Dysplasia—Optical Biopsy

When performing endoscopy, light emitted from the endoscope's light source is reflected back from the luminal gastrointestinal tract to optical fibers or charged-coupled devices (CCDs, i.e. CCD video-chips) and projected onto video-monitors. During each procedure, the endoscopist can evaluate indirectly the color and brightness of the gastrointestinal tract and thereby distinguish normal mucosa from abnormal tissue. Spectroscopy follows the same principle by objectively quantifying the color and brightness of light. This information can be used to detect changes within the gastrointestinal mucosa that are too fine to be noticed by the normal eye. Because of its ability to make histological-like characterizations of tissue by using light, spectroscopic techniques have been referred to as "optical biopsy."

Although spectroscopy is unlikely to replace tissue biopsy anytime soon, many aspects of spectroscopy offer advantages over standard histopathology. By providing a more quantitative measure of features, such as nuclear size and number, or changes in collagen, porphyrin or tryptophan concentrations, spectroscopy may enhance the current qualitative measures used in pathologic diagnosis. Different spectroscopic techniques can be used to provide information about tissue biochemistry and oxygenation. The ability to extract *in vivo* information about specific biochemical changes that take place during the development of neoplasia could provide a rich source of diagnostic information, and further our understanding of some of the basic processes involved. In addition, spectroscopic analysis during endoscopic procedures has the potential to overcome the limitations of sampling error by directing the endoscopist to biopsy areas of the gastrointestinal mucosa that are most likely to contain dysplasia.

Interaction Between Light and Tissue

Light of any source directed towards a mucosal surface may undergo one of the following interactions based on the physical properties of light and tissue: (a) reflection by the tissue, as it occurs when the endoscopist visualizes the mucosa by fiberoptic or video-endoscopy; (b) absorption by the tissue and conversion to another form of energy such as heat; or (c) absorption by the tissue and re-emission as another wavelength (color) of light. This last property is referred to as fluorescence. Finally photons of light can be scattered within the tissue and return (termed "backscattering") or they can be transmitted through the tissue. The time required for a photon to contact the tissue and return to a collecting device can be also measured, allowing two-dimensional (or tomographic) details to be elicited. Lastly, photons of light cause most tissue molecules to vibrate, thus transferring some energy to the molecules and reducing the energy and wavelength of the light; hence the Raman shift. Many of the properties of light–tissue interaction can be exploited to infer tissue characteristics or create anatomic images during endoscopic procedures.

Types of Spectroscopy

Although many types of spectroscopy have been applied for examining gastrointestinal disease, the ones that have been used for examining dysplasia are point-probe spectroscopy with diffuse reflectance spectroscopy, laser- or light-induced fluorescence spectroscopy, light-scattering spectroscopy (LSS), and fluorescence imaging.

Point-Probe Spectroscopy

Diffuse Reflectance Spectroscopy

Reflectance spectroscopy measures quantitatively the color and intensity of reflected light. Unlike autofluorescence spectroscopy, the reflected light always maintains the same wavelength, although differed wavelengths are absorbed and reflected to different degrees. A typical example is provided by hemoglobin. When illuminated with white light, oxygenated hemoglobin absorbs much of the blue light, and reflects back only the red light, give blood its characteristic color (Fig. 16.1). De-oxygenated hemoglobin absorbs a higher degree of red light, thus appears bluer when illuminated with white light. Reflectance spectroscopy thus provides information about tissue hemoglobin concentrations and oxygenation status, of interest because of the property of malignant tissue to promote angiogenesis.

Laser- or Light-Induced Fluorescence Spectroscopy

All tissues exhibit endogenous fluorescence (autofluorescence) when exposed to light of a certain wavelength. Fluorescence spectroscopy is based on the principle that certain molecules of gastrointestinal cells, called fluorophores, emit light when stimu-

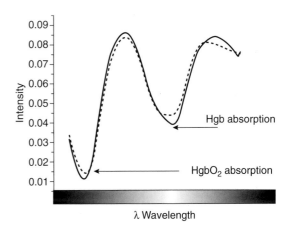

Fig. 16.1 Reflectance spectra. Diffuse white light has an equal intensity of each color in the visible spectrum. When white light encounters tissue, some wavelengths are absorbed and others are reflected. Hemoglobin (Hbg) is the most significant absorber of light, creating the "dips" seen in this figure due to absorption of blue light by oxygenated hemoglobin. This gives blood its characteristic red color (white light less the blue component). Key: solid line, predicted by mathematical model; dashed line, actual reflectance spectrum.

Table 16.1 Fluorescence characteristics of endogenous fluorophores.

Fluorophore	Peak excitation (nm)	Peak emission (nm)
NADH	340	470
FADH	460	520
Collagen	335	390
Porphyrin	390	630–680
Elastin	285	350
Tryptophan	305	340

FADH, flavine adenine dinucleotide; NADH, nicotinamide adenine denucleotide.

lated by light (excitation). During this process energy is transferred to the molecule, hence the wavelength of the emitted light is longer (lower energy) than the excitation wavelength. Among the most relevant fluorophores in the gastrointestinal tract are the reduced form of nicotinamide adenine denucleotide (NADH), flavine adenine dinucleotide (FADH), collagen, porphyrins, and tryptophan. Each of these fluorophores has its characteristic excitation and emission spectrum (Table 16.1). The success of autofluorescence spectroscopy as a technique for detecting dysplastic changes is based on the observation that the development of dysplasia is accompanied by modification in the biochemical composition of tissue and consequently changes of the concentration of certain fluorophores. Autofluorescence of tissue is induced by monochromatic light, mostly generated by lasers, or by filtered white light.

In contrast to endogenous fluorophores which give off a weak signal, exogenous fluorophores, such as porphyrin compounds, can be administered topically or intravenously to enhance the fluorescence effect. Exogenous fluorophores are specifically retained in neoplastic tissue and exhibit an induced fluorescence signal of much higher intensity. Among different sensitizers, porphyrins have been best studied for application in fluorescence spectroscopy. Porphyrins are products of the heme biosynthetic pathway. The major limitation of exogenous sensiti-

zation with porphyrins is their photosensitizing property with prolonged skin photosensitivity. Newer agents with shorter half-life are more promising (e.g. 5-aminolevulinic acid [5-ALA]).

One major difficulty in measuring fluorescence spectra is the background generated by scattering and absorption. To remove these distortions, some investigators analyze the fluorescence spectra in combination with information from the corresponding reflectance spectra, which allows "subtraction" of this background to leave "intrinsic fluorescence" [4]. The success of this simple model is predicated on the fact that fluorescence and reflectance spectra collected from a specific site using the same light delivery/collection geometry undergo similar distortions. By extracting the intrinsic (undistorted) tissue fluorescence, changes in tissue biochemistry can be isolated in a more sensitive and specific manner.

Multiexcitation Fluorescence Spectroscopy
Different fluorophores are excited by different wavelengths of light. The optimal excitation wavelength for detecting dysplasia and discriminating dysplasia from non-dysplastic or normal mucosa remains unknown. A significant technical advance in fluorescence spectroscopy was made with the development of a fast multiexcitation system capable of exciting the tissue with up to 11 different wavelengths in less than 1 s [4,5]. The excitation light source of this rapid multiexcitation system pumps 10 dye cuvettes precisely mounted on a rapidly rotating wheel. In this manner, 11 different excitation wavelengths are obtained and delivered to the optical fiber-probe. The researchers are now able to collect a wide array of fluorescence spectra and determine the optimal excitation wavelength or combination of wavelengths.

Time-Resolved Fluorescence Spectroscopy
In addition to specific excitation and emission wavelengths, different fluorophores fade or decay their fluorescence at different rates. Hence, the difference between normal and abnormal tissue can be enhanced by measuring fluorescence at different times (often measured in nanoseconds) after excitation. This technique, termed "time-resolved fluores-

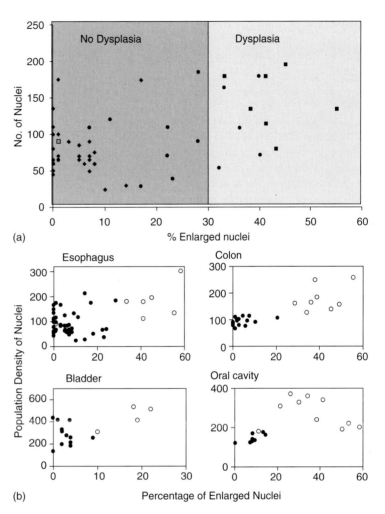

Fig. 16.2 (a) Light-scattering spectroscopy (LSS) in patients with Barrett's esophagus. Each point represents a single biopsy site. The number of nuclei and percentage of enlarged (>10 μm) is plotted. The color indicates the consensus pathological diagnosis. The graph demonstrates that LSS can accurately detect dysplasia by the fact that dysplastic sites have increased number and size of nuclei (upper right corner) compared to non-dysplastic sites (lower left corner). Key: (◆) normal histological diagnosis; (▨) indefinite histological diagnosis; (■) dysplasia. Reproduced with permission from Wallace *et al.* [9]. (b) The same principal can be applied to detect dysplasia at other sites such as the colon, bladder, and oral cavity. Key: (●) no dysplasia; (○) dysplasia or CIS. Reproduced with permission from Backman *et al.* [8]

cence," has been used to increase the accuracy of detecting dysplasia in Barrett's esophagus [6].

Light-Scattering Spectroscopy

Light propagation in tissue is governed by scattering and absorption. LSS measures the extent to which the angular path of photons of light is altered by structures (scatterers) they encounter. Like a steel ball in a pinball machine, photons encounter many structures in their way and bounce forward, backward, up, down, and sideways. The scattering in tissue depends on the scatterer's size, the number of the scatterers, and the wavelength of the incident light. The primary scattering centers are thought to be the collagen fiber network of the extracellular matrix,

the mitochondria, cell nuclei, and other intracellular structures. By mathematical modeling, the number, size, and optical density of cellular structures (such as nuclei), can be determined by measuring the diffuse reflected light from epithelial surfaces [7]. This phenomenon has been exploited during endoscopic procedures to determine the number of nuclei, the size of nuclei, and the degree of crowding of nuclei in patients with dysplastic changes in Barrett's esophagus, colon polyps, bladder, and oral cavity [4,8,9] (Fig. 16.2). These studies have demonstrated that light scattering can accurately measure nuclear size, detected increased nuclear size and variability in dysplasia, and accurately and reliably characterize different grades of dysplasia with less interobserver variability than routine pathology. Unlike fluorescence, LSS uses a broad range of light, such as white light, to detect changes over the entire visible spectrum.

Trimodal Spectroscopy

Reflectance spectroscopy, laser-induced autofluorescence spectroscopy, and LSS provide quantitative information that characterizes either biochemical or morphological aspects of tissue that can be significantly altered during the development of neoplasia. The ability to characterize dysplastic and non-dysplastic tissue is improved by combining the information provided by each of the spectroscopic techniques, obtained simultaneously with one system (Plate 16.1; color plate section falls between pp. 148–9) an approach named *trimodal spectroscopy*. When a spectroscopic classification is consistent with at least two of the three analysis methods, HGD is identified with very high sensitivity and specificity.

Raman Spectroscopy

Raman spectroscopy measures the vibration that light can induce in most molecules in the tissue. Since some of the light energy is transferred to the molecule in this process, the light emitted back from the tissue is reduced in energy and has a longer wavelength. This "shift" was first described by Dr. C. V. Raman in 1928, hence the name. Near-infrared light is typically used to excite the tissue. There are several advantages to Raman spectroscopy compared with other methods including: (i) decreased background signal from the tissue; (ii) less laser-induced photo-thermal degradation; and (iii) deeper penetration into soft tissues. Raman spectroscopy has recently been applied to the detection of Barrett's associated dysplasia with very promising results [10]. An excellent review is provided by Wong Kee Song and Marcon [11].

Fluorescence Imaging

Analogous to point-probe spectroscopy, fluorescence imaging (or fluorescence endoscopy) can use the detection of autofluorescence or exogenous induced fluorescence. In contrast to point-probe spectroscopy, fluorescence imaging permits full inspection of the area at risk. In that way, large areas of tissue surface are screened in a blue-light modus. Whenever selective fluorescence of abnormal tissue (red) appears, optical-guided biopsies can be taken in the white-light mode. Several endogenous fluorophores can be used to detect specific autofluorescence of dysplastic or malignant tissue. They can be used either systemically (by intravenous injection or oral ingestion) or by applying the solution directly on Barrett's mucosa with the help of a special spray catheter. The advantage of drug-induced fluorescence is that the fluorescent signal generated by these exogenous fluorophores is typically stronger than autofluorescence and can be detected by simpler and cheaper instruments. Among exogenous fluorophores, 5-ALA is the most interesting substance for fluorescence diagnosis. 5-ALA is converted intracellularly into the photoactive compound protoporphyrin IX (PPIX). PPIX is associated with a significantly higher tumor selectivity compared to other exogenous fluorophores used in fluorescence imaging (e.g. photophrin) [12]. Furthermore, compared to other exogenous fluorophores skin sensitivity is reduced to 24–48 h [13,14].

Technical Background of Spectroscopy
Point-Probe Spectroscopy

Spectroscopic systems require an excitation light source and a detector or spectrometer to analyze the light that returns from the tissue. Standard desktops or laptop computers are coupled to the system to store, analyze, and display the resulting spectra.

Light Sources   For reflectance spectroscopy and LSS, standard white-light lamps, such as Xenon-flash lamps, are used. For laser-induced autofluorescence spectroscopy, light of a single color (monochromatic light) is used to excite the tissue. Monochromatic light is best achieved by laser light, although light of a narrow range of wavelengths can also be produced by filtered white light. Some fluorophores, such as collagen, are best excited by ultraviolet of blue light (337–370 nm). Others are better excited by longer wavelengths (see Table 16.1). Commonly used lasers in spectroscopy are helium cadmium lasers (325 nm) and nitrogen lasers (337 nm). Using single wavelengths provides only information regarding specific tissue molecules. A significant technical advance was made with the development of a multiexcitation laser capable of exciting the tissue with up to 11 different wavelengths (from 337 to 505 nm) in less than 1 s (Plate 16.1; color plate section falls between pp. 148–9). Lasers used for spectroscopy do deliver very low energies, so tissue is generally not damaged by the spectroscopic investigation.

Optical Fibers Point-probe spectroscopy can either use a single optical fiber with a beam splitter to separate the excitation light from the light returning from the tissue or a bundle of 7–10 optical fibers with dedicated excitation and collection fibers. The array of optical fibers in the bundle is typically designed with a central excitation fiber, which delivers light to the tissue, surrounded by 6–9 collection fibers that transmit light back to a detector. An outer plastic sheath protects the optical fiber. Both ends are usually polished to reduce internal reflection and light scattering. The entire apparatus consisting of fibers, protective sheath, and polished ends is referred to as an optical probe. These probes are 1–2 mm in diameter, and fit easily through the instrument channel of standard diagnostic endoscopes.

Detection Devices A light detector or spectrometer is used to measure the intensity of the light emitted from the tissue. In order to characterize a broad array of wavelengths, a grating splits the emission light from the tissue onto the detector surface. The detector usually consists of an array of diodes coupled with an optical multichannel analyzer, which measure the intensity of each emission wavelength. Because the intensity of the excitation wavelength is exponentially greater than all other emission wavelengths, a filter is used to obscure the signal produced at the excitation wavelength. For example, if 337 nm excitation light is used, then the 337 nm emission light is blocked by the long-pass filter (allows passage of all longer wavelengths), and all longer wavelengths are analyzed.

Fluorescence Imaging

Fluorescence endoscopy is performed with special endoscopes, which are connected to a light source delivering white and blue light. During endoscopy, it is possible to easily switch between the conventional white-light mode and the blue-light mode, permitting a rapid survey of wide areas of the mucosa. To date, there are two devices commercially available for the gastrointestinal tract (D-Light; Storz, Germany, and LIFE-GI; Xillix, Canada). Both of these systems require the use of glass-fiber endoscopes. The development of video-endoscopes is underway.

The LIFE-GI system uses blue-light excitation (400–450 nm) provided by a filtered high-pressure mercury lamp. Fluorescence is picked up by two intensified CCD cameras for detection of selected fluorescence emission bands in the green (490–560 nm) and in the red (630–750 nm). The fluorescence information is processed and displayed as a real-time, false-color image in which normal mucosa appears green and abnormal tissue appears red. In a newer GI-prototype (LIFE II system) the wavelength ranges of excitation and fluorescence processing have been modified [13]. In addition to blue-light illumination, the tissue is excited simultaneously with red-near-infrared light. This red-near-infrared reflectance image serves as reference to correct non-uniform illumination distribution and unequal fluorescence collection caused by irregular tissue surface and changing endoscope angles. Preliminary experience demonstrated better contrast between diseased and normal tissue.

The D-Light system uses violet-blue-light excitation (375–440 nm) provided by a short-arc xenon lamp. Fluorescence imaging detection makes use of a special observation filter and a CCD camera with three channels in the green, red, and blue wavelength ranges. The main application field of this system is photodynamic diagnosis using 5-ALA. The system can also be modified for use in the autofluorescence diagnosis.

Clinical Results of Spectroscopy

Point-Probe Spectroscopy

Different authors have investigated the use of spectroscopy in the detection of neoplastic changes of the esophagus (Table 16.2 [4,6,9,15–22]). Light-induced autofluorescence spectroscopy [15,16]

Table 16.2 Clinical data of point-probe spectroscopy in neoplastic disease of the esophagus.

Author	Setting	Patients (n)	Specimen (n)	Technique	Sensitivity (%)	Specificity (%)
Panjehpour et al. [17]	Normal esophagus vs. esophageal cancer	32	134	Laser-induced autofluorescence spectroscopy	100	98
Von-Dinh et al. [19]	Normal esophagus vs. esophageal cancer	48	>200	Laser-induced autofluorescence spectroscopy	n.c.	n.c.
Stael von Holstein et al. [21]	Normal esophagus vs. BE vs. esophageal cancer (in vitro)	7	145	Laser-induced fluorescence spectroscopy (Photofrin)	n.c.	n.c.
Mayinger et al. [15]	Normal esophagus vs. esophageal cancer	11		Light-induced autofluorescence spectroscopy	n.c.	n.c.
Vo-Dinh et al. [20]	Normal esophagus vs. BE or vs. esophageal carcinoma	70	114	Laser-induced autofluorescence spectroscopy	n.c.	n.c.
Panjehpour et al. [18]	Non-dysplastic BE vs. BE with HGD	36	308	Laser-induced autofluorescence spectroscopy	n.c.	96
	BE with LGD vs. BE with HGD	36	308	Laser-induced autofluorescence spectroscopy	n.c.	100
	Non-dysplastic BE and LGD vs. LGD with focal HGD	36	308	Laser-induced autofluorescence spectroscopy	28	n.c.
	Non-dysplastic BE and LGD vs. HGD	36	308	Laser-induced autofluorescence spectroscopy	90	n.c.
Bourg-Heckly et al. [16]	Normal esophagus and BE vs. dysplastic BE and cancer	24	218	Light-induced autofluorescence spectroscopy	86	95
Wallace et al. [9]	Non-dysplastic BE vs.dysplastic BE	13	76	Light-scattering	90	90
Georgakoudi et al. [4]	Non-dysplastic BE vs. dysplastic BE	16	40	Trimodal spectroscopy	93	100
	Non-dysplastic BE and LGD vs. BE with HGD	16	40	Trimodal spectroscopy	100	100
Brand et al. [22]	Non-dysplastic BE vs. BE with HGD	20	97	Laser-induced fluorescence spectroscopy (5-ALA)	77	71
Ortner et al. [6]	Non-dysplastic BE vs. dysplastic BE	53	141	Time-resolved fluorescence spectroscopy (5-ALA)	76	63

5-ALA, 5-aminolevulinic acid; BE, Barrett's esophagus; LGD, low-grade dysplasia; HGD, high-grade dysplasia; n.c., not calculated.

and laser-induced autofluorescence spectroscopy [17–20], laser-induced fluorescence spectroscopy with exogenous fluorophores [21,22], LSS [4,9] and trimodal spectroscopy [4], and time-resolved fluorescence spectroscopy [6] were evaluated. Early reports concentrated on the distinction between normal and cancerous changes of the esophageal mucosa. More recent studies showed the potential of spectroscopy in the detection of dysplasia in Barrett's esophagus.

Panjehpour *et al.* used laser-induced autofluorescence with a wavelength of 410 nm and could distinguish normal esophagus from malignant esophageal tissue with high accuracy [17]. With the help of a different spectral analysis technique Von-Dinh *et al.* could diagnose esophageal malignancy with a high degree of reliability [20].

The same group of investigators found laser-induced autofluorescence spectroscopy to be sensitive for the detection of diffuse HGD in Barrett's esophagus and adenocarcinoma. However, only 28% of the specimens with LGD and focal HGD were classified as abnormal by this technique [18]. Mayinger *et al.* replaced the expensive laser with filtered ultraviolet-blue-light source and showed specific differences in the emitted autofluorescence spectra of esophageal carcinoma with normal mucosa [15]. In another study, Bourg-Heckly *et al.* demonstrated the ability of light-induced autofluorescence to identify HGD in Barrett's esophagus and early cancer and reported a sensitivity and specificity of 86% and 95%, respectively [16]. The spectral distribution of normal esophageal mucosa and Barrett's mucosa were similar.

Some authors used exogenous fluorophores to enhance the spectroscopic characteristics of neoplastic tissues. In an *in vitro* study, Stael von Holstein *et al.* demonstrated the feasibility of laser-induced fluorescence measurements after sensitizing with Photofrin to distinguish normal and malignant tissue in surgical specimen from the esophagus [21]. Brand *et al.* used oral 5-ALA and showed a sensitivity of 77% and specificity of 71% [22]. Ortner *et al.* combined time-resolved fluorescence spectroscopy and topical application of 5-ALA to enhance the spectroscopic characteristics of dysplastic Barrett's esophagus [6].

LSS and trimodal spectroscopy are novel techniques and few data is published so far [4,8,9]. Perelman *et al.* and Backman *et al.* described the use of LSS to determine the size distribution of epithelial cell nuclei *in vitro* and *in vivo* [7,8]. Wallace *et al.* presented a prospective validation study of LSS to identify dysplasia in a cohort of patients with Barrett's esophagus [9]. The sensitivity and specificity of LSS for detecting dysplasia (either LGD or HGD) were 90% and 90%, respectively, with all HGD and 87% of LGD sites correctly classified. In a consecutive study, Georgakoudi *et al.* stated that the combination of laser-induced autofluorescence, reflectance, and LSS (called trimodal spectroscopy) results in a superior sensitivity and specificity for separating HGD versus non-HGD in Barrett's esophagus (100% and 100%) and dysplastic versus non-dysplastic Barrett's esophagus (93% and 100%) [4].

Fluorescence Imaging

With the development of the fluorescence imaging systems, scientific interest concentrated mostly on the esophagus, not least because of the increasing clinical significance of Barrett's esophagus. Different authors investigated the use of fluorescence imaging in the detection of neoplastic changes of the esophagus (Table 16.3 [14,23–29]). Most of the studies dealing with fluorescence imaging in patients with Barrett's esophagus investigated patients with long segment Barrett's esophagus. Studies of fluorescence imaging in patients with short segment Barrett's esophagus are rare. Early reports showed the feasibility and usefulness of both fluorescence imaging systems in the detection of dysplasia and neoplasms in patients with Barrett's esophagus and other gastrointestinal diseases [23–25]. In a study of 47 patients with Barrett's esophagus, HGD, or carcinoma was found in 14 of 113 biopsies taken from areas that exhibited fluorescence [12]. HGD was found in only 3 of 130 fluorescence-negative biopsy specimens. Another study correctly diagnosed two cases of HGD and 20 cases of non-dysplastic intestinal metaplasia [26]. However, out of eight cases with LGD, only five and three cases of LGD were correctly diagnosed by fluorescence imaging and standard white-light endoscopy, respectively. A recent study demonstrated the good diagnostic performance of

Table 16.3 Clinical data of fluorescence imaging in neoplastic disease of the esophagus.

Author	Setting	Patients (n)	Specimen (n)	Technique	Sensitivity (%)	Specificity (%)
Van Ierland-van Leeuwen & Tytgat [23]	Normal esophagus vs. BE/esophageal cancer	15	—	LIFE-GI	100	93
Du Vall et al. [24]	Normal esophagus vs. BE/esophageal cancer	43	—	LIFE-GI	83	84
Messmann et al. [25]	Non-dysplastic BE vs. BE with LGD/HGD	2	—	D-Light (5-ALA systemically*)	n.c.	n.c.
Haringsma & Tytgat [28]	Non-dysplastic BE and LGD vs. BE with HGD	111	—	LIFE-GI	90	89
Endlicher et al. [14]	Non-dysplastic BE vs. dyplastic BE	47	273	D-Light (5-ALA locally)	60	70
				D-Light (5-ALA systemically†)	80–100	27–56
Haringsma et al. [29]	Non-dysplastic BE vs. BE with HGD	2	—	LIFE II-GI	n.c.	n.c.
Stepinac et al. [26]	Non-dysplastic BE vs. dysplastic BE	30	178	D-Light (5-ALA systemically*)	100	63
Niepsuj et al. [27]	Non-dysplastic BE and LGD vs. BE with HGD‡	34	109	LIFE-GI	n.c.	n.c.

5-ALA, 5-aminolevulinic acid; BE, Barrett's esophagus; LGD, low-grade dysplasia; HGD, high-grade dysplasia; n.c., not calculated.
* 20 mg/kg
† 5, 10, 20, or 30 mg/kg
‡ Detection of HGD with white-light endoscopy vs. fluorescence imaging (0.7 vs. 8.3%, $P = 0.016$)

autofluorescence imaging in the detection of HGD in patients with known Barrett's esophagus [27].

Future Directions

The very promising and substantial results demonstrate the ability of spectroscopic techniques to provide useful information for disease classification in a non-invasive manner. Although each of the techniques discussed in this article shows great potential, their combination should allow us to create a comprehensive picture of the biochemical and morphologic state of tissue. Development of software for performing data analysis in real time at endoscopy will allow us to test the applicability of these techniques as a guide to performing biopsies.

Although spectroscopic techniques have advanced substantially from their initial *in vitro* and animal studies, there remains much work to be done before these systems can be integrated into routine endoscopy. The diagnostic ability of combined techniques has to be validated in different organ systems and in larger patient cohorts. Major efforts are needed to build smaller, more reliable, and less expensive instruments. Under these circumstances, we hope to have a new technique in the near future that can substantially reduce the sampling error inherent in random biopsy, and thus improve the sensitivity for detecting dysplasia in patients at risk or with premalignant disorders.

References

1. Reid BJ, Haggitt RC, Rubin CE *et al.* Observer variation in the diagnosis of dysplasia in Barrett's esophagus. *Hum Pathol* 1988;**19**:166–78.
2. Petras RE, Sivak MV, Rice TW. Barrett's esophagus. A review of the pathologists role in diagnosis and management. *Pathol Annu* 1991;**26**:1–32.
3. Haggit RC. Barrett's esophagus, dysplasia, and adenocarcinoma. *Hum Pathol* 1994;**25**:982–93.
4. Georgakoudi I, Jacobson BC, Van dam J *et al.* Fluorescence, reflectance, and light-scattering spectroscopy for evaluating dysplasia inpatients with Barrett's esophagus. *Gastroenterology* 2001;**120**:1620–9.
5. Zangaro R, Silveira L, Manoharan R *et al.* Rapid multi-excitation fluorescence spectroscopy for *in vivo* tissue diagnosis. *Appl Optics* 1996;**35**:5211–9.
6. Ortner MEJ, Ebert B, Hein E *et al.* Time gated fluorescence spectroscopy in Barrett's oesophagus. *Gut* 2003;**52**:28–33.
7. Perelman LT, Backman V, Wallace MB *et al.* Observation of periodic fine structure in reflectance from biological tissue: a new technique for measuring nuclear size distribution. *Phys Rev Lett* 1998;**80**:627–30.
8. Backman V, Wallace MB, Perelman LT *et al.* Detection of preinvasive cancer cells. *Nature* 2000;**406**:35–6.
9. Wallace MB, Perelman LT, Backman V *et al.* Endoscopic detection of dysplasia in patients with Barrett's esophagus using light-scattering spectroscopy. *Gastroenterology* 2000;**119**:677–82.
10. Kendall C, Stone N, Shepherd N *et al.* Raman spectroscopy, a potential tool for the objective identification and classification of neoplasia in Barrett's oesophagus. *J Pathol* 2003;**200**:602–9.
11. Wong Kee Song LM, Marcon NE. Fluorescence and Raman spectroscopy. *Gastrointest Endosc Clin N Am* 2003;**13**:279–96.
12. el-Sharabasy MM, el-Waseef AM, Hafez MM *et al.* Porphyrin metabolism in some malignant disese. *Br J Cancer* 1992;**65**:409–12.
13. Regula J, MacRobert AJ, Gorchein A *et al.* Photosensitisation and photodynamic therapy of oesophageal, duodenal, and colorectal tumours using 5 aminolaevulinic acid induced protoporphyrin IX—a pilot study. *Gut* 1995;**36**:67–75.
14. Endlicher E, Knuechel R, Hauser T *et al.* Endoscopic fluorescence detection of low and high grade dysplasia in Barrett's oesophagus using systemic or local 5-aminolaevulinic acid sensitisation. *Gut* 2001;**48**:314–9.
15. Mayinger B, Horner P, Jordan M *et al.* Endoscopic fluorescence spectroscopy in the upper GI tract for the detection of GI cancer: initial experience. *Am J Gastroenterol* 2001;**96**:2616–21.
16. Bourg-Heckly G, Blais J, Padilla JJ *et al.* Endoscopic ultraviolet-induced autofluorescence spectroscopy of the esophagus: tissue characterization and potential for early cancer diagnosis. *Endoscopy* 2000;**32**:756–65.
17. Panjehpour M, Overholt BF, Schmidhammer JL *et al.* Spectroscopic diagnosis of esophageal cancer: new classification model, improved measurement system. *Gastrointest Endosc* 1995;**41**:577–81.
18. Panjehpour M, Overholt BF, Vo-Dinh T *et al.* Endoscopic fluorescence detection of high-grade dysplasia in Barrett's esophagus. *Gastroenterology* 1996;**111**:93–101.
19. Von-Dinh T, Panjehpour M, Overholt BF *et al.* *In vivo* diagnosis of the esophagus using differential norma-

lized fluorescence (DNF) indices. *Lasers Surg Med* 1995;**16**:41–7.

20. Von-Dinh T, Panjehpour M, Overholt BF. Laser-induced fluorescence for esophageal cancer and dysplasia diagnosis. *Ann N Y Acad Sci* 1998;**838**:116–22.

21. Stael von Holstein C, Nilsson AM, Andersson-Engels S *et al.* Detection of adenocarcinoma in Barrett's oesophagus by means of laser induced fluorescence. *Gut* 1996;**39**:711–6.

22. Brand S, Wang TD, Schomacker KT *et al.* Detection of high-grade dysplasia in Barrett's esophagus by spectroscopy measurement of 5-aminolevulinic acid-induced protoporphyrin IX fluorescence. *Gastrointest Endosc* 2002;**56**:479–87.

23. Van Ierland-van Leeuwen ML, Tytgat GNJ. Detection of dysplasia using fluorescence *in vivo* using the Xillix-LIFE-GI-System [abstract]. *Endoscopy* 1996;**28**: 44.

24. Du Vall GA, Saidi R, Kost J *et al.* Real time fluorescence endoscopy (LIFE) in the gastrointestinal (GI) tract [abstract]. *Gastrointest Endosc* 1997;**45**:AB28.

25. Messmann H, Knuechel R, Baeumler W *et al.* Endoscopic fluorescence detection of dysplasia in patients with Barrett's esophagus, ulcerative colitis, or adenomatous polyps after 5-aminolevulinic acid-induced protoporphyrin IX sensitization. *Gastrointest Endosc* 1999;**49**:97–101.

26. Stepinac T, Felley C, Jornod P *et al.* Endoscopic fluorescence detection of intraepithelial neoplasia in Barrett's esophagus after oral administration of aminolevulinic acid. *Endoscopy* 2003;**35**:663–8.

27. Niepsuj K, Niepsuj G, Cebula W *et al.* Autofluorescence endoscopy for detection of high-grade dysplasia in short-segment Barrett's esophagus. *Gastrointest Endsoc* 2004;**58**:715–9.

28. Haringsma J, Tytgat GNJ. Fluorescence imaging of high-grade dysplasia in Barrett's esophagus [abstract]. *Gastrointest Endosc* 2001;**53**:AB148.

29. Haringsma J, Tytgat GNJ, Yano H *et al.* Autofluorescence endoscopy: feasibility of detection of GI neoplasms unapparent to white light endoscopy with an evolving technology. *Gastrointest Endosc* 2001;**53**: 642–50.

CHAPTER 17

Emerging Techniques: Optical Coherence Tomography, Confocal Imaging, and Others

Thomas D. Wang and Jacques Van Dam

Introduction

Recent advances in technology have allowed for the development of new techniques for optical imaging of the esophagus with unprecedented resolution and tissue penetration that extend beyond the capabilities of conventional white-light endoscopy. The use of optical methods to detect disease is promising because the intensity, wavelength, and phase of light can be manipulated to extract biochemical and morphological information from the mucosa with techniques such as reflectance, fluorescence, and coherence tomography. Moreover, data can be acquired without physical excision of tissue so that the natural history of esophageal disease can be studied over time without risk of bleeding. Several emerging techniques that will be discussed in this chapter include: optical coherence tomography (OCT), confocal imaging, and others (endocytology and fluorescence imaging). All of these imaging techniques involve the use of an optical fiber to transmit light between the instrument and the tissue. The main impetus driving these developments is to provide better surveillance of the esophagus for neoplastic changes. In particular, the detection of dysplasia in the setting of Barrett's esophagus has drawn great interest because of the alarming rise in incidence of esophageal adenocarinoma, the fastest growing cancer in the USA [1]. The current biopsy surveillance standards suffer from sampling error, increased procedure time, and cost. The detection of disease in the esophagus is challenging for several reasons: (i) subcellular resolution is required to distinguish morphological changes associated with neoplasia; (ii) diseased glands may be present below the mucosal surface; and (iii) the surface area of potential involvement can be most of the esophagus.

Some of the clinical endpoints for optical imaging in the esophagus are shown in Table 17.1, and include: (i) detection of high-grade dysplasia in Barrett's esophagus for removal by physical biopsy; (ii) identification of metaplastic glands beneath neosquamous re-epithelialized mucosa following endoscopic ablation; (iii) assessment of tumor invasion depth prior to endoscopic mucosal resection (EMR); (iv) localization of cancer margins prior to surgical resection; (v) evaluation of effectiveness of pharmacological therapy; and (vi) reduction in number of physical biopsies and frequency of surveillance. Potential emerging techniques presented in this chapter that are most relevant are shown in the adjacent column. In the esophagus, methods of high-resolution imaging as well as wide area surveillance are needed in order to achieve many of these clinical goals. A comprehensive evaluation of the mucosa requires visualization of subcellular features, such as nuclei (size, number, chromatin content) and organelles, thus axial (perpendicular to mucosal surface) and transverse (parallel to mucosal surface) resolution on the micron scale is needed. The transverse resolution improves with the inverse of the numerical aperture of the objective (angle at which the beam converges), and the axial resolution improves with the inverse of the square of the numerical aperture. Thus, it is much easier to achieve a high transverse resolution than axial. Moreover, premalignant

Table 17.1 Clinical endpoints for high-resolution imaging in the esophagus.

Clinical endpoints	Potential technique
High-grade dysplasia in Barrett's esophagus	OCT, confocal, endocytoscopy, fluorescence imaging
Metaplastic glands beneath re-epithelialized mucosa	OCT, confocal
Submucosa tumor invasion prior to EMR	OCT, confocal
Preoperative identification of tumor margins	OCT, confocal, endocytoscopy, fluorescence imaging
Effectiveness of pharmacological therapy	Confocal, endocytoscopy, fluorescence imaging
Minimal number of biopsies/frequence of surveillance	OCT, confocal, endocytoscopy fluorescence imaging

EMR, endoscopic mucosal resection; OCT, optical coherence tomography.

mucosa may exhibit dysplastic glands and microarchitectural distortions up to 1 mm or more below the mucosal surface, thus techniques of vertical cross-sectional imaging (plane perpendicular to mucosal surface) are necessary. Furthermore, identification of the boundary between carcinoma and normal mucosa requires horizontal cross-sectional imaging (plane parallel to mucosal surface). Finally, dysplasia may be present within a segment of Barrett's mucosa that may extend 10 cm or more in length, thus imaging of large surface areas are also critical.

Optical Coherence Tomography

OCT is a method of imaging that is analogous to endoscopic ultrasound. The principle of operation is based on use of low-coherence interferometry to measure the intensity and time delay of photons backscattered from tissue microstructures [2,3]. Hence, OCT produces a vertical cross-sectional reflectance image of the esophagus with depth below the submucosa. Because OCT uses light rather than sound, it can achieve much higher resolution over a tissue penetration depth of several millimeters, which is adequate to evaluate many mucosal diseases seen in the esophagus [4,5]. The axial resolution of current clinical OCT systems is ~10 μm, a level that approaches cellular resolution [6,7]. Thus, the presence of disease on OCT images is revealed by abnormalities in mucosal morphology rather than by subcellular changes. However, ultrahigh-resolution OCT systems are being developed that promise a fac-

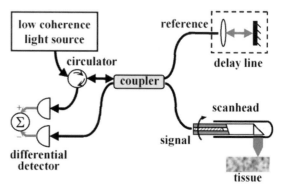

Fig. 17.1 Optical coherence tomography (OCT) schematic. A low-coherence source delivers infrared light to a fiber-optic interferometer and is separated into a signal and reference path. Light is focused by the scanhead into the tissue, and backscattered light is collected and returned to the coupler. An optical circulator recovers some of the returning light for improved collection efficiency. Light entering the reference path is scanned by the delay line to identify the position of the signal photons. Returning light from both paths is recombined at the differential detector. Reproduced with permission from Rollins *et al* [9].

tor of 10 or more improvement in resolution [8]. A limitation of OCT is that contrast is dependent on differences in the index of refraction of cellular and tissue structures, which are typically less than a factor of two, and may limit detection sensitivity.

Principle of Operation

Light from a low-coherence source enters a fiber-optic interferometer, as shown in Fig. 17.1, where it passes through an optical circulator and coupler that creates a signal and reference path [9]. Infrared light is used because it is less sensitive to scattering by tissue than visible, thus can penetrate more deeply into tissue [10]. The light in the signal path goes to the scanhead, where it is focused by the objective lens into the tissue. A fraction of the backscattered light is refocused by the same objective back into the optical fiber, and passes through the coupler. The optical circulator recovers half of the returning light split by the coupler for better collection efficiency. Light in the reference path enters a delay line where it reflects off a mirror whose location is precisely known. Returning light from both the signal and reference paths are recombined by the coupler to the differential detector. Interference between the signal and reference beams occurs only when the difference between the path lengths traveled is less than the coherence length of the light source. By scanning the reference mirror in the delay line, the magnitude of the backscattered light from the signal arm can be determined as a function of axial depth. For clinical imaging, the OCT catheter consists of a single mode optical fiber that is coupled to a low numerical aperture objective lens and a prism that directs the beam into the tissue [11]. The assembly is contained within a flexible conduit that extends the entire length of the catheter probe and is protected by a sealed, transparent outer sheath with an outer diameter of ~2 mm.

Linear Scanning

In the linear scanning mode, a translator is attached to the conduit at the proximal end of the catheter, and moves the optical assembly under computer control in a longitudinal direction along the axis of the probe. The catheter is manipulated within the instrument channel while the operator steers the distal tip of the endoscope to accurately place the probe onto the desired location on the mucosa with light pressure for stability against motion created by esophageal peristalsis, heart beats, and respiration. Because infrared light used for imaging is not visible to the operator, a separate red beam is provided to assist with aiming. Linear scanned OCT images are displayed in Cartesian coordinates, and are rectangular in dimensions with uniform pixel spacing. More-

over, these images have less distortion and less motion artifact than radial scanned OCT images with similar pixel density. This image format is well suited for imaging discrete structures such as patches of Barrett's or ulcers, but the resulting field of view is usually much smaller than the surfaces of clinical interest, and sampling of the mucosa at multiple sites is needed to adequately evaluate the extent of disease. Clinical OCT imaging systems with linear scanning have demonstrated an axial and transverse resolution of ~10 μm and ~25 μm, respectively [11]. *In vivo* images have been acquired with dimensions of 5.5 mm (512 pixels) in length and 2.5 mm (256 pixels) in depth with a frame rate of 4 images/s. The optical power incident on tissue is 5.0 mW at a wavelength of 1300 nm.

Radial Scanning

In the radial scanning mode, the optical assembly rotates within the sheath in a circular fashion to obtain a vertical cross-sectional image of the entire circumference of the esophagus, as shown in Fig. 17.2 [7,9]. The catheter is placed in the center of the lumen, and suctioning collapses the wall of the esophagus onto the probe surface. This technique is done to minimize the effect of motion artifact, and to improve the coupling of light between the catheter and mucosal surface. Radial scanned images are displayed in polar coordinates, and the transverse pixel spacing increases with distance from the probe. Because of the larger field of view, radial scanning is more sensitive than linear to any movement. Moreover, if the catheter probe drifts out of the center of the lumen, only a limited sector of the full esophageal circumference can be seen. Because of the larger area of tissue imaged, radial scanning benefits from the use of a power efficient interferometer for improved light collection efficiency and from a Fourier-domain rapid scan delay line for increased effective scanning speed of the reference arm of the interferometer. Clinical OCT imaging systems with radial scanning have demonstrated an axial and transverse resolution of ~10 μm and ~25 μm, respectively [7]. Radial images have been acquired with depth of ~2.5 mm from the probe with a frame rate of 4 images/s. The optical power incident on the tissue is 22 mW at a wavelength of 1310 nm. More power is needed for

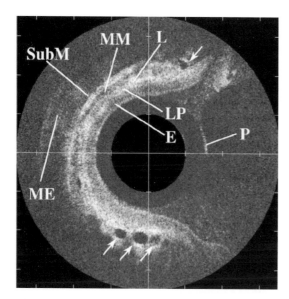

Fig. 17.2 Optical coherence tomography (OCT) images of normal esophagus collapsed around the probe (P) is taken with radial scanning, and reveals the epithelium (E), lamina propria (LP), muscularis mucosa (MM), submucosa (SubM), and muscularis externa (ME). Circular structures (three arrows) in the submucosa represent blood vessels. Concentrated regions of high intensity in the lamina propria have identified as lymph nodes (L). Reproduced with permission from Rollins *et al* [9].

radial scanning than for linear because of the larger field of view.

Clinical OCT Imaging

OCT images of normal squamous esophagus with a depth of ~2.5 mm appear as a well-defined, layered structure, as shown by the radial scanned image in Fig. 17.2 (distance between separator marks is 1 mm) [9]. The esophageal wall has been collapsed onto the surface of the probe (P). The epithelium (E) is the most superficial layer, consists primarily of squamous cells with low nucleus-to-cytoplasm ratio, and appears with relatively weak backscatter intensity. The next layer is the lamina propria (LP), which consists primarily of connective tissue, and appears bright. Below is the muscularis mucosa (MM), composed of a layer of muscle cells, and appears with minimal backscatter intensity. One layer deeper is the submucosa (SubM), which is quite bright, followed by the muscularis externa (ME),

which is dark. Circular structures (three arrows) with low intensity can be seen in the submucosa represent blood vessels. Concentrated regions of high intensity in the lamina propria have identified as lymph nodes (L). The contrast between each layer is determined by the difference in average index of refraction. In addition, backscattered light appears with an exponentially decreasing intensity with depth into the mucosa because of greater tissue absorption and scattering along both the illumination and collection paths.

Barrett's esophagus is distinguished from normal on OCT images by features that include the absence of the normal layered structure of squamous epithelium, disorganized mucosal architecture, heterogeneous contrast, irregular mucosal surface, and presence of submucosal glands [11–13]. In a prospective study, OCT was found to be 97% sensitive and 92% specific for detection of Barrett's [11]. The presence of glands within Barrett's mucosa appeared as a disruption of the well-defined layered architecture of normal mucosa, and revealed decreased intensity pockets beneath the epithelial surface. Furthermore, there is a larger variability in image features from Barrett's than from normal esophagus among different patients. At this time, the sensitivity of OCT for the detection of dysplasia has not been established. However, studies have noted that the presence of dysplasia on OCT was found to have greater glandular irregularity and altered reflectance characteristics. Current limitations in the resolution and contrast of clinical OCT imaging systems prevent clear identification of nuclear changes and goblet cells, the key features necessary for detecting dysplasia and Barrett's, respectively. These limitations are being addressed by the next generation OCT imaging systems.

OCT images of esophageal adenocarcinoma arising from Barrett's esophagus appear with a total loss of the layered structure of normal esophagus, replaced by a heterogenous layer [12,13]. Regions of bright alternating with poor scattering are visible, possibly representing the lamina propria and crypts, respectively. The tissue penetration depth of light is noticeably less than that of normal squamous esophagus and Barrett's mucosa, possibly because of greater number and more dense intra-cellular packing of malignant cells. Images of ulcer in the tumor revealed a homogeneous pattern with bright intensity from the underlying connective tissue in the stroma. OCT images of squamous cell carcinoma appeared similar to that of adenocarcinoma, demonstrating loss of well-defined, layered structure of normal esophagus, heterogeneous pattern with alternating brightly and poorly scattering regions, and poor tissue penetration depth.

Future Advancements

While OCT has demonstrated impressive results, continued development of this technique promises significant improvement in imaging performance. Limitations in the resolution of current clinical systems are being addressed by the development of ultra-short pulse lasers that emit pulses with a bandwidth up to 350 nm, compared to 68 nm in current clinical systems [14]. Using these sources, ultrahigh-resolution images of Barrett's esophagus have been collected *in vitro* with an axial resolution of ~1 μm. A transverse resolution of ~5 μm was achieved by increasing the numerical aperture of the objective lens. However, this change in optics reduces the working distance of the probe. In order to achieve a significant image depth, multiple images were collected at different focal distances and then tiled together to create the final image. With these improvements, it was still unclear if subcellular features could be resolved, but localized foci of high backscatter intensity suggest the presence of nuclei.

Doppler OCT is an extension of this technique being developed to visualize the dynamics of blood flow [15,16]. This method is based on the principle that backscattered light from a moving particle, such as a blood cell flowing through a vessel, is Doppler shifted by a frequency that is proportional to the particle's velocity. This velocity can be extracted from the backscattered light in the signal path of the interferometer by frequency shifting the reference path, a process known as heterodyne detection. This concept has been demonstrated in the lab, and is being developed for *in vivo* use. When adequately advanced, Doppler OCT can potentially be used to measure flow in esophageal varices, locate and assess significance of bleeding sources within ulcers, and monitor angiogenesis in esophageal tumors.

Confocal Imaging

Confocal imaging is performed routinely in the lab using a bulk optics instrument to image cells and tissues with subcellular resolution by performing optical sectioning [17]. This process uses a pinhole between the object and detector to reject light from planes out of focus, thus providing a clear in focus image of a thin section within the specimen. Conventional confocal microscopes can achieve submicron resolution using a high numerical aperture objective lens to tightly focus the illumination and collection beams. The main limitation of confocal microscopy for *in vivo* imaging is the large physical dimensions of the objectives lenses needed to achieve subcellular resolution. Recently, high quality microlenses have become available with the millimeter dimensions necessary for endoscope compatibility, but this reduced size is achieved at a cost of less working distance and axial resolution. For example, the working distance of confocal microendoscopes is on the order of several hundred microns, which limits the tissue penetration depth to a factor of 10 less than that of OCT. Moreover, the dynamic range, or sensitivity to orders of magnitude changes in light intensity, is only on the order of 20–30 dBs, representing a factor of only two to three orders. This limitation allows for horizontal cross-sectional imaging, but not vertical. However, confocal imaging, which is not coherence based, is sensitive to fluorescence, thus can potentially achieve much better contrast than OCT. Currently, confocal microendoscopy is at a very early stage of development. The available clinical prototypes are designed with a single axis configuration that uses a single fiber and objective assembly to deliver the illumination and light collection. These instruments use 488 nm for excitation, and collect fluorescence from intra-vital dyes either sprayed onto the mucosal surface or injected intravenously. *In vivo* images have been collected that demonstrate subcellular details with high contrast. The emergence of the dual axes architecture has demonstrated the potential to overcome some of the limitations in working distance and dynamic range of the single axis prototypes.

Principle of Operation

Confocal microendoscopy is based on the use of a single mode optical fiber to act as a pinhole and to deliver light between the objective lens and detector [18]. The size of the fiber core defines the volume below the mucosal surface from which backscattered light can originate and become collected. Backscattered light from all other regions does not have the correct trajectory to enter the optical fiber, and thus is spatially filtered. This arrangement is combined with a method of scanning to create an image from a thin section of tissue, known as optical sectioning. Confocal microendoscopes use optical fibers to transmit the collected light to the detector with the fiber core functioning as a pinhole. Confocal microendoscopy is sensitive to fluorescence, which can be from endogenous biomolecules or from exogenous biomarkers. In addition, reflectance can be collected at the same time as fluorescence with complete image registration, thus, the morphology of cells and tissues can be directly related to the underlying biochemistry and molecular properties.

Distal Scanning

Confocal microendoscopy has been developed with the scanning mechanism located in the distal end using a tuning fork mechanism that vibrates the optical fiber at resonance (Optiscan Imaging Ltd, Victoria, Australia) [19,20]. The size of the scanner is not sufficiently small for the microscope to pass through the instrument channel of the endoscope, and instead, it is built into the insertion tube. The diameter of the endoscope (Pentax EC3870K) is 12.8 mm, which is approximately the same size as that of therapeutic endoscopes. In the optical assembly, the fiber is coupled to a high numerical aperture objective and achieves a transverse and axial resolution of 0.7 and 7 μm, respectively, at a wavelength of 488 nm. Horizontal cross-sectional images are collected with parameters that include a frame rate of 1.6 images/s, penetration depth of up to 250 μm below the mucosal surface, and a field of view of 320 μm, using a maximum laser power of 1 mW. Fluorescence images are collected with use of intra-vital dyes, including fluorescein sodium and acriflavin hydrochloride for contrast enhancement. While clinical studies have not been performed in the

esophagus at this time, it has been used in 27 patients undergoing colonoscopy to reveal clear images of cells and subcellular structures. Intraepithelial neoplasia in the colon from a total of 390 sites was detected with a sensitivity of 97.4% and specificity of 99.4% [19].

Proximal Scanning

Confocal microendoscopy has also been developed with scanning is performed over the proximal surface of the catheter probe (Mauna Kea Technologies, Paris, France) [21]. The microendoscope consists of a fiber-optic bundle that contains several tens of thousands of individual fibers coupled to a micro-lens objective. For scanning, two separate mirrors located in the instrument unit oscillate the fast and slow axes at 4 and 12 Hz, respectively, focusing a 488 nm laser beam into each fiber of the bundle in sequence. Prior to image collection, the fiber-optic bundle is first calibrated to remove the contributions from autofluorescence and to adjust for differences in the transmission efficiency of each individual fiber. Fluorescence is generated by the use of intra-vital dyes, such as fluorescein, cresyl violet, and rhodamine, and images are acquired at a frame rate of 12 images/s. Because the scanning mechanism is located external to the probe, a much smaller catheter diameter can be achieved than for that of the distal scanning instruments. Currently available probes have diameters that range from 0.3 to 1.8 mm. The smaller probes have a transverse and axial resolution of 5 and 15 μm, respectively, with a field of view of 400 × 280 μm. However, the working distance for these probes is 0 μm, thus they must be in contact with the mucosa to image. Currently, this system has been used to collect fluorescence images in small animals such as transgenic mice. Clinical studies are in progress.

Dual Axes Architecture

A novel dual axes confocal architecture is being developed to overcome some of the limitations in working distance and dynamic range exhibited by the single axis design [22,23]. In this configuration, two low numerical aperture objectives are oriented with the illumination and collection beams crossed at an angle θ, as shown in Fig. 17.3. The transverse

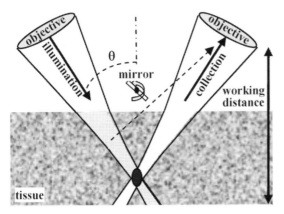

Fig. 17.3 Dual axes confocal schematic. Two low numerical aperture objectives are oriented with the illumination and collection beams crossed at an angle, and the transverse and axial resolution is determined by the overlap between the two beams. Light scattered along the illumination path (checkered region) arrives at the collection lens at the angle that is unlikely to be collected (dashed line). The long working distance allows for a scanning mirror to be placed on the tissue side of the objective to create a large field of view. Reproduced with permission from Rollins *et al* [9].

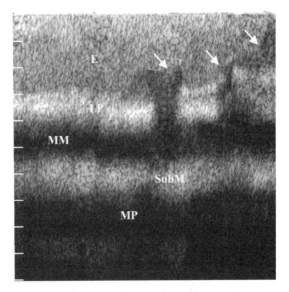

Fig. 17.4 A dual axes reflectance image from esophagus collected *ex vivo* with 1345 nm light is shown. The mucosa on the left half of the image appears to be organized into well-defined, layered structures that correspond to epithelium (E), lamina propria (LP), muscularis mucosa (MM), submucosa (SubM), and muscularis propria (MP). The epithelium on the right half is disrupted by invaginating structures (three arrows) that appear to be glands associated with the pit epithelium of Barrett's esophagus. Reproduced with permission from Rollins *et al* [9].

and axial resolution is determined by the dimension of the overlap between the two beams. In addition, this configuration achieves a dynamic range that allows for the collection of vertical cross-sectional image over 1 mm deep [24]. Furthermore, light scattered along the illumination path (checkered region) arrives at the collection lens at the angle that reduces its chances of being collected (dashed line), resulting in improved image contrast. In addition, the long working distance allows for a micro–electro–mechanical systems (MEMS) scanning mirror to be placed on the tissue side of the objective and creates a large field of view [25]. A tabletop prototype using this approach has been demonstrated with 6 μm resolution at 1345 nm. An *ex vivo* reflectance image, shown in Fig. 17.4, was collected from a freshly excised biopsy specimen at the neo-squamocolumnar junction (Z line) of a patient with Barrett's esophagus [24]. The mucosa on the left half of the image appears to be organized into horizontal layers, which by direct comparison to histology, correspond to epithelium (E), lamina propria (LP), muscularis mucosa (MM), submucosa (SubM), and muscularis

propria (MP). The epithelium on the right half is disrupted by invaginating structures (three arrows) that appear to be glands associated with the pit epithelium of Barrett's esophagus.

Future Advancements

While confocal microscopy has made tremendous scientific contributions as a laboratory instrument, the clinical impact of this imaging modality will be determined by future advances in: (i) scaling down the instrument size while preserving subcellular resolution and image contrast; (ii) achieving clinically relevant tissue penetration depths; (iii) obtaining a useful field of view; (iv) minimizing laser power requirements to avoid mucosal damage; and (v) realizing an affordable cost for mass production, distribution, and clinical use. With regard to these endpoints, confocal microendoscopy is at a very early stage of development, but recent technological advances in optical fibers, light sources, detectors, MEMS fabrication techniques, and molecular biology suggest that the future for this technology is promising. The combination of confocal microendoscopy with novel methods of wide area surveillance promises to significantly improve the ability of the endoscopist to visualize and evaluate the mucosa and submucosa of the gastrointestinal tract. A particularly promising direction is the use of fluorescence tagged reagents that have high binding affinity for cell surface and intra-cellular molecules unique to precancerous mucosa. In addition, the use of near infrared light, which is much less sensitive to tissue scattering and hemoglobin absorption, will achieve deeper tissue penetration. Advancements in these areas will significantly broaden the set of endoscopic tools available for detecting, monitoring, and treating mucosal disease.

Furthermore, clinical studies are needed to validate the use of confocal microendoscopy to detect premalignant lesions in the gastrointestinal tract, particularly in the setting of mucosa at high risk for developing adenocarcinoma, such as Barrett's esophagus and ulcerative colitis. Moreover, as confocal probes are scaled down in size, their use in pancreatic duct and biliary tract epithelium will be investigated. The parameters for confocal images collected in horizontal and vertical cross-sections and three-dimensional images will be defined, and databases of these images will be standardized. In addition, the use of fluorescence-tagged reagents must be evaluated for safety and non-toxicity, in addition to efficacy. The clinical use of confocal microendoscopy will identify early, treatable precancerous and cancerous lesions, reduce the number of biopsy specimens taken, increase the quality of histology, lower the costs of pathology, and ultimately produce better patient outcomes.

Others

Endocytoscopy

While confocal imaging requires a laser for sufficient intensity to image below the mucosal surface, endoscytoscopy can image the surface with subcellular resolution with just a white-light source. These instruments are designed to perform cytology *in vivo*.

Two prototypes (Olympus Corp., Tokyo, Japan) have been developed with magnifications of 450× and 1125×, and provide a field of view of 300 and 120 μm, respectively [26]. These flexible instruments are 380 cm long and 3.2 mm in diameter, and can pass through the instrument channel of a therapeutic endoscope, using a standard white-light source and video-processor. Endocytoscopic images are collected as follows: (i) the mucosal surface is sprayed with 5 mL of 1% methylene blue, and then approximately 20 s is allowed for absorption of the intra-vital stain; (ii) the plastic hood attached to the distal end of the endoscope is placed in contact with the mucosal surface; (iii) the endocytoscopy probe is inserted into the instrument channel of the endoscope until contact is made with the target mucosa; (iv) light pressure is applied to achieve image stability because slight movements from esophageal peristalsis heart beats, and respiration can create motion artifact.

An endocytoscopic image at 450× magnification with methylene blue staining is shown in Plate 17.1 (color plate section falls between pp. 148–9). The image is acquired at the boundary between esophageal cancer (top half) and normal squamous mucosa (bottom half). The region of cancer appears to stain darker overall, and has a much higher density of nuclei than that of normal. Images collected at 1125× magnification image (not shown), reveal an irregular distribution of cells and heterogeneous morphology. Nuclei appeared with different degrees of staining, sizes, and shapes, and the nuclear-to-cytoplasm ratio was quite variable. Nuclear inclusion bodies and nucleoli could be distinguished, but mitotic activity could not. In normal esophagus stained with methylene blue, the first two to three layers of squamous epithelial cells were seen with the 450× magnification probe. Nuclei appeared with regular staining, shape, and size characteristics, and the nucleus-to-cytoplasm ratio was small. Nucleoli were observed in some cases with the 1125× magnification endoscope. In addition, staining with toluidine blue has been used to visualize squamous epithelium, and the degree of cell staining was similar to that of methylene blue. The surface layer of the squamous epithelial cells and the nuclei were clearly visible.

Fluorescence Imaging

While the emerging optical techniques discussed so far are limited to fields of view of a few millimeters or less, wide area imaging on the centimeter scale can be performed with fluorescence endoscopy [27]. Fluorescence is a process where biomolecules absorb light, and elevate electrons to higher energy levels. Subsequent relaxation of these electrons to the energy ground state results in the emission of fluorescence at longer wavelengths. Methods based on fluorescence have been developed to interrogate the biochemistry of the mucosa to reveal differences in cell and tissue metabolism. Autofluorescence in particular is an attractive approach because it takes advantage of changes in concentrations of endogenous fluorophores, such as collagen, nicotinamide adenine dinucleotide (NADH), and flavine adenine dinucleotide (FADH), and has demonstrated the potential to localize dysplasia [28]. These approaches avoid the use of exogenous contrast agents that may produce undesired side effects. The application of fluorescence to imaging exploits the differences in the peak wavelength and intensity between normal and dysplastic mucosa resulting from variations in the concentration and distribution of these metabolically active biomolecules and to changes in the tissue microarchitecture.

The LIFE system (Xillix Corp., Richmond, BC) uses the blue light (425–455 nm) from a Xenon lamp for excitation, a fiber-optic endoscope to transmit fluorescence, and intensified charge-coupled device (CCD) cameras for detection. Fluorescence is spectrally divided into two color regimes by a dichroic mirror and then filtered into the green (480–580 nm) and red (620–720 nm) regions. Intensified cameras are needed because of the relatively weak fluorescence intensity. The white-light image can be imaged in the conventional fashion. A ratio of the red-to-green images is determined to compensate for variations in the distance and angles from various sites of the mucosa. An example of a ratio fluorescence image of Barrett's esophagus collected *in vivo* is shown in Plate 17.2 (color plate section falls between pp. 148–9) [27]. The region of red enhancement (within arrowheads) was found to contain high-grade dysplasia. Clinical evidence for the usefulness of endogenous fluorescence endoscopy as a guide for biopsy is beginning to emerge with mixed results. A recent study using targeted biopsy performed first under endogenous fluorescence imaging with the LIFE system in 34 patients with short segment Barrett's esophagus found a greater number of sites of high-grade dysplasia than under subsequent conventional endoscopy (9 vs. 1, $P = 0.016$) [29]. In another study, 35 patients with Barrett's esophagus were evaluated first by autofluorescence endoscopy and then by random four-quadrant biopsy. However, fluorescence imaging was found to have a collective sensitivity of 21% for the detection of neoplastic lesions, including 88, 19, and 12 specimens of low-grade dysplasia, high-grade dysplasia, and cancer, respectively [30].

Comparison of Emerging Techniques

A summary of the performance parameters for the emerging techniques of OCT, confocal, endocytology, and fluorescence imaging, shown in Table 17.2, compares the strengths and limitations of each method. These parameters include transverse and axial resolution, field of view, tissue penetration depth, frame rate, and contrast mechanism. OCT is the furthest developed of these imaging modalities, and the key feature is high dynamic range to perform vertical cross-sectional imaging with tissue penetration well below the submucosa of the esophagus. Also, large fields of view of several millimeters can be achieved in both the linear and radial scanning modes. Currently, the resolution of clinical systems is limited to changes in mucosal morphology; however, future ultrahigh-resolution instruments promise to reach the subcellular regime. Unfortunately, this coherence technique is not sensitive to non-coherent light, such as fluorescence; thus, contrast is limited to the inherent differences in refractive index between normal and diseased tissues. Confocal microendoscopy is in an early stage of development, and can achieve subcellular resolution and high contrast with fluorescence images. However, the single axis confocal architecture has limited dynamic range that allows for horizontal cross-sectional imaging only, and the high numerical aperture optics needed to achieve good resolution limits the working distance and field of view to several

Table 17.2 Summary of imaging parameters for emerging techniques.

Imaging parameter	OCT	Confocal	Endocytoscopy	Fluorescence imaging
Type of light	Reflectance	Fluorescence reflectance	Fluorescence reflectance	Fluorescence
Wavelengths	830–1300 nm	488–1300 nm	400–700 nm	450–700 nm
Axial resolution	10 μm	<1 μm	<1 μm	>50 μm
Transverse resolution	25 μm	7 μm	N/A	N/A
Contrast mechanism	Δ Refractive index Δ Refractive index	Fluorescence dyes	Intra-vital stains	Fluorescence dyes
Field of view	>1 mm	0.3 mm	0.3 mm	>100 mm
Tissue penetration	2–3 mm	0.25 mm	0 mm	0 mm
Frame rate (per second)	4	2	30	30

N/A, not applicable; OCT, optical coherence tomography.

hundred microns. Future development of the dual axes configuration may overcome some of these limitations. Furthermore, endoscytoscopy uses a standard white-light source to provide submicron transverse resolution horizontal cross-sectional images. Images collected with intra-vital stains can reveal nuclear and organelle details, but this technique is limited to the mucosal surface and does not perform optical sectioning. Finally, fluorescence imaging makes use of conventional fiber-optic endoscopes to achieve a large field of view to image biochemical activity of the mucosal surface. This technique complements the subcellular imaging instruments previously discussed.

Future Directions

These emerging optical imaging techniques promise to equip gastroenterologists with the future ability to more thoroughly evaluate the esophageal mucosa for the presence of disease. These methods add deep tissue penetration, subcellular resolution, and biochemical activity to the capabilities of conventional white-light endoscopy, and can potentially be combined together with a clever design. An example imaging strategy may include the use of fluorescence imaging to survey the entire distal esophagus for sus-

picious regions of disease, followed by OCT to assess the full mucosal depth for subsurface abnormalities, and concluded with confocal microendoscopy or endocytology to provide subcellular details of nuclear and cytoplasmic structures. Furthermore, breakthroughs in the molecular biology of cancer transformation can be incorporated into the imaging strategy with use of fluorescence tagged reagents to bind neoplastic biomarkers. These advances promise to provide earlier detection of precancerous changes in the mucosa in a non-destructive manner that will allow for the natural history of esophageal disease to be observed. These new strategies of "optical biopsy" are unlikely to replace conventional biopsy with histopathological interpretation of excised tissue anytime soon. Rather, they are more likely to provide a more accurate and efficient approach to target biopsy of diseased tissue, thus reducing the number of conventional biopsies required, increasing surveillance intervals, reducing cost, and ultimately improving patient care.

References

1. American Cancer Society. *Cancer Facts and Figures, 2005.* Atlanta: American Cancer Society, 2005.

2. Huang D, Swanson EA, Lin CP *et al.* Optical coherence tomography. *Science* 1991;**254**:1178–81.

3. Tearney GJ, Brezinski ME, Bouma BE *et al. In vivo* endoscopic optical biopsy with optical coherence tomography. *Science* 1997;**276**:2037–9.

4. Tearney GJ, Brezinski ME, Southern JF *et al.* Optical biopsy in human gastrointestinal tissue using optical coherence tomography. *Am J Gastroenterol* 1997; **92**(10):1800–4.

5. Kobayashi K, Izatt JA, Kulkarni MD, Willis J, Sivak MV, Jr. High-resolution cross-sectional imaging of the gastrointestinal tract using optical coherence tomography: preliminary results. *Gastrointest Endosc* 1998;**47**:515–23.

6. Bouma BE, Tearney GJ, Compton CC, Nishioka NS. High resolution of the human esophagus and stomach *in vivo* using optical coherence tomography. *Gastrointest Endosc* 2000;**51**: 467–74.

7. Sivak MV, Jr, Kobayashi K, Izatt JA *et al.* High-resolution endoscopic imaging of the GI tract using optical coherence tomography. *Gastrointest Endosc* 2000;**51**:474–9.

8. Drexler W, Morgner U, Kaertner FX *et al. In vitro* ultrahigh-resolution optical coherence tomography. *Opt Lett* 1999;**24**:1221–3.

9. Rollins AM, Ung-arunyawee R, Chak A *et al.* Real-time *in vivo* imaging of human gastrointestinal ultrastructure by use of endoscopic optical coherence tomography with a novel efficient interferometer design. *Opt Let* 1999;**24**:1358–60.

10. Richards-Kortum R, Sevick-Muraca E. Quantitative optical spectroscopy for tissue diagnosis. *Annu Rev Phys Chem* 1996;**47**:555–606.

11. Poneros JM, Brand S, Bouma BE *et al.* Diagnosis of specialized intestinal metaplasia by optical coherence tomography. *Gastroenterology* 2001;**120**:7–12.

12. Zuccaro G, Gladkova N, Vargo J *et al.* Optical coherence tomography of the esophagus and proximal stomach in health and disease. *Am J Gastroenterol* 2001;**96**:2633–9.

13. Jackle S, Gladkova N, Feldchtein F *et al. In vivo* endoscopic optical coherence tomography of esophagitis, Barrett's esophagus, and adenocarcinoma of the esophagus. *Endoscopy* 2000;**32**:750–5.

14. Li XD, Boppart SA, Van Dam J *et al.* Optical coherence tomography: advanced technology for the endoscopic imaging of Barrett's esophagus. *Endoscopy* 2000;**32**: 921–30.

15. Chen Z, Milner TE, Dave D, Nelson JS. Optical Doppler tomographic imaging of fluid flow velocity in highly scattering media. *Opt Let* 1997;**24**:64–6.

16. Wong RC, Yazdanfar S, Izatt JA *et al.* Visualization of subsurface blood vessels by color Doppler optical coherence tomography in rats: before and after hemostatic therapy. *Gastrointest Endosc* 2002;**55**:88–95.

17. Pawley J, ed. *Handbook of Biological Confocal Microscopy*, 3rd edn. New York: Plenum, 1996.

18. Delaney PM, Harris MR, King RG. Fiber-optic laser scanning confocal microscope suitable for fluorescence imaging. *Opt Let* 1994;**33**:573–7.

19. Kiesslich R, Burg J, Vieth M *et al.* Confocal laser endoscopy for diagnosing intraepithelial neoplasias and colorectal cancer *in vivo. Gastroenterology* 2004; **127**:706–13.

20. Kiesslich R, Goetz M, Burg J *et al.* Diagnosing *Helicobacter pylori in vivo* by confocal laser endoscopy. *Gastroenterology* 2005;**128**(7):2119–23.

21. Laemmel E, Genet M, Le Goualher G *et al.* Fibered confocal fluorescence microscopy (Cell-viZio) facilitates extended imaging in the field of microcirculation. A comparison with intravital microscopy. *J Vasc Res* 2004;**41**:400–11.

22. Wang TD, Mandella MJ, Contag CH, Kino GS. Dual axes confocal microscope for high resolution *in vivo* imaging. *Opt Let* 2003;**28**:414–6.

23. Wang TD, Contag CH, Mandella MJ, Kino GS. Dual axes confocal microscope with post-objective scanning and low coherence heterodyne detection. *Opt Let* 2003;**28**:1915–7.

24. Wang TD, Contag CH, Mandella MJ, Chan NY, Kino GS. Confocal fluorescence microscope with dual-axis architecture and biaxial postobjective scanning. *J Biomed Opt* 2004;**9**:735–42.

25. Dickensheets DL, Kino GS. A micromachined scanning confocal optical microscope. *Opt Let* 1996;**21**:764–6.

26. Kumagai Y, Monma K, Kawada K. Magnifying chromoendoscopy of the esophagus: *in-vivo* pathological diagnosis using an endocytoscopy system. *Endoscopy* 2004;**36**:590–4.

27. Haringsma J, Tytgat GN, Yano H *et al.* Autofluorescence endoscopy: feasibility of detection of GI neoplasms unapparent to white light endoscopy with an evolving technology. *Gastrointest Endosc* 2001;**53**:642–50.

28. Zonios GI, Cothren RM, Arendt JT *et al.* Morphological model of human colon tissue fluorescence. *IEEE Trans Biomed Eng* 1996;**43**:113–22.

29. Niepsuj K, Niepsuj G, Cebula W *et al.* Autofluorescence endoscopy for detection of high-grade dysplasia in short-segment Barrett's esophagus. *Gastrointest Endosc* 2003;**58**:715–9.

30. Egger K, Werner M, Meining A *et al.* Biopsy surveillance is still necessary in patients with Barrett's oesophagus despite new endoscopic imaging techniques. *Gut* 2003;**52**:18–23.

CHAPTER 18
Medical Management of Barrett's Esophagus

Ernst J. Kuipers

Introduction

Within the gastrointestinal tract, there is no shorter segment with a higher cancer incidence than the gastroesophageal junction. This exceptionally high incidence is due to a combination of factors, which include being the transitional zone between squamous and columnar epithelium, and between neutral and severely acidic pH; the influence of acid and bile reflux; the presence of *Helicobacter pylori* colonization within the cardia; and the exposure to reactive nitrogen substances resulting from the local interaction between saliva and acid [1]. The sharply rising incidence of esophageal adenocarcinoma is perhaps related to an increased incidence of Barrett's esophagus [2]. In a recent cohort follow-up study of 500 000 subjects followed between 1996 and 2003, we observed an increased incidence of Barrett's esophagus from 15.1 to 24.6/100 000/year [3]. Investigators from Scotland reported a rise in newly diagnosed Barrett's esophagus from 1/100 000 population in 1980 to 48/100 000 in 1992 [4]. A similar increase was noted in the USA from 22/100 000 in 1987 to 80/100 000 in 1998 [5], as well as an increased incidence of Barrett's esophagus from 0.37/100 000/year in 1965–1969 to 10.5/100 000/year in 1995–1997 [6]. In contrast to the other observations, the increases in the USA were fully attributable to a similar increase in the number of upper gastrointestinal endoscopies performed during the same time interval. The increased incidence of Barrett's esophagus may partly be due to higher awareness among endoscopists and the more common use of endoscopy and esophageal biopsy sampling, but this is unlikely to completely explain

the changing epidemiology of Barrett's esophagus and Barrett's carcinoma. The increased incidence of Barrett's esophagus is related to the high incidence of gastroesophageal reflux disease (GERD) in Western countries. A recent Canadian study performed diagnostic endoscopy in untreated patients with dyspepsia and showed that 43% of these patients had signs of erosive esophagitis [7]. The incidence of reflux disease, Barrett's esophagus, and esophageal adenocarcinoma is significantly lower in Asian countries, but an increasing trend has already been observed [8]. Endoscopy is required for adequate assessment of the condition of the esophageal mucosa in an individual patient, in particular to evaluate for the presence of erosive esophagitis and Barrett's esophagus. Once a diagnosis of Barrett's esophagus is established, further medical management predominantly consists of drug therapy, and endoscopic surveillance and treatment if needed. Endoscopic surveillance and treatment aim at early detection and treatment of Barrett's neoplasia. Drug treatment aims at symptom control, healing of esophagitis, and possible prevention of progression of Barrett's esophagus to dysplasia and adenocarcinoma.

Symptom Control and Healing of Esophagitis

Prevalence and Severity of Symptoms and Esophagitis

Most patients with Barrett's esophagus have symptomatic GERD with heartburn, regurgitation, retrosternal pain, and sometimes with other extra-esophageal symptoms such as chronic cough, laryngeal disorders, and asthma. Patients with long segment Barrett's esophagus often have remarkably few symptoms, despite severe reflux [9] (Plate 18.1; color plate section falls between pp. 148–9). The Barrett's segment then functions as mechanism for symptom control, with the columnar epithelium being less sensitive to acid than the squamous epithelium that it replaced. In a study comparing 74 patients with Barrett's esophagus with 216 GERD patients without Barrett's esophagus, Barrett's patients with normal esophageal motility had more severe acid reflux, but nevertheless a lower symptom index than GERD patients without Barrett's esophagus [10]. Barrett's patients with abnormal esophageal motility had even higher esophageal acid exposure, and similar symptom scores as the GERD patients. This reduced esophageal sensitivity has been supported by other studies [11,12]. However, in an individual patient, the severity and character of reflux symptoms does not allow reliable prediction of the presence of esophagitis nor of Barrett's epithelium. Two large studies of respectively 6215 and 10 294 patients with GERD only identified severity and duration of symptoms as weak predictors for the presence of erosive esophagitis [13,14]. Similarly, a matched case-control study of 79 patients with Barrett's esophagus and 180 GERD patients without Barrett's esophagus found that Barrett's patients had a history of longer symptom duration [15]. In line with this observation, the duration of reflux symptoms has also been associated with the risk of development of esophageal adenocarcinoma [16]. In a nation-wide, population-based case-control study in Sweden including 189 patients with esophageal adenocarcinoma and 820 controls, persons with recurrent reflux symptoms had an odds ratio of 7.7 for development of esophageal adenocarcinoma. This risk increased with more frequent, more severe, and longer-lasting symptoms to 43.5. Together, these data demonstrate that duration and severity of symptoms predict, albeit weakly, the presence of erosive esophagitis and its complications. Barrett's patients generally have had symptoms of longer duration than patients with uncomplicated reflux disease, but the severity of symptoms is often limited in view of the severity of pathological reflux.

Proton Pump Inhibitor Therapy

The first aim in the medical management of patients with a Barrett's esophagus is therefore to alleviate reflux symptoms. Proton pump inhibitors (PPIs) have become the mainstay of therapy for this purpose because of their high efficacy and excellent safety profile. Standard doses equivalent to 20 mg omeprazole heal esophagitis and eliminate symptoms in 80–95% of GERD patients. Specific data on symptom relief and healing of esophagitis in Barrett's patients are limited and mainly come from small series of patients. However, they suggest that the response of Barrett's patients to PPI treatment is inferior compared to patients with mild reflux disease. This is related to the more severe reflux in Barrett's patients, in particular in patients with long segment Barrett's esophagus [17,18]. Symptom improvement and healing of esophagitis can be achieved in nearly all patients with Barrett's metaplasia with a higher PPI dose, but pathologic reflux often remains even in asymptomatic patients. In a randomized study, 105 patients with Barrett's esophagus were treated with 30 mg lansoprazole once daily or 150 mg ranitidine twice daily. After 4 weeks, esophagitis had healed in 86% of the lansoprazole-treated patients, compared to 48% of the ranitidine-treated patients [19]. In another group of 13 Barrett's patients, treatment with 60 mg lansoprazole once daily led to symptom improvement and healing of erosive esophagitis in all, but 24-h intra-esophageal pH recordings showed that five patients (38%) continued to have pathological gastroesophageal reflux [20]. In another study, 25 patients with Barrett's esophagus underwent 24-h esophageal pH and Bilitec 2000 monitoring while being treated with 40–60 mg omeprazole daily. Five patients (25%) had pathological esophageal acid reflux, and fifteen (60%) had evidence of abnormal bile reflux [21]. Others have observed persistent pathological acid reflux in 50% of 48 asymptomatic Barrett's patients while treated with up to 80 mg of daily esomeprazole [22]. Symptom control is thus a poor predictor of persistent acid reflux in patients with Barrett's esophagus. Together, these data show that PPIs are effective for symptom control and healing of esophagitis in Barrett's patients, but at the same time that a considerable proportion of these patients continue to have pathologic gastroesophageal reflux even when symptoms are adeqately controlled.

H2-Receptor Antagonists, Prokinetics, and Other Drugs

Many patients with Barrett's esophagus require potent acid suppression. PPIs suit this purpose better than other drugs; nevertheless, there is some role for treatment with H2-receptor antagonists, prokinetics, and other drugs. A proportion of Barrett's patients have adequate symptom control with H2-blocker treatment in a dose equivalent to 300 mg of ranitidine daily [23,24], but many require high-dose treatment in doses equivalent to 600–3000 mg of ranitidine daily [23]. In a randomized 2-year follow-up study comparing omeprazole and ranitidine, 33 patients with Barrett's esophagus were allocated to treatment with twice daily ranitidine 150 mg [24]. This treatment reduced esophageal acid exposure (determined by the percentage of time over 24 h with a pH < 4.0) from 14.3% to 9.4%, whereas treatment with twice daily omeprazole 40 mg reduced acid reflux from 19.7% to 0.1% of time. In the ranitidine arm, six (18%) patients changed therapy to open-label omeprazole because of insufficient control of reflux symptoms, the remainder continued ranitidine treatment [24]. This confirms that most patients with Barrett's esophagus have severe pathological reflux, with discrepant symptom severity. In a group of 42 Barrett's patients treated with ranitidine, 24 (58%) required 300 mg daily for healing of esophagitis and symptom relief, the remainder, however, needed on average a four-times higher dose with a dose-range between 600 and 2400 mg daily [25]. For these reasons there is, with the current wide availability of PPIs, a minor role for H2-blocker mono-therapy in patients with Barrett's esophagus. However, patients who suffer from persistent acid reflux on PPI treatment in particular have reflux episodes at night [26]. This nocturnal acid breakthrough usually occurs after 23.00 with single daily PPI dosing and after 01.00 with twice daily dosing of PPI and can be treated by addition of an H2-blocker at night, starting at a dose equivalent to 150 mg ranitidine. This had been hypothesized to decrease nightly acid reflux, although tolerance can develop and clinical data are lacking [27,28].

The role for prokinetic therapy in patients with Barrett's esophagus is poorly studied, and appears limited. Treatment with cisapride alone as well as in combination with a PPI has little effect, other than some reduction of bile reflux and perhaps somewhat more rapid clearance of supine acid reflux, which may be beneficial for some patients [29,30]. This is in line with a study showing that the combination of cisapride 10 mg twice daily and omeprazole 20 mg daily was more effective than either treatment alone for the maintenance of remission in patients with reflux esophagitis [31]. However, the current preference for patients with Barrett's esophagus and persistent pathological reflux is to increase the PPI dose and start twice daily dosing before considering a combination with a prokinetic. When symptoms and esophagitis persist despite high-dose twice-daily PPI therapy, 24-h pH-metry and Bilitec measurements help to diagnose persistent acid reflux, nocturnal acid breakthrough, or the presence of bile reflux, or both. If duodenogastric bile reflux predominates, the addition of another drug should be considered. Apart from a prokinetic, potentially effective compounds include baclofen, a GABA-B receptor agonist with an effect on transient lower esophageal sphincter relaxations, a mucosal-protective compound such as sucralfate, or a bile salt binder such as cholestyramine. Data in Barrett's patients are however lacking.

Finally, newer drugs with more potent acid suppressive capacities may in the near future offer new treatment opportunities in particular for patients with Barrett's esophagus and severe gastroesophageal reflux. These drugs may ideally have a more rapid onset of action, a stronger suppressive effect, and longer duration of activity. They should enable a more complete elimination of acid reflux to the Barrett's esophagus with once daily dosing.

Prevention of Symptomatic Relapse

Studies on maintenance use of PPIs have shown that these drugs are also very effective for the prevention of symptomatic relapse of GERD. In the largest study on PPI maintenance therapy in 230 patients with severe reflux disease, maintenance treatment up to 11 years with omeprazole in variable dose was initialised depending upon symptoms and endoscopical presence of esophagitis [32]. During 1490

Table 18.1 Cohort studies into the effect of proton pump inhibitor (PPI) maintenance therapy on Barrett's epithelium.

Study	Design	Medication	Patients (n)	Duration (months)	Outcome
Neumann et al. [38] 1995	Open	Omeprazole 20 mg o.d.	24	12–24	Appearance of squamous islands
Malesci et al. [37] 1996	Open	Omeprazole 60 mg o.d.	14	12	Reduction in length
Sharma et al. [20] 1997 and Sampliner [39] 1994	Open	Lansoprazole 60 mg o.d.	27	48–72	Appearance of squamous islands
Cooper et al. [35] 1998	Open	Omeprazole 20 mg o.d.	47	24–60	Appearance of squamous islands
Peters et al. [24] 1999	Randomized, double-blind	Omeprazole 40 mg b.d./ ranitidine 150 mg b.d.	65	24	Reduction in length and appearance of islands with omeprazole No change with ranitidine
Wilkinson et al. 1999 [33] and Gore et al. [36] 1993	Open	Omeprazole 40 mg o.d.	23	60	Appearance of squamous islands
Srinivasan et al. [34] 2001	Open	Omeprazole 20 mg o.d./ lansoprazole 30 mg o.d./ additional H2-blocker when symptomatic	9	13–118	Reduction in length Appearance of squamous islands

b.d., twice daily; o.d., once daily

treatment years, 158 relapses of esophagitis were observed, corresponding with one relapse per 9.4 treatment years. In another study on 27 Barrett's patients, treatment with 60 mg lansoprazole daily for an average of 5.7 years led to persistent disease remission without recurrent esophagitis [20]. Other studies also indicate that long-term PPI treatment is effective in Barrett's patients to prevent symptomatic relapse [24,33,34].

Regression of Barrett's Epithelium

As columnar metaplasia of the distal esophagus is largely confined to subjects with pathological gastroesophageal acid reflux, the question comes forward whether profound acid suppressive therapy can lead to regression of Barrett's metaplasia. This hypothesis has been tested in various studies [20,24,33–39] (Table 18.1). Only one of these studies had a randomized, double-blind design [24]. In this study, 68 Barrett's patients were treated for 24 months with either omeprazole 40 mg twice daily, or with ranitidine 150 mg twice daily. Endoscopy was performed at 0, 3, 9, 15, and 24 months with measurement of length and surface area of Barrett's esophagus; pH-metry was performed at 0 and 3 months. There was a small, but statistically significant regression of Barrett's esophagus in the omeprazole group, both in length and in surface area, with the latter showing a small reduction of 8% after 24 months. No change was observed in the ranitidine group. The difference between the regression in the omeprazole and ranitidine group was statistically significant for the area of Barrett's esophagus ($P = 0.02$), and showed a trend in the same direction for the length of Barrett's esophagus ($P = 0.06$) [24].

All other studies had an open, uncontrolled design and included fewer patients, although some had a longer duration of follow-up. All of these studies consistently reported that PPI maintenance therapy leads to the appearance of islands of squamous epithelium within the Barrett's segment [20,33–39] (see Table 18.1), but only the two smallest studies reported results similar to Peters *et al.* [24], i.e. a reduction in length of the Barrett's segment [34,37]. The consistent report of the appearance of islands of squamous epithelium supports the concept that columnar metaplasia can be replaced by squamous epithelium under persistent long-term non-acidic conditions, but several critical remarks are justified. First of all, only a few of these studies performed 24-h esophageal pH-metry studies during PPI therapy [20,24,34,37], confirming a esophageal pH < 4.0 for less than 4% of time in all patients in all studies except for one [20]. In the latter study, five (38%) patients still had an esophageal pH below 4.0 for 10.6% of time. Secondly, only one of the open studies had a control group treated with an H2-receptor antagonist [38], and the open design in all these studies makes observer bias an important potential confounder. Thirdly, foci of intestinal metaplasia may be present underneath these squamous islands. Finally, the repeated endoscopical evaluation of a Barrett's segment is subject to considerable inter and intraobserver variation. This interferes with the repeated evaluation of a Barrett's segment in an individual patient. With these remarks in mind, the available data suggest that high-dose PPI maintenance therapy may lead to islands of squamous epithelium with an area of Barrett's metaplasia. If Barrett's mucosa is ablated endoscopically by endoscopic mucosal resection, photodynamic therapy or another treatment, profound acid suppressive maintenance therapy is needed for persistent re-epithelialization with squamous epithelium [40].

Prevention of Neoplasia

Profound Acid Suppressive Therapy

This brings the question forward whether PPI maintenance therapy can prevent the development of neoplasia in patients with a Barrett's esophagus. Data on this issue are scarce and inconclusive. First,

two cohort studies on long-term PPI therapy for GERD demonstrated that this therapy cannot prevent the new development of Barrett's esophagus. In one study of 230 patients with severe GERD treated with 20–120 mg omeprazole for an average of 6.9 years, 12% of the study population was newly diagnosed with Barrett's metaplasia during follow-up [32]. In a second study, 14.5% of 83 GERD patients developed Barrett's metaplasia during maintenance treatment with 20–80 mg of omeprazole [41]. These data suggest that PPI therapy may not be adequate in all patients to prevent the development of intestinal metaplasia of the distal esophagus as a first step in the cascade that can lead to esophageal adenocarcinoma. Nevertheless, other data support the hypothesis that PPI therapy can slow the progression of this process. In a cohort of 236 Barrett's patients followed for an average 5 years, the annual incidence of dysplasia was 4.7%. Multivariate analysis revealed that the use of PPI was independently associated with a reduced risk of dysplasia with a hazards ratio of 0.25 (95% clearance interval [CI] 0.13–0.47) [42]. Another cohort study followed 350 Barrett's patients for a median of 4.7 years. Patients who had not used a PPI for at least 2 years during follow-up had 5.6 times (95% CI 2.0–15.7) the risk of developing low-grade dysplasia [43]. These results with respect to low-grade dysplasia may have been influenced by the effect of PPI treatment on inflammation within Barrett's mucosa. Such inflammation is common in the presence of pathological acid reflux, and interferes with the interpretation of low-grade dysplasia. If patients, who do not receive adequate acid suppression, are diagnosed with low-grade dysplasia in Barrett's mucosa, repeated biopsy sampling after 6–8 weeks of adequate acid suppression should be considered. However, the same series also reported that PPI treatment reduced the risk of developing high-grade dysplasia or adenocarcinoma (hazard ratio 20.9; 95% CI 2.8–158.0) [42,44]. This is in line with studies showing that profound acid suppression increases the epithelial differentiation and decreases proliferation within Barrett's mucosa [44,45].

These encouraging results are however tempered by others. Profound acid suppression decreases gastroesophageal acid reflux, but short pulses of acid esophageal acid exposure often persist. *In vitro* studies show that these short pulses may increase cell proliferation in Barrett's mucosa [46]. Apart from these acid pulses, many patients with Barrett's metaplasia suffer from duodenogastric bile reflux [47]. Exposure to bile can induce or suppress proliferation, depending on the pH and thus on the level of ionisation of bile salts and their capability to enter the mucosal cell lining [48]. This capability is maximal in the pH range from 3.0 to 6.0, the range that is usually reached during PPI therapy. These *in vitro* data question whether PPI therapy has an unequivocal preventive effective on neoplasia development in Barrett's epithelium. This is supported by clinical observations. A cohort study including 417 patients with Barrett's esophagus did not find any effect of 4 years of omeprazole treatment on the incidence of esophageal adenocarcinoma [49]. In the absence of other data, we have to interpret the widespread use of PPIs and the increasing incidence of Barrett's metaplasia and neoplasia as independent phenomena with the first having no demonstrated effect on the latter. This means that PPIs should be prescribed to Barrett's patients to control symptoms and esophagitis, but there is as yet no evidence that high-dose maintenance treatment adequately prevents neoplasia.

Aspirin and Cyclooxygenase-2 Inhibitors

A second approach for the chemoprevention of esophageal adenocarcinoma aims at the use of aspirin and cyclooxygenase-2 (COX-2) inhibitors. Reflux esophagitis and its complication of Barrett's metaplasia are chronic inflammatory conditions. Intervention in this inflammatory process either by selective COX-2 inhibition or combined COX-1 and COX-2 inhibition by aspirin, may offer a mechanism for chemoprevention. Chemoprevention is discussed in detail in Chapter 24.

Conclusions

The gastroesophageal junction is an important zone within the gastrointestinal tract, with a high incidence of neoplasia. The medical management of patients with Barrett's esophagus includes drug therapy in most patients. Barrett's patients have a strong indication for maintenance treatment with a PPI, primarily to improve symptoms of acid reflux, and for healing and prevention of recurrence of esophagitis. Many patients suffer from severe acid reflux, even though symptoms may be relatively mild. Elimination of reflux often requires high-dose, twice daily PPI treatment. Whether PPI therapy, treatment with aspirin, or a selective COX-2 inhibitor reduces the risk for esophageal dysplasia and adenocarcinoma in patients with Barrett's metaplasia remains to be shown.

References

1. McColl KE. When saliva meets acid: chemical warfare at the oesophagogastric junction. *Gut* 2005;**54**:1–3.
2. Pohl H, Welch HG. The role of overdiagnosis and reclassification in the marked increase of esophageal adenocarcinoma incidence. *J Natl Cancer Inst* 2005;**97**:142–6.
3. van Soest E, Dieleman J, Siersema PD, Sturkenboom M, Kuipers EJ. Increasing incidence of Barrett's esophagus in the general population. *Gut* 2005;**54**:1062–6.
4. Prach AT, MacDonald TA, Hopwood DA, Johnston DA. Increasing incidence of Barrett's oesophagus: education, enthousiasm, or epidemiology? *Lancet* 1997;**350**:933.
5. Conio M, Cameron AJ, Romero Y *et al.* Barrett's esophagus and adenocarcinoma. Prevalence and incidence in Olmsted's county, Minnesota. *Gastroenterology* 1999; **116**:A384.
6. Locke GR, III, Talley NJ, Fett SL, Zinsmeister AR, Melton LJ, III. Prevalence and clinical spectrum of gastroesophageal reflux: a population-based study in Olmsted County, Minnesota. *Gastroenterology* 1997; **112**:1448–56.
7. Thomson AB, Barkun AN, Armstrong D *et al.* The prevalence of clinically significant endoscopic findings in primary care patients with uninvestigated dyspepsia: the Canadian adult dyspepsia empiric treatment —prompt endoscopy (CADET-PE) study. *Aliment Pharmacol Ther* 2003;**17**:1481–91.
8. Hongo M. Review article: Barrett's oesophagus and carcinoma in Japan. *Aliment Pharmacol Ther* 2004; **20**(suppl 8):50–4.
9. Brandtmg, Darling GE, Miller L. Symptoms, acid exposure and motility in patients with Barrett's esophagus. *Can J Surg* 2004;**47**:47–51.
10. Byrne PJ, Mulligan ED, O'Riordan J, Keeling PW, Reynolds JV. Impaired visceral sensitivity to acid reflux in patients with Barrett's esophagus. The role of esophageal motility. *Dis Esophagus* 2003;**16**:199–203.

11. Fletcher J, Gillen D, Wirz A, McColl KE. Barrett's esophagus evokes a quantitatively and qualitatively altered response to both acid and hypertonic solutions. *Am J Gastroenterol* 2003;**98**:1480–6.

12. Mulligan ED, Purcell T, Lawlor P, Reynolds JV, Byrne PJ. Symptoms are a poor indication of severity of reflux in Barrett's oesophagus. *Br J Surg* 2000;**87**: 362–73.

13. Labenz J, Jaspersen D, Kulig M *et al*. Risk factors for erosive esophagitis: a multivariate analysis based on the ProGERD study initiative. *Am J Gastroenterol* 2004; **99**:1652–6.

14. El-Serag HB, Johanson JF. Risk factors for the severity of erosive esophagitis in *Helicobacter pylori*-negative patients with gastroesophageal reflux disease. *Scand J Gastroenterol* 2002;**37**:899–904.

15. Eisen GM, Sandler RS, Murray S, Gottfried M. The relationship between gastroesophageal reflux disease and its complications with Barrett's esophagus. *Am J Gastroenterol* 1997;**92**:27–31.

16. Lagergren J, Bergstrom R, Lindgren A, Nyren O. Symptomatic gastroesophageal reflux as a risk factor for esophageal adenocarcinoma. *N Engl J Med* 1999;**340**: 825–31.

17. Frazzoni M, De Micheli E, Savarino V. Different patterns of oesophageal acid exposure distinguish complicated reflux disease from either erosive reflux oesophagitis or non-erosive reflux disease. *Aliment Pharmacol Ther* 2003;**18**:1091–8.

18. Fass R, Hell RW, Garewal HS *et al*. Correlation of oesophageal acid exposure with Barrett's oesophagus length. *Gut* 2001;**48**:310–3.

19. Sontag SJ, Schnell TG, Chejfec G *et al*. Lansoprazole heals erosive reflux oesophagitis in patients with Barrett's oesophagus. *Aliment Pharmacol Ther* 1997;**11**: 147–56.

20. Sharma P, Sampliner RE, Camargo E. Normalization of esophageal pH with high-dose proton pump inhibitor therapy does not result in regression of Barrett's esophagus. *Am J Gastroenterol* 1997;**92**:582–5.

21. Todd JA, Basu KK, de Caestecker JS. Normalization of oesophageal pH does not guarantee control of duodenogastro-oesophageal reflux in Barrett's oesophagus. *Aliment Pharmacol Ther* 2005;**21**:969–75.

22. Gerson LB, Boparai V, Ullah N, Triadafilopoulos G. Oesophageal and gastric pH profiles in patients with gastro-oesophageal reflux disease and Barrett's oesophagus treated with proton pump inhibitors. *Aliment Pharmacol Ther* 2004;**20**:637–43.

23. Collen MJ, Johnson DA, Sheridan MJ. Basal acid output and gastric acid hypersecretion in gastroesophageal reflux disease. Correlation with ranitidine therapy. *Dig Dis Sci* 1994;**39**:410–7.

24. Peters FT, Ganesh S, Kuipers EJ *et al*. Endoscopic regression of Barrett's oesophagus during omeprazole treatment; a randomised double blind study. *Gut* 1999;**45**:489–94.

25. Collen MJ, Johnson DA. Correlation between basal acid output and daily ranitidine dose required for therapy in Barrett's esophagus. *Dig Dis Sci* 1992;**37**: 570–6.

26. Basu KK, Bale R, West KP, de Caestecker JS. Persistent acid reflux and symptoms in patients with Barrett's oesophagus on proton-pump inhibitor therapy. *Eur J Gastroenterol Hepatol* 2002;**14**:1187–92.

27. Xue S, Katz PO, Banerjee P, Tutuian R, Castell DO. Bedtime H2 blockers improve nocturnal gastric acid control in GERD patients on proton pump inhibitors. *Aliment Pharmacol Ther* 2001;**15**:1351–6.

28. Fackler WK, Ours TM, Vaezi MF, Richter JE. Long-term effect of H2RA therapy on nocturnal gastric acid breakthrough. *Gastroenterology* 2002;**122**:625–32.

29. Smythe A, Bird NC, Troy GP, Ackroyd R, Johnson AG. Does the addition of a prokinetic to proton pump inhibitor therapy help reduce duodenogastro-oesophageal reflux in patients with Barrett's oesophagus? *Eur J Gastroenterol Hepatol* 2003; **15**:305–12.

30. Smythe A, Bird NC, Troy GP, Globe J, Johnson AG. Effect of cisapride on oesophageal motility and duodenogastro-oesophageal reflux in patients with Barrett's oesophagus. *Eur J Gastroenterol Hepatol* 1997;**9**:1149–53.

31. Vigneri S, Termini R, Leandro G *et al*. A comparison of five maintenance therapies for reflux esophagitis. *N Engl J Med* 1995;**333**:1106–10.

32. Klinkenberg-Knol EC, Nelis F, Dent J *et al*. Long-term omeprazole treatment in resistant gastroesophageal reflux disease: efficacy, safety, and influence on gastric mucosa. *Gastroenterology* 2000;**118**:661–9.

33. Wilkinson SP, Biddlestone L, Gore S, Shepherd NA. Regression of columnar-lined (Barrett's) oesophagus with omeprazole 40 mg daily: results of 5 years of continuous therapy. *Aliment Pharmacol Ther* 1999;**13**: 1205–9.

34. Srinivasan R, Katz PO, Ramakrishnan A *et al*. Maximal acid reflux control for Barrett's oesophagus: feasible and effective. *Aliment Pharmacol Ther* 2001;**15**:519–24.

35. Cooper BT, Neumann CS, Cox MA, Iqbal TH. Continuous treatment with omeprazole 20 mg daily for up to 6 years in Barrett's oesophagus. *Aliment Pharmacol Ther* 1998;**12**:893–7.

36. Gore S, Healey CJ, Sutton R *et al*. Regression of columnar lined (Barrett's) oesophagus with continuous omeprazole therapy. *Aliment Pharmacol Ther* 1993;**7**:623–8.

37. Malesci A, Savarino V, Zentilin P *et al*. Partial regression of Barrett's esophagus by long-term therapy with high-dose omeprazole. *Gastrointest Endosc* 1996;**44**:700–5.

38. Neumann CS, Iqbal TH, Cooper BT. Long term continuous omeprazole treatment of patients with Barrett's oesophagus. *Aliment Pharmacol Ther* 1995;**9**:451–4.

39. Sampliner RE. Effect of up to 3 years of high-dose lansoprazole on Barrett's esophagus. *Am J Gastroenterol* 1994;**89**:1844–8.

40. Kahaleh M, Van Laethem JL, Nagy N, Cremer M, Deviere J. Long-term follow-up and factors predictive of recurrence in Barrett's esophagus treated by argon plasma coagulation and acid suppression. *Endoscopy* 2002;**34**:950–5.

41. Wetscher GJ, Gadenstaetter M, Klingler PJ *et al*. Efficacy of medical therapy and antireflux surgery to prevent Barrett's metaplasia in patients with gastroesophageal reflux disease. *Ann Surg* 2001;**234**:627–32.

42. El-Serag HB, Aguirre TV, Davis S *et al*. Proton pump inhibitors are associated with reduced incidence of dysplasia in Barrett's esophagus. *Am J Gastroenterol* 2004;**99**:1877–83.

43. Hillman LC, Chiragakis L, Shadbolt B, Kaye GL, Clarke AC. Proton-pump inhibitor therapy and the development of dysplasia in patients with Barrett's oesophagus. *Med J Aust* 2004;**180**:387–91.

44. Ouatu-Lascar R, Fitzgerald RC, Triadafilopoulos G. Differentiation and proliferation in Barrett's esophagus and the effects of acid suppression. *Gastroenterology* 1999;**117**:327–35.

45. Peters FT, Ganesh S, Kuipers EJ *et al*. Effect of elimination of acid reflux on epithelial cell proliferative activity of Barrett esophagus. *Scand J Gastroenterol* 2000;**35**:1238–44.

46. Fitzgerald RC, Omary MB, Triadafilopoulos G. Dynamic effects of acid on Barrett's esophagus. An *ex vivo* proliferation and differentiation model. *J Clin Invest* 1996;**98**:2120–8.

47. Stein HJ, Kauer WK, Feussner H, Siewert JR. Bile reflux in benign and malignant Barrett's esophagus: effect of medical acid suppression and nissen fundoplication. *J Gastrointest Surg* 1998;**2**:333–41.

48. Kaur BS, Ouatu-Lascar R, Omary MB, Triadafilopoulos G. Bile salts induce or blunt cell proliferation in Barrett's esophagus in an acid-dependent fashion. *Am J Physiol Gastrointest Liver Physiol* 2000;**278**:G1000–9.

49. Bateman DN, Colin-Jones D, Hartz S *et al*. Mortality study of 18 000 patients treated with omeprazole. *Gut* 2003;**52**:942–6.

CHAPTER 19

Thermal Endoscopic Therapy of Barrett's Esophagus

Jacques Deviere

Introduction

Barrett's esophagus is defined as the replacement of squamous esophageal epithelium by intestinal metaplasia (IM) in the distal esophagus. It is a fairly frequent complication of gastroesophageal reflux disease (GERD): 5–10% of patients with GERD are diagnosed with Barrett's esophagus and GERD. GERD appears to be essential for the development of Barrett's esophagus [1]. IM is a premalignant lesion that may further develop into dysplasia and lead to adenocarcinoma of the esophagus [2]. The latter now accounts for almost 50% of esophageal cancer cases in Western countries, and the largest increase in its incidence was recorded during the past two decades [3]. Patients with Barrett's esophagus have a 2–25% risk of developing low- to high-grade dysplasia and a 0.5–1.0% risk of having adenocarcinoma, namely 30–150 times higher than the general population. Forty to fifty percent of Barrett's esophagus patients with high-grade dysplasia may develop adenocarcinoma within 5 years [4,5].

Medical therapies using high doses of proton pump inhibitors (PPIs) or surgical therapies (e.g. fundoplication) have been proposed to reverse Barrett's esophagus and abrogate the trigger event in the cascade of the metaplasia–dysplasia–cancer sequence, namely GERD. Retrospective surgical therapies have, however, failed to demonstrate a significant benefit in Barrett's esophagus regression and on the development of adenocarcinoma [6–8]. Similarly, high doses of PPIs offer only a modest remission with partial restoration of squamous islands within the IM [9–15].

The risk of surgery for patients with Barrett's esophagus who develop esophageal adenocarcinoma is very high with an operative mortality varying between 1.6% and 9.4% [16]. These patients are very often older, overweight with significant cardiac and respiratory problems. Moreover, the surgical resection for high-grade dysplasia and early cancer still has an early morbidity of more than 50% and a late morbidity of 26% with an actuarial survival at 5 years of 79% [17]. Surgery is offering a "massive macroscopic morbid solution for a microscopic mucosal problem" [18] in this setting. Therefore, there is clearly a place for an alternative, less invasive treatment that could offer curative treatment to nearly every patient. Photodynamic therapy (PDT) and, even more impressively, mucosal resection have reached a major place in this indication and are discussed in other chapters.

Thermal endoscopic modalities are relatively cheap, technically easier than mucosal resection, and have been directed towards:

1 The destruction of non-dysplastic IM, leading to its replacement by squamous epithelium, in the hope of having a direct impact on the risk of tumor development.

2 The treatment of Barrett's esophagus associated with low-grade dysplasia with the same purpose.

3 The treatment of high-grade dysplasia or intramucosal adenocarcinoma in patients who present for a potential indication for surgical resection.

Destruction of Non-Dysplastic Barrett's Esophagus

Ablation of Barrett's esophagus stands as an attractive alternative treatment that could directly impact on the risk of tumor development. Recent studies using laser therapy (Nd : YAG), argon plasma coagulation (APC), and multipolar electrocoagulation (MPEC) demonstrate, when combined with profound acid suppression, significant Barrett's esophagus regression with eradication of IM and squamous re-epithelialisation of the targeted lesions [19–22]. APC and MPEC have been the most studied in this particular indication.

In an uncontrolled study, MPEC, associated with profound acid suppression (omeprazole, 80 mg/day), was able to induce visual reversal of Barrett's esophagus (assessed by lugol staining) in 85% of the cases, and complete reversal (no IM demonstrated at biopsy) in 78% of the cases at 6 months follow-up [21].

Although less studied than APC, MPEC has been recently revitalized with a prospective randomized trial showing a similar efficacy of MPEC and APC (in combination with high-dose PPI) in achieving endoscopic and histologic ablation [23]. Simple MPEC using a Goldprobe (Boston Sc., Natick, MA) was also reported as less time consuming than APC. On the other hand, there is now ongoing development of balloon-based bipolar electrodes [24], which might render circumferential coagulation of long Barrett's segments technically much easier.

APC is the most extensively studied technique for the ablation of non-dysplastic Barrett. This is a technique that is easy to use and allows the treatment of large surface areas. The APC device consists of a contact-free monopolar high frequency probe that delivers electrical energy through ionized plasma of argon gas to the target tissue, engendering tissue surface coagulation. The coagulation depth is reported to be controlled to 1–3 mm due to the physical properties of the electrically insulating zone of tissue dessication, which confers increased electrical resistance and contributes to the limited depth of coagulation. Depth of injury is however dependent on generator power setting (0–155 W, i.e. 30–90 W for Barrett's esophagus ablation), argon gas flow rate (0.5–7 L/min, i.e. 1–2 L for Barrett's esophagus ablation), probe–tissue distance (2–8 mm) and duration of application (0.5–2.0 s or continuous) [25]. When applied in Barrett's esophagus, APC generates a white coagulum either circumferentially, point by point for a short segment, or by achieving longitudinal strips in a backward direction during withdrawal of the endoscope.

Like for MPEC, short-term results of studies evaluating the effectiveness of APC in combination with PPI treatment for patients having non-dysplastic esophagus have shown that, after one to six APC sessions, a success rate of complete histological Barrett's esophagus eradication ranging from 55% to 100% could be achieved [26–34] (Table 19.1). Partial regression could also be observed in some patients with a significant Barrett's esophagus length reduction. Higher success rates appear to be observed by upgrading the APC power setting from 30–90 W, but with increased incidence of strictures [31,32].

Endoscopic thermal ablation of Barrett's esophagus (61–100%) was not always associated with histological eradication of IM (55–100%). In fact, remaining buried glands and persisting IM under the squamous re-epithelialisation were reported with a frequency of 0–44% in areas where Barrett's esophagus was endoscopically eliminated (see Table 19.1). For APC, the use of higher power setting (resulting in a deeper injury) and higher PPI doses as suggested in some studies may account for the very low incidence of residual buried glands observed in some of the trials.

It is amazing to notice that it is more than 10 years after the first reports on clinical application of APC in non-dysplastic Barrett's that level 1 evidence of its ability to induce partial or complete replacement of IM by squamous mucosa has become available [35]. This was done in an interesting study of patients with Barrett's esophagus undergoing APC or surveillance after surgery. Overall, at 1 year complete "ablation" was achieved in 63% of the treated group and 15% of the surveillance group ($P < 0.01$). None of the patients had dysplasia at the end of follow-up and, interestingly, in this subgroup of patients, they noticed a reduction of the frequency of buried glands between 1 month to 1 year of follow-up (a feature at the opposite of that known after APC application without surgical fundoplication). This is clearly an area which deserves more investigation since it might become one of the few indications for endoscopic ablation of non-dysplastic IM.

Table 19.1 Studies on argon plasma coagulation (APC) and multipolar electrocoagulation (MPEC) in non-dysplastic Barrett's esophagus: short-term results.

Authors	Patients	APC/MPEC sessions (median, range)	APC power setting (W)	Length of Barrett's (cm) (range)	PPI doses during treatment	Endoscopic ablation (%)	Residual intestinal metaplasia (%)
MPEC							
Sampliner et al. [21] 2001	58	Mean 3.5 (1–6)	—	Median 3 (2–6)	Omeprazole 80 mg/day	85.0	22
Dulai et al. [23] 2005	24	Mean 3.1	—	≥2 (<7)	Pantoprazole 80 mg/day	88.0	19
APC							
Mork et al. [29] 1998	15	4 (1–8)	60	Median 4 (2–8)	Omeprazole 60 mg/day	86.7	0
Van Laethem et al. [33] 1998	31	2.4 (1–4)	60	Mean 4.5 (3–11)	Omeprazole 40 mg/day	81.0	24
Byrne et al. [27] 1998	30	4 (2–7)	60	Median 5 (3–17)	Omeprazole 20–40 mg/day	100.0	30
Grade et al. [28] 1999	9	Mean 1.7	60	Mean 3.5 (U/K)	Lansoprazole 60–90 mg/day	100.0	22
Pereira-Lima et al. [31] 2000	33	Mean 1.9	65–70	Median 4 (0.5–7.0)	Omeprazole 60 mg/day	100.0	0
Schultz et al. [32] 2000	73	2 (1–4)	90	Median 4 (1–12)	Omeprazole 120 mg/day	98.6	0
Morris et al. [30] 2001	53	Mean 3	U/K	Mean 6 (3–15)	Omeprazole 20–60 mg/day	U/K	30
Basu et al. [26] 2002	50	4 (1–8)	30	Mean 5.9 (3–19)	Omeprazole 20 mg/day	68.0	44
Kahaleh et al. [34] 2002	39	3 (1–4)	60	Mean 4.7 (2–11)	Omeprazole 40 mg/day	70.0	18
Dulai et al. [23] 2005	24	Mean 3.6	60	≥2 (<7)	Pantoprazole 80 mg/day	81.0	35

PPI, proton pump inhibitor; U/K, unknown.

Complications of thermal ablation (APC and MPEC) treatment include chest discomfort and odynophagia, which are very frequent. Although unusual, severe complications are not negligible and include strictures [21,31–33], fever [21–31], bleeding [21–33], or even perforation and death [27–31] (the latter two were only reported with APC). When APC was used, strictures were associated with higher power setting and usually responded well to one to three balloon dilatations. Fever with pleural effusions was quite frequent in one study and may be related to microperforations [31]. Perforations ($n = 5$) were the most serious complications; two of them resolved with conservative medical treatment and parenteral nutrition; three required thoracotomy and drainage, two of which died postoperatively [27,30,31]. This is of course a major concern with this technique, and is difficult to justify in these patients with non-dysplastic Barrett's for whom endoscopic surveillance is effective. This is one of the reasons why routine use of thermal ablation should be ruled out for this indication, outside a careful prospective study approved by the local ethics committees.

Long-term results have been somewhat disappointing with relapse of IM with positive biopsies ranging from 0% to 68% when performing endoscopic follow-up in patients successfully treated (Table 19.2). Kahaleh *et al.* examined 39 patients with a median follow-up of 36 months (range 12–46 months) in order to identify the predictive factors of Barrett's esophagus remission [34]. Multivariate analysis revealed that short Barrett's esophagus and normalization of acid exposure with PPI treatment (as demonstrated by 24-h pH-metry) were the only independent predictive factors for sustained long-term re-epithelialisation. Recently more optimistic results were reported [36] at a median of 51 months (range 9–85 months) after APC ablation with a relapse rate of IM evaluated at 3% per year.

That the length of Barrett's esophagus is a predictive factor is already reported in previous studies, and is an obvious factor: short IM areas are easier to eradicate than larger areas. Incomplete endoscopic eradication with the persistence of residual buried glands may indeed be responsible for early relapse of Barrett's esophagus. Adequate and optimal acid sup-

pression should have been guessed when clinical trials demonstrated almost no Barrett's esophagus relapse with very high doses of PPI (omeprazole 60–120 mg) [32–36]. In the Kahaleh study, patients with normal pH monitoring relapsed less than patients with abnormal monitoring results (12.5% vs. 83%) while receiving PPIs [34]. Along the same line, Basu *et al.* observed a higher rate of Barrett's esophagus recurrence in patients who had reduced their PPI use [26]. This suggests that, once the eradication is obtained, it should be followed by a life-long treatment with high doses of PPIs to avoid recurrence. However, it is worth mentioning that patients taking PPIs with normal pH monitoring may still relapse. Indeed, both acid and biliary reflux are significantly higher in patients with Barrett's esophagus than in controls or patients with GERD [37,38]. Interestingly, a trend for more severe biliary reflux was observed among patients with persistent Barrett's esophagus at the end of treatment in the Basu study [26]. This emphasizes that acid reflux is surely not the only factor to be considered when looking for the mechanisms affecting outcome of such treatment [39]. Also interestingly, the immunohistochemical expression of *p53*, a potential biomarker of carcinogenesis, when present in Barrett's esophagus, remains unchanged after ablation in the new squamous mucosa [40].

Another concern with thermal ablation is the description of two cases of adenocarcinoma arising under the squamous re-epithelialization [41,42]. This adenocarcinoma may have progressed during follow-up from residual buried glands and may have been missed by routine surveillance biopsies. Such discovery is concerning when considering the high percentage of residual buried glands after treatment and the relapse rates of IM on longer follow-up. After a total follow-up of 173 and 280 patients per year, Morris *et al.* and Madisch *et al.* did not observe the development of dysplasia or adenocarcinoma in their group of treated non-dysplastic patients [30,36]. This suggested a potential benefit of such treatment when compared to the overall incidence of cancer in untreated Barrett's esophagus patients. In the long-term follow-up of our cases [34], we observed two adenocarcinomas, which represents an incidence very similar to the one observed in the general

Table 19.2 Studies on argon plasma coagulation (APC) in non-dysplastic Barrett's esophagus: long-term results.

Authors	Patients	APC power setting (W)	PPI doses maintenance	Median follow-up (months)	Intestinal metaplasia on follow-up (%)
Mork et al. [29] 1998	15	60	Omeprazole 20–60 mg/day	6.0–13.0	7.6
Van Laethem et al. [33] 1998	31	60	Omeprazole 10 or 40 mg/day	12.0	47.0
Byrne et al. [27] 1998	30	60	Omeprazole 20 mg/day	9.0	30.0
Pereira-Lima et al. [31] 2000	33	65–70	Omeprazole 30 mg/day	10.6	3.0
Schultz et al. [32] 2000	73	90	Omeprazole 20 or 40 mg/day	12.0	0.0
Morris et al. [30] 2001	53	U/K	Omeprazole 20–60 mg/day	38.5	U/K
Basu et al. [26] 2002	50	30	Omeprazole 20–60 mg/day	14.0	68.0
Kahaleh et al. [34] 2002	39	60	Omeprazole 20 or 40 mg/day	36.0	62.0
Madisch et al. [36] 2005	66	90	Omeprazole 120 mg/day	51.0	12.0

PPI, proton pump inhibitor; U/K, unknown.

Barrett's esophagus population not undergoing ablation. This not only suggests that surveillance and biopsies targeting could not be avoided but even could become more difficult after treatment completion, since the lesion may be covered by squamous epithelium. This also questions the final objective of such ablative therapy: cancer prevention.

Whether PDT could provide better results than thermal therapy is unlikely, as suggested by a recent prospective study where APC appears more effective than 5-aminolevulinic acid (5-ALA) PDT [43].

Cost-effectiveness of these treatments has not been studied but is highly questionable. If successful in every patient, the cost of a median of three endoscopic therapy sessions is not minor. Moreover, the cost of potential complication management must be considered, and may be very high. Furthermore, lifelong maintenance therapy with high doses of PPI will also dramatically enhance the cost of this ablative therapy. This might be justified if no further follow-up was needed, which is far to be demonstrated Currently, available data suggest that thermal ablation increases the cost of management/surveillance of non-dysplastic Barrett, and is associated with potential complication without any demonstrated clinical benefit. Therefore, not only should it not be performed outside of rigorous clinical trials, but the potential usefulness of new trials should be carefully analyzed, maybe focusing on subgroups of patients such as those having had previous fundoplication.

Barrett's esophagus associated with low-grade dysplasia represents a group of patients for whom there is no consensus about treatment. Although almost all the ablative therapies have been shown to eradicate low-grade dysplasia, and most of the series included some patients with this condition, the potential impact on the development of adenocarcinoma is not known. This is, however, the first group of patients where a level 1 evidence for potential reversal of IM became available [44], and it was with PDT and not with thermal therapy. Using 5-ALA PDT in combination with omeprazole, versus omeprazole alone, the authors were able to achieve regression of low-grade dysplasia in 100% in the 5-ALA group versus 33% in the omeprazole group at 1 year. Long-term follow-up of these patients would be of major interest. In addition, since this group recently

showed [43] that thermal ablation with APC is slightly better than PDT in ablating dysplastic Barrett's esophagus, APC, which is easier to use and more widely available, would deserve to be specifically studied in this indication.

Endoscopic Ablation of High-Grade Dysplasia or Early Cancer (Mucosal Type)

This is the area where local endoscopic therapy is currently the most interesting since it challenges surgical resection and provides a lower morbidity and mortality. Mucosal type early cancers are known as having almost no risk of lymph node metastases. Unfortunately, there are mainly two techniques that are used successfully in this indication, namely PDT and mucosectomy, and thermal therapy plays only a minor role, if any [45,46]. It is however occasionally used, in combination with mucosal resection, to remove the small areas of residual IM [47].

Conclusion

Thermal therapy for ablating Barrett's epithelium has been widely studied in non-dysplastic Barrett's esophagus, but no evidence is currently available that sustains its potential routine use in this indication. There is, however, some niches of indications that deserve further investigations such as the destruction of Barrett's esophagus after surgical fundoplication (or endoscopic treatment of GERD) and destruction of IM associated with low-grade dysplasia. Long-term data (with a special focus on the development of high-grade dysplasia or cancer) on all patients having been included in the currently published trials would also be of major interest.

References

1. Katzka DA, Rustgi AK. Gastroesophageal reflux disease and Barrett's esophagus. *Med Clin North Am* 2000; **84**:1137.
2. Hameeteman W, Tytgat GN, Houthoff HJ, van den Tweel JG. Barrett's esophagus: development of dysplasia and adenocarcinoma. *Gastroenterology* 1989; **96**:1249.

3. Lagergren J, Bergstrom R, Lindgren A, Nyren O. Symptomatic gastroesophageal reflux as a risk factor for esophageal adenocarcinoma. *N Engl J Med* 1999;**340**:825.

4. Spechler SJ. Barrett's esophagus: diagnosis and management. *Baillires Best Pract Res Clin Gastroenterol* 2000;**14**:857.

5. Spechler SJ. Clinical practice. Barrett's esophagus. *N Engl J Med* 2002;**346**:836.

6. Attwood SE, Barlow AP, Norris TL, Watson A. Barrett's oesophagus: effect of antireflux surgery on symptom control and development of complications. *Br J Surg* 1992;**79**:1050.

7. Williamson WA, Ellis FH, Gibb SP, Shahian DM, Aretz HT. Effect of antireflux operation on Barrett's mucosa. *Ann Thorac Surg* 1990;**49**:537.

8. Sagar PM, Ackroyd R, Hosie KB *et al*. Regression and progression of Barrett's oesophagus after antireflux surgery. *Br J Surg* 1995;**82**:806.

9. Bozymski EM, Shaheen NJ. Barrett's oesophagus: acid suppression, but no regression. *Am J Gastroenterol* 1997;**92**:556.

10. Cooper BT, Neumann CS, Cox MA, Iqbal TH. Continuous treatment with omeprazole 20 mg daily for up to 6 years in Barrett's oesophagus. *Aliment Pharmacol Ther* 1998;**12**:893.

11. Devière J, Buset M, Dumonceau JM, Rickaert F, Cremer M. Regression of Barrett's epithelium with omeprazole. *N Engl J Med* 1989;**320**:1497.

12. Gore S, Healey CJ, Sutton R *et al*. Regression of columnar lined (Barrett's) oesophagus with continuous omeprazole therapy. *Aliment Pharmacol Ther* 1993;**7**:623.

13. Malesci A, Savarino V, Zentilin P *et al*. Partial regression of Barrett's esophagus by long-term therapy with high-dose omeprazole. *Gastrointest Endosc* 1996;**44**:700.

14. Neumann CS, Iqbal TH, Cooper BT. Long term continuous omeprazole treatment of patients with Barrett's oesophagus. *Aliment Pharmacol Ther* 1995;**9**:451.

15. Wilkinson SP, Biddlestone L, Gore S, Shepherd NA. Regression of columnar-lined (Barrett's) oesophagus with omeprazole 40 mg daily: results of 5 years of continuous therapy. *Aliment Pharmacol Ther* 1999;**13**:1205.

16. Bollschweiler E, Schorder W, Holscher AH *et al*. Postoperative risk analysis in patient with adenocarcinoma or squamous cell carcinoma of the oesophagus. *Br J Surg* 2000;**87**:1106.

17. Zaninotto, Parenti AR, Ruol A *et al*. Oesophageal resection for high-grade dysplasia in Barrett's oesophagus. *Br J Surg* 2000;**97**:1002.

18. Barr H. Ablative mucosectomy is the procedure of choice to prevent Barrett's cancer. *Gut* 2003;**52**:14.

19. Barham CP, Jones RL, Biddlestone LR *et al*. Photothermal laser ablation of Barrett's oesophagus: endoscopic and histological evidence of squamous re-epithelialisation. *Gut* 1997;**41**:281.

20. Overholt BF, Panjehpour M, Haydek JM. Photodynamic therapy for Barrett's esophagus: follow-up in 1000 patients. *Gastrointest Endosc* 1999;**49**:1.

21. Sampliner RE, Faigel D, Fennerty MB *et al*. Effective and safe endoscopic reversal of nondysplastic Barrett's esophagus with thermal electrocoagulation combined with high-dose acid inhibition: a multicenter study. *Gastrointest Endosc* 2001;**53**:554.

22. Sharma P, Jaffe PE, Bhattacharyya A, Sampliner RE. Laser and multipolar electrocoagulation ablation of early Barrett's adenocarcinoma: long-term follow-up. *Gastrointest Endosc* 1999;**49**:442.

23. Dulai GS, Jensen DM, Cortina G, Fontana L, Ippoliti A. Randomized trial of APC vs. multipolar electrocoagulation for ablation of Barrett's esophagus. *Gastrointest Endosc* 2005;**61**:232–40.

24. Ganz RA, Utley DS, Stern RA *et al*. Complete ablation of esophageal epithelium with a balloon-based bipolar electrode: a phased evaluation in the porcine an in the human esophagus. *Gastrointest Endosc* 2004;**60**:1002–10.

25. Ginsberg GG, Barkun AN, Bosco JJ *et al*. The argon plasma coagulator: February 2002. *Gastrointest Endosc* 2002;**55**:807.

26. Basu KK, Pick B, Bale R, West KP, De Caestecker JS. Efficacy and 1 year follow up of argon plasma coagulation therapy for ablation of Barrett's oesophagus: factors determining persistence and recurrence of Barrett's epithelium. *Gut* 2002;**51**:776.

27. Byrne JP, Armstrong GR, Attwood SE. Restoration of the normal squamous lining in Barrett's esophagus by argon beam plasma coagulation. *Am J Gastroenterol* 1998;**93**:1810.

28. Grade AJ, Shah IA, Medlin SM, Ramirez FC. The efficacy and safety of argon plasma coagulation therapy in Barrett's esophagus. *Gastrointest Endosc* 1999;**50**:18.

29. Mork H, Barth T, Kreipe HH *et al*. Reconstitution of squamous epithelium in Barrett's oesophagus with endoscopic argon plasma coagulation: a prospective study. *Scand J Gastroenterol* 1998;**33**:1130.

30. Morris CD, Byrne JP, Armstrong GR, Attwood SE. Prevention of the neoplastic progression of Barrett's oesophagus by endoscopic argon beam plasma ablation. *Br J Surg* 2001;**88**:1357.

31. Pereira-Lima JC, Busnello JV, Saul C *et al*. High power setting argon plasma coagulation for the eradication of Barrett's esophagus. *Am J Gastroenterol* 2000;**95**:1661.

32. Schulz H, Miehlke S, Antos D *et al*. Ablation of Barrett's epithelium by endoscopic argon plasma coagulation in combination with high-dose omeprazole. *Gastrointest Endosc* 2000;**51**:659.

33. Van Laethem JL, Cremer M, Peny MO, Delhaye M, Devière J. Eradication of Barrett's mucosa with argon plasma coagulation and acid suppression: immediate and mid term results. *Gut* 1998;**43**:747.

34. Kahaleh M, Van Laethem JL, Nagy N, Cremer M, Devière J. Long term follow-up and factors predictive of recurrence in Barrett's esophagus treated by argon plasma therapy and acid suppression. *Endoscopy* 2002;**12**:950.

35. Ackroyd R, Tam W, Schoeman M, Devitt PG, Watson DI. Prospective randomized controlled trial of argon plasma coagulation ablation vs. endoscopic surveillance in patients with Barrett's esophagus after antireflux surgery. *Gastrointest Endosc* 2004;**59**:1–7.

36. Madisch A, Michlke S, Bayerdorffer E *et al*. Long term follow up after ablation of Barrett's esophagus with argon plasma coagulation. *World J Gastroenterol* 2005; **11**:1182–6.

37. Martinez de Haro L, Ortiz A, Parrilla P *et al*. Intestinal metaplasia in patients with columnar lined esophagus is associated with high levels of duodenogastroesophageal reflux. *Ann Surg* 2001;**233**:34.

38. Menges M, Muller M, Zeitz M. Increased acid and bile reflux in Barrett's esophagus compared to reflux esophagitis, and effect of proton pump inhibitor therapy. *Am J Gastroenterol* 2001;**96**:331.

39. Ouatu-Lascar R, Fitzgerald RC, Triadafilopoulos G. Differentiation and proliferation in Barrett's esophagus and the effects of acid suppression. *Gastroenterology* 1999;**117**:327.

40. Lopes CV, Pereira-Luma J, Hartmann AA. *p53* immunohistochemical expression in Barrett's esophagus before and after endoscopic ablation by argon plasma coagulation. *Scand J Gastroenterol* 2005;**40**:259–63.

41. Shand A, Dallal H, Palmer K, Ghosh S, MacIntyre M. Adenocarcinoma arising in columnar lined oesophagus following treatment with argon plasma coagulation. *Gut* 2001;**48**:580.

42. Van Laethem JL, Peny MO, Salmon I, Cremer M, Devière J. Intramucosal adenocarcinoma arising under squamous re-epithelialisation of Barrett's oesophagus. *Gut* 2000;**46**:574.

43. Kelthy CJ, Ackroyd D, Brown NJ *et al*. Endoscopic ablation of Barrett's esophagus: a randomized controlled trial of photodynamic therapy vs. argon plasma coagulation. *Aliment Pharmacol Ther* 2004;**20**:1289–96.

44. Ackroyd R, Brown NJ, Davis MF *et al*. Photodynamic therapy for dysplastic Barrett's oesophagus: a prospective, double blind, randomised, placebo controlled trial. *Gut* 2000;**47**:612.

45. Gossner L, May A, Stolte G *et al*. KTP laser destruction of dysplasia and early cancer in columnar-lined Barrett's esophagus. *Gastrointest Endosc* 1999;**49**:8–12.

46. Van Laethem JL, Jagodzinski R, Peny MO, Cremer M, Devière J. Argon plasma coagulation in the treatment of Barrett's high grade dysplasia and *in-situ* adenocarcinoma. *Endoscopy* 2001;**33**:257–61.

47. May A, Gossner L, Pech O *et al*. Intraepithelial high grade neoplasia and early adenocarcinoma in short-segment Barrett's esophagus (SSBE): curative treatment using local endoscopic techniques. *Endoscopy* 2002;**34**:604.

CHAPTER 20

Ablation of Barrett's Esophagus with Laser and Photodynamic Therapy

Kenneth K. Wang and Navtej S. Buttar

Background

The field of ablation therapy for Barrett's esophagus has been markedly changed by the completion of a prospective randomized trial that for the first time has demonstrated that photodynamic therapy (PDT) can significantly reduce the risks of cancer development as compared to observation [1]. This is the first non-surgical therapy for Barrett's esophagus that has been shown to decrease cancer risk. Because of this, it is important for anyone interested in the treatment of Barrett's esophagus to be familiar with PDT and laser ablation.

Endoscopic therapy for Barrett's esophagus is controlled by two major factors. The first is the control of chronic gastroesophageal reflux disease that has been previously discussed in Chapter 14. Acid suppression is necessary, but the degree of control needed to ablate tissue has yet to be established. Prospective randomized trials have shown that less than normal degrees of acid suppression do not decrease the effectiveness of ablative therapies. The second issue in treatment of Barrett's esophagus is the elimination of the metaplastic mucosa. PDT has been thought to be almost optimal for this because of the ability of endoscopists to treat large segments of mucosa with a single application of light and drug. However, before any treatment course is taken for Barrett's esophagus, it is important to address patient issues, physician issues, and the physical characteristics of the Barrett's esophagus. Patient-related issues would include factors such as whether or not the patient is anticipated to enjoy a long quality life. Patients who are of advanced age or have multiple comorbidities that would severely limit their sur-

vival would definitely be less likely to require any intervention. On the other hand, young patients without any comorbidities might well benefit from surgical options since a lifetime of future surveillance might not be necessary. The factors that are related to the physical characteristics of Barrett's esophagus include the detection of dysplasia or cancer. If only non-dysplastic Barrett's is found, most esophagologists would not consider doing PDT or any other ablative therapy because of the low risk of cancer. Although there is some benefit for decreasing the need for surveillance and alleviating patient anxiety, thus far, no therapy targeted towards non-dysplastic Barrett's has actually been able to find any long-term benefit in terms of decreased cancer risk or increased survival with these therapies. In patients who are in between these two groups, endoscopic therapies might well be the preferred choice. Other physical characteristics might also include the presence of nodules within a Barrett's esophagus with dysplasia, which would increase the risk of cancer being present. These lesions should be fully characterized by endoscopic ultrasound or hopefully removed with endoscopic mucosal resection in order to exclude the possibility of cancer being present.

Thermal Laser Therapy for Barrett's Esophagus

Laser (light amplification by stimulated emission of radiation) refers to light energy that has the properties of coherence, collimation, and monochromaticity. Coherence refers to the fact that all the photons from the laser are in the same phase. Collimation refers to the non-divergence of the light. This means that even when the light is shining long distances, the beam remains very tight rather than diffusing to wider diameters over distance. These properties account for the use of lasers as pointers, as the laser spot remains focused despite great distances. Monochromaticity indicates that all photons have the same wavelength (or color). If a prism were applied to laser light, only one color would be seen through the prism [2]. A thermal laser system consists of an excitation source that provides the energy for stimulation, a substrate (medium) that is stimulated and produces the photons, and lastly a resonator system that produces the collimated beam of light. The laser type is defined by the substrate that is used to produce laser light, which may be solid, liquid, or gas. The substrate type also determines the wavelength of the laser light that is produced, although adjustment of the wavelength can be done with optical techniques.

In 1960, Maiman constructed the first laser that could produce visible light by using a synthetic ruby crystal [3]. This was followed by use of several other substrates including neodymium (Nd), praseodymium (Pr), thulium (Tm), holmium (Ho), erbium (Er), ytterbium (Yb), gadolinium (Gd), and complex molecules such as yttrium–aluminum–garnet (YAG). The energy produced by a thermal laser is focused on a very small area which can produce significant tissue damage.

Special terms are used to measure the laser energy. *Irradiance* is the power used to deliver energy to tissues and expressed as power per unit of surface area (watts per square centimeter). *Fluence* is the total amount of energy applied to a tissue and is determined by multiplying the irradiance by the duration of light exposure. Fluence is expressed typically as joules per square centimeter. The laser and tissue interaction are affected by wavelength of the light, the power of the laser light, the mode of emission of laser energy (pulsed vs. continuous), and the optical properties of the tissue (absorption and scattering).

Laser energy can produce various effects depending on the degree of thermal injury to protein. Denaturation of protein occurs with moderate tissue heating (>40°C), protein coagulation occurs when temperatures reach >60°C, vaporization of tissue water occurs at 100°C, tissue charring occurs with temperatures reached that are over >250°C, and finally tissue vaporization occurs at >300°C. The thermal lasers that have been used in Barrett's esophagus have had a wide range of abilities to injure tissue.

The Nd : YAG laser with a wavelength of 1060 nm has a relatively deep tissue penetration of 4–6 mm that results in more extensive tissue injury [4–6]. Similarly, semiconductor diode lasers (805–980 nm) can penetrate up to 10 mm and cause coagulation. Argon lasers (455–515 nm) have a penetrance of 1 mm and KTP : YAG lasers (532 nm) have penetration from 0.3 to 1.0 mm. These are laser types with the least ability to cause deep tissue injury and have been selected to avoid complications such as perforation or stricture. Pulse dye laser (504 nm) can cause "plasma" bubbles. The expansion of these plasma bubbles changes the ultrastructure of tissue and disrupts it along stress lines [7].

In the mid 1960s, the use of the laser was explored in the management of cancer on experimental basis [8–10]. In 1984 Boyce and Swain *et al.* used endoscopic laser techniques to palliate advanced esophageal adenocarcinoma [11,12]. Several other studies in the late 1980s and early 1990s, mainly using the Nd : YAG laser, were also directed toward unresectable tumors of esophagus [11,13–17]. The experimental studies on animals and the initial use of laser for the management of Barrett's was initially reported in 1992 [18–20]. The experimental use of thermal lasers in Barrett's esophagus in the last decade can be divided into three indications. The first indication is Barrett's with low-grade or no dysplasia. The use of laser in this group can be considered preventive as this may eradicate Barrett's and therefore potentially prevent the development of high-grade dysplasia (HGD) and cancer. The second group is Barrett's with HGD with or without superficial cancer. The conventional treatment for this group is esophagectomy as the risk for malignancy is high. When only HGD is present and these patients are managed by periodic surveillance without surgery for 5–7 years, about 30% develop cancers and about another 30% of patients have persisting HGD; and in 30% of patients the HGD regresses [21,22]. Laser use in this group can be considered therapeutic and is intended to eliminate both HGD and occult carcinoma. The third indication is for palliation of patients with advanced-stage esophageal cancers arising in the background of Barrett's esophagus. This indication has not been clinically successful, given the popularity of expandable metal stents, so it will not be discussed further.

Use of Thermal Lasers as a Preventative Therapy in Barrett's Esophagus

The use of lasers to treat Barrett's mucosa began about a decade ago. The primary problem with thermal lasers has been the residual intestinal glands that remain underlying the endoscopically normal appearing squamous mucosa. Brandt and Kauvar reported treatment of a patient with Barrett's esophagus by the use of Nd:YAG in 1992 (Fig. 20.1) [19]. The patient was noted to only have a transient regression of Barrett's that reappeared after 14 weeks. Suppression of acid and repeat treatment with Nd:YAG subsequently eliminated the Barrett's mucosa [19]. This became the basis of the perceived need for a degree of acid suppression to generate squamous epithelium. In 1993, Sampliner et al. reported another case in which only a half of the Barrett's esophagus was ablated, demonstrating that the squamous re-epithelization was limited only to the ablated area [23]. Later in 1993, Berenson et al. reported a case series of 10 patients with Barrett's esophagus (two patients with low-grade dysplasia [LGD]) treated with an argon laser every 2–5 weeks [24]. Each patient had 1–8 areas of treatment, ranging from 0.5 to 12.0 cm^2. After a follow-up period of 2–9 months, 38/40 treatment areas showed partial or complete squamous epithelization. This study indicated that complete re-epithelization was more likely if the ablated segment of Barrett's tissue was adjacent to squamous epithelium. In fact, the more contact the segment had with squamous tissue, the better the re-epithelialization. The summary of the most recent laser series is outlined in Table 20.1 [24–29].

Barham et al. have used the KTP:YAG to ablate 16 patients with non-dysplastic Barrett's esophagus [25]. Omeprazole (40 mg a day) was used for acid suppression and 20 mg for maintenance. After a period of 3–18 months; 13 patients had surface epithe-

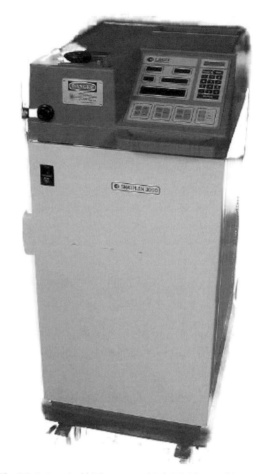

Fig. 20.1 A typical high-powered Nd:YAG laser. This device requires special power and water cooling systems such that, even though it is portable, rooms have to be equipped with 220 V three-way current to power this unit.

lization with squamous epithelium. In 11 patients, 23/53 biopsies showed persistence of Barrett's under squamous. No significant complications occurred. Another study by Biddlestone et al. using a similar KTP:YAG in 10 patients showed small islands of squamous epithelium in six patients [26]. Longer stretches of surface squamous epithelium were found overlying glandular tissue in nine patients, superficial squamous metaplasia of Barrett's glands in six patients, and squamous lining of deeper parts of Barrett's gland in only two patients [26]. Gossner et al. treated four patients with Barrett's esophagus and LGD using a KTP:YAG [27]. A non-contact semicircular technique was used in two separate

Table 20.1 Lasers for eradication of Barrett's esophagus with or without low-grade dysplasia.*

Diagnosis	Patients (*n*)	Laser	No. of treatments	Squamous epithelization	Follow-up (months)	Comments	Ref.
BE ± LGD†	10	Argon	1–8	38/40 segments	2–9	Partial remission	[24]
BE	4	Nd:YAG	5–6	0	6	No difference compared to acid suppression alone	[28]
BE	16	KTP	1–6	13 on surface	3–18	Persistence at depth in 11	[25]
BE†	11	Nd:YAG	1–8	9	8–52	Metaplasia of cardia in 2	[29]
BE†	10	KTP	1–6	9 on surface	4	Persistence at depth in 8	[26]
BE + LGD	4	KTP	2	4	6–12	Barrett's length 2–4 cm	[27]

BE, Barrett's esophagus; LGD, low-grade dysplasia.
*Acid suppression.
† Some patients had fundoplication; others on proton pump inhibitors.

procedures. Adequate acid suppression was ensured by 24-h pH monitoring and proton pump inhibitors (doses as high as 80 mg daily). All patients had elimination of dysplasia on a short follow-up of 6–12 months. Patients in this study had Barrett's length ranging between 2 and 4 cm [27].

These positive results have been encouraging; however, a negative study has been reported as well. Luman *et al.* published a randomized pilot trial of eight patients comparing acid suppression with proton pump inhibitors versus acid suppression and additional Nd:YAG treatment [28]. According to their report, the extent of Barrett's remained unchanged in both groups. In addition, surgical fundoplication has been used for acid control. Salo *et al.* used Nd:YAG after fundoplication for acid control and reported the complete eradication of esophageal Barrett's in 9/11 patients, with a follow-up period ranging from 8 to 52 months [29]. Two patients had persistent specialized intestinal metaplasia of cardia. There were no reported complications.

The eradication of Barrett's esophagus with or without LGD is feasible using various forms of thermal lasers. Theoretically, Nd:YAG can cause deep injury and thus has the best chance to eradicate the deeper Barrett's glands, but this can potentially increase complications including perforation and stricture formation. Perforation can occur in upward of 7% cases, as has been noted during palliative laser of esophageal cancer [30–32]. The power levels used in the treatment of Barrett's esophagus are much smaller and are probably less likely to cause this degree of complication but caution should be exercised.

The trials reported to date have not reported any significant complications, although the number of cases is limited. KTP laser therapy causes more superficial injury and may lead to less complications. There is a suggestion that these therapies may be associated with increased persistence of Barrett's epithelium underlying the neosquamous lining, which can complicate surveillance after the procedure.

Lasers in the Treatment of HGD and Adenocarcinoma

Laser use in Barrett's esophagus with HGD or superficial adenocarcinoma is limited. In 1995, Ertan *et al.*

Table 20.2 Thermal lasers used in Barrett's esophagus with high-grade dysplasia or superficial adenocarcinoma.

Diagnosis	Patients (n)	Laser	No. of treatments	Results	Follow-up (months)	Comments	Ref.
HGD + sACA	1	Nd : YAG	5.0	Eradication in 1	30	Second focus of cancer	[33]
HGD + sACA	4 + 2	KTP	2.4	Eradication in 6	9–15	Residual Barrett's in 1	[27]
sACA	6	Nd : YAG + MPEC	2.8 + 3.3	Initial eradication in 6	9–86	Recurrence of sACA in 1	[34]
HGD + sACA	17	Nd : YAG	–	Eradication in 11	–	–	[35]

HGD, high-grade dysplasia; MPEC, multipolar electrocoagulation; sACA, superficial adenocarcinoma.

reported a single case of Barrett's with HGD and intramucosal adenocarcinoma that was treated with Nd : YAG [33]. The patient declined surgery and underwent five treatment sessions. Acid suppression was achieved with omeprazole (40 mg). At 18 months there was complete squamous epithelization, which persisted up to 30 months. The patient did develop a new focus of cancer contiguous to the first site, required repeat treatment, and remained tumor free at 12 months after the last treatment. Small pilot trials involving three to six patients have recently been reported (Table 20.2) [27,33–35]. The studies used KTP and a combination of Nd : YAG and multipolar coagulation with limited success. It is difficult to assess the use of this technology given the limited number of patients treated. One trial with 17 patients with superficial cancers and HGD had 100% elimination of cancer or dysplasia, but did have strictures develop in 12% of patients and one episode of gastrointestinal bleeding from an esophageal ulcer.

PDT and Barrett's Esophagus

PDT is the result of an interaction between three separate distinct components. First, a drug termed a photosensitizer is administered intravenously in the case of sodium porfimer and is selectively taken up by Barrett's esophagus 48 h prior to photoradiation with light of a specific wavelength to activate the photosensitizer. Photoradiation is done with a light of 630 nm wavelength. The light activates the photosensitizer, which causes the photosensitizer to enter triplet state, which in turn interacts with molecular oxygen producing singlet oxygen that causes cell damage. This effect was first credited to Oscar Raab who was working on developing antimalarial compounds in 1897. Raab found that drugs such as acridine were much more toxic in sunlight to paramecia. A Nobel prize was actually awarded to Niels Finsen in 1903 who found that ultraviolet light could treat cutaneous tuberculosis and smallpox. The work with PDT in human neoplasia only began in 1960 at the Mayo Clinic.

The delay between administration of drug and photoradiation is to allow the drug to diffuse out of normal tissues. It is found that at 48 h, there is the largest difference in concentration between neoplastic and normal tissues. There are other agents, such as aminolevulinic acids (ALAs), which can be administered orally just 4 h prior to photoradiation. ALA is a prodrug that must be converted to protoporphyrin IX within the cell mitochondria. The protoporphyrin IX is what serves as the photosensitizer. The advantage of using ALA is that this is predominately a mucosal agent, so esophageal strictures are very uncommon. In addition, the drug itself is eliminated rapidly so there is not the prolonged duration of cutaneous photosensitivity that is seen with sodium porfimer, which persists in the skin for upwards of 30–90 days after drug administration. Newer agents have been evolved, but not yet clinically approved in the gastrointestinal tract. These agents generally can be activated by light of longer wavelengths for deeper tissue penetration and much shorter degrees of cutaneous photosensitivity often lasting only a day. These photosensitizes include m-tetrahydroxyphenylchlorin (m-THPC), lutetium texaphyrin, polyvinylpyrroolidene, Ester-analogs of ALA, Redachlorin, hydroxybacteriopheophorbide, and talaporphyrin. Of course, with this rapid drug clearance, the treatment window in which photoradiation must be applied is also vastly decreased to typically about 2 h. However, treatment can also be given much closer to drug injection allowing clinicians to truly make PDT a 1-day procedure.

Photoradiation can be conducted at 630 nm with sodium porfimer because this is the deepest penetrating light than can be used with the drug. Although shorter wavelengths of light (blue–green light) can be used to activate the drug, red light is preferred since it can penetrate the tissue and it is less absorbed by hemoglobin which is obviously present in large amounts in tissue.

This is the principle behind using shorter wavelengths of light to diagnose intrapapillary capillary loops in narrow band imaging. In this technology, the shorter wavelengths of light are heavily absorbed by hemoglobin; therefore, the areas that contain blood are enhanced because they become dark areas that absorb light.

Light sources used for PDT are usually lasers because the light needs to be delivered within body cavities. It should be recognized that a wide variety of light sources can be used to activate sodium porfimer. For instance, a broad band light source, even such as that within the endoscope, can activate the drug. Lasers have definitely evolved from tunable dye lasers that require specialized water cooling and high voltage, 220 V, three-way outlets, to solid-state diode lasers that can be operated from standard 110 V outlet current sources and are air cooled. The future of photoradiation will probably be higher power light admitting diodes (LEDs) that can be coupled to probes, which can provide light energy to tumors with even greater ease and decreased cost.

The dosimetry involved in photoradiation must be carefully calculated for photodynamic effect. Ideally, the dose should be calculated based upon the surface area treated. However, in the case of esophageal therapy, this is usually judged to be a fixed amount of light per length of diffusing fiber inserted. The bare fiber was initially used as shown in Plate 20.1 (color plate section falls between pp. 148–9). The problem with this was the positioning of the fiber was often not within the center of the lumen of the esophagus and unequal radiation would occur. The US Food and Drug Administration (FDA) approved this dose method for PDT using a photoradiating balloon at 130 J/cm of fiber (Plate 20.2; color plate section falls between pp. 148–9) which helped to center the balloon. The power output is recommended to be 400 mW/cm of fiber. Therefore, treatment times are generally around 365 s or 6 min for the average photoradiation session.

The effect of PDT is delayed for about 8 h after light application. After photoradiation, there is no mucosa effect but gradual mucosal ischemia, necrosis, and apoptosis occurs creating an eschar that can be viewed in 24 h (Plate 20.3a,b; color plate section falls between pp. 148–9). Patients also usually do not experience pain or other side effects until 8 or more hours after photoradiation.

The initial application of PDT in the gastrointestinal tract was primarily palliation of unresectable cancers which involved bare cylindrical diffusing fibers that allow the light to be distributed perpendicular to the axis of the endoscope. Balloons were later introduced to allow more uniform treatment of the flat mucosa found in Barrett's esophagus. Balloons theoretically allow the mucosa to be flattened out to prevent the protruding area of mucosa from casting shadows producing islands of untreated Barrett's mucosa. The first use of PDT in Barrett's esophagus was reported by the group from Roswell Park in abstract form in 1990 when two patients that were treated for early esophageal cancer also had elimination of their Barrett's segment. Since then, PDT has been used in a number of reports in Barrett's esophagus.

PDT for Barrett's with or without LGD

The evidence for the use of PDT for eradication of Barrett's without dysplasia or LGD is limited. Laukka and Wang reported the use of low-dose PDT in management of Barrett's esophagus [37]. Five patients were treated with 1.5 mg/kg of hematoporphyrin derivative (HpD); 48 h later they were photoradiated (at 630 nm) and delivered a total energy of 175 J/cm. The Barrett's area decreased by 10–50%, the LGD persisted, and Barrett's buried under neosquamous epithelium was noted. None of the five patients developed stricture. The study used proton pump inhibitors for acid suppression.

Overholt et al. reported the use of PDT in 14 patients [36]. Porfimer sodium was used as a photosensitizer (2 mg/kg) and light was delivered using an esophageal centering balloon (energy 175–200 J/cm). The post-treatment follow-up period ranged from 4 to 84 months. One patient developed HGD, and 13 patients had no dysplasia. The Barrett's mucosa was completely ablated in seven patients. Contact thermal therapy using the Nd:YAG laser was combined with PDT in the majority of these patients. Islands of persistent Barrett's mucosa were treated with thermal cautery. Overall, a 75–80% reduction in Barrett's surface area was reported. Strictures occurred in 34% of the patients treated. The study used proton pump inhibitors for acid suppression.

A long-term follow-up study in 40 patients with LGD treated with ALA-based PDT has recently found that macroscopic reduction in the amount of Barrett's mucosa occurred in 88%. More importantly, eradication of dysplasia was found in all patients, which has persisted for a mean of 53 months.

To date, only one study has directly compared the use of PDT with laser ablation. Biddlestone et al. did not find any difference between PDT using ALA as the photosensitizer and KTP laser-based mucosal ablation [26]. Theoretically, PDT may be safer because it does damage the connective tissue matrix and therefore is non-perforating. Although the reported data suggest that PDT may produce more strictures than thermal therapies, this may be a dose-related phenomenon. In our experience, if the drug and light dosages are decreased, stricture formation is an uncommon event.

PDT in Treatment of HGD and Adenocarcinoma

In a large multicenter trial a total of 208 patients were randomized 2:1 to either PDT with 20 mg twice a day of omeprazole or to 20 mg of omeprazole alone a day [1]. Patients were followed using a four-quadrant jumbo biopsy protocol for a period of 2 years. All biopsies were read at a single center. What is very remarkable about this study is that 485 patients were initially screened for this study of which only 208 qualified on re-biopsy. Over half of the patients that were screened actually were not found to have HGD on follow-up endoscopy. Of the 208, 138 patients were treated with PDT versus 70 treated with omeprazole alone. The mean age of the patients was 66 years, 85% were male, and 99% were Caucasian, which is fairly representative of the Barrett's population. This trial involved 27 sites throughout the USA, Canada, UK, and France. The patients were similar in the sense that two-thirds had HGD at multiple levels. Using an intention to treat analysis, 77% of the patients in the treatment group had elimination of HGD during the 2-year interval. Unfortunately, esophageal strictures were reported to occur in one-third of the patients treated. A number of additional observational studies have been reported using PDT for Barrett's esophagus. These are listed in Table 20.3. Different agents and application techniques (centering balloons and other devices) make it very difficult to compare the results.

PDT has recently been reported to eliminate HGD for long periods of observation [39]. In one series that used sodium porfimer based PDT and Nd:YAG laser therapy for residual Barrett's mucosa, 103 patients with HGD, LGD, or early cancer have been followed for a mean of 51 months. HGD was eliminated in 60/65 patients, although three of these (5%) did develop subsquamous non-dysplastic metaplastic epithelium. Intention-to-treat analysis showed that the success rates were about 44% for those with early stage cancer and 78% for patients with HGD.

Table 20.3 Photodynamic therapy (PDT) for high-grade dysplasia or cancer in Barrett's esophagus.

Study	Diagnosis	Patients (n)	Agent	No. of Rx	Results	Follow-up (months)	Year
PhoBar [1]	HGD	208	Sodium Porfimer	3	77% HGD	24	2005
Pech [47]	HGD, CA	66	ALA	1–2	97–100% response	37	2005
Wang [48]	LGD, HGD, CA	169	Porfimer, HpD	2	50% complete ablation	54	2005
Wolfsen [49]	HGD, CA	102	Sodium Pofimer	1	56% complete ablation	19	2004
Etienne [50]	HGD, CA	12	m-THPC	1	100% complete ablation	34	2004
Overholt [41]	LGD,HGD,CA	103	Sodium Porfimer	N/A	44% CA, 78% HGD	51	2003
Gossner [51]	HGD, CA	27	ALA	2	100% HGD, 55% CA	17	1999

ALA, aminolevulinic acid; CA, cancer; HGD, high-grade dysplasia; LGD, low-grade dysplasia; m-THPC, m-tetrahydroxyphenylchlorin; N/A, not applicable.

LGD responded the best with 93% of patients having elimination of dysplasia.

In addition, multiple studies have been reported using Markov modeling to determine the most cost-effective way of managing Barrett's esophagus with HGD considering such strategies as surgical resection, continued careful observation with surgery if cancer is found, or PDT with continued surveillance. These studies have all found that PDT with efficacy as defined in the literature is the most cost-effective strategy that dominates both surgery and observation [42,43]. The incremental cost-benefit of doing endoscopic ablative therapy with PDT was a reasonable $25,621 when compared with no therapy [42]. The typically accepted amount for clinically reasonable procedures is $50,000 or less. Surgery only became cost-effective on sensitivity testing if the incidence of cancer exceeded 30% a year which has never been reported to occur.

There are still some caveats to mention in the treatment of HGD with PDT. One is the persistence of genetic abnormalities in any residual tissue after PDT. This was originally reported in three patients that despite initial down-staging of dysplasia for a minimum duration of 18 months, re-developed HGD and were all found to have persistence of genetic abnormalities such as *p53* or ploidy [44]. This has also been reported recently in a much larger cohort of 29 patients who had either PDT or argon plasma coagulation of dysplastic or non-dysplastic Barrett's mucosa. Abnormal chromosome number and increased *p53* expression were found in areas of residual Barrett's mucosa [45]. This implies that any ablative therapy for Barrett's esophagus should attempt to eliminate all areas of Barrett's mucosa. The first reported death using PDT for ablation therapy in Barrett's esophagus was described in a randomized trial using ALA PDT at different dosages of light as well as argon plasma coagulation for non-dysplastic and LGD [46]. One patient who received ALA 3 days prior died of unknown causes. This is worrisome since ALA is known to cause hemodynamic instability especially in dehydrated patients. This reported case raises the spector that this vascular instability may persist for longer periods of time with ALA.

Conclusions

Thermal laser therapy has been shown to be relatively effective in localized lesions. However, this technology is not routinely available anymore because of limited clinical utility and cost. PDT appears to be increasing in popularity, although it still is not available at most medical centers. Recent completed trials suggest that it is effective in decreasing HGD and cancer risk compared to surveillance alone. Cost-efficacy analysis suggests that this may be the best strategy for HGD. However, ablative therapy should be able to completely eliminate the metaplastic mucosa in order to eliminate cancer risk. The future of this therapy will reside in the development of new agents that can be applied on the day of therapy and that can markedly reduce the duration of cutaneous photosensitivity. A decrease in stricture rates should also be possible with better dosimetry.

References

1. Overholt BF, Lightdale CJ, Wang KK, *et al*. Photodynamic therapy with porfimer sodium for ablation of high-grade dysplasia in Barrett's Esophagus, international partially blinded, randomized phase III trial. *Gastrointest Endosc* 2005;**62**:488–98.

2. van Hillegersberg R. Fundamentals of laser surgery. *Euro J Surg* 1997;**163**:3–12.

3. Maiman T. Stimulated optical radiation in ruby. *Nature* 1960;**187**:493–4.

4. Mordon S. Laser–tissue interaction. *IEEE Trans Biomed Eng* 1989;**361**:145–243.

5. McKenzie AL. Physics of thermal processes in laser–tissue interaction. *Phys Med Biol* 1990;**35**:1175–209.

6. Dederich DN. Laser/tissue interaction. *Alpha Omegan* 1991:**84**:33–6.

7. Floratos DL, de la Rosette JJ. Lasers in urology. *BJU Int* 1999;**84**:201–11.

8. Hume R, Ketcham AS, Minton JP. Light-absorption characteristics of tumor tissue at ruby and neodymium laser energy wavelengths. *J Surg Res* 1966;**6**:531–5.

9. McGuff PE, Gottlieb LS, Katayama I, Levy CK. Comparative study of effects of laser and/or ionizing radiation therapy on experimental or human malignant tumors. *Am J Roentgenol Radium Ther Nucl Med* 1966;**96**:744–8.

10. Naveau S, Poitrine A, Poynard T *et al*. Palliative treatment of cancers of the esophagus and cardia with YAG neodymium laser (preliminary noncontrolled trial) [in French]. *Gastroenterol Clin Biol* 1984;**8**:545–50.

11. Boyce HW, Jr. Palliation of advanced esophageal cancer. *Semin Oncol* 1984;**11**:186–95.

12. Swain CP, Brown SG, Edwards DA *et al*. Laser recanalization of obstruction foregut cancer. *Br J Surg* 1984;**71**:112–5.

13. Wood JW, Innes JW. Tumor ablation by endoscopic Nd : YAG laser. *Am J Gastroenterol* 1985;**80**:715–8.

14. Tenchini P, Breda B, Abrescia F *et al*. Nd–YAG laser disobstruction of esophageal endoprostheses occluded by neoplastic development in the palliative treatment of esophagea cancer [in Italian]. *Chir Ital* 1986;**38**:44–53.

15. Pifano E, Chavez R, Pino G, Jiron A. Effects of YAG-laser on the mucosa of the upper digestive tract. *In vitro* study [in Spanish]. *GEN* 1986;**40**:30–1.

16. Rontal E, Rontal M, Jacob HJ, Klass A. Laser palliation for esophagea carcinoma. *Laryngoscope* 1986;**96**:846–50.

17. Loizou LA, Grigg D, Atkinson M *et al*. A prospective comparison of laser therapy and intubation in endoscopic palliation for malignant dysphagia. *Gastroenterology* 1991;**100**:1303–10.

18. Schaarschmidt K, Stratmann U, Lehmann RR *et al*. The rat esophagus: ultrastructure and radiological aspects of tissue response after 1 320 nm Nd : YAG laser irradiation. *Exp Toxicol Pathol* 1992;**38**:619–22.

19. Brandt LJ, Kauvar DR. Laser-induced transient regression of Barrett's epithelium. *Gastrointest Endosc* 1992; **44**:239–44.

20. Stratmann U, Schaarschmidt K, Lehmann RR *et al*. The cell response of rat esophagus after intraluminal irradiation with Nd–YAG-laser (1 064 nm) after various postoperative times: a light and electron microscopic study [in German]. *Anat Anz* 1993;**175**:95–100.

21. Wright TA. High-grade dysplasia in Barrett's oesophagus. *Br J Surg* 1997;**84**:760–6.

22. Cameron AJ. Management of Barrett's esophagus. *Mayo Clin Proc* 1998;**73**:457–61.

23. Sampliner RE, Hixson LJ, Fennerty MB, Garewal HS. Regression of Barrett's esophagus by laser ablation in an antacid environment. *Dig Dis Sci* 1993;**38**:365–8.

24. Berenson MM, Johnson TD, Markowitz NR *et al*. Restoration of squamous mucosa after ablation of Barrett's esophageal epithelium. *Gastroenterology* 1993; **104**:1686–91.

25. Barham CP, Jones RL, Biddlestone LR *et al*. Photothermal laser ablation of Barrett's oesophagus: endoscopic and histological evidence of squamous re-epithelialization. *Gut* 1997;**41**:281–4.

26. Biddlestone LR, Barham CP, Wilkinson SP *et al*. The histopathology of treated Barrett's esophagus: squamous reepithelialization after acid suppression and laser and photodynamic therapy. *Am J Surg Pathol* 1998;**22**:239–45.

27. Gossner L, May A, Stolte M *et al*. KTP laser destruction of dysplasia and early cancer in columnar-lined Barrett's esophagus. *Gastrointest Endosc* 1999;**49**:8–12.

28. Luman W, Lessels AM, Palmer KR. Failure of Nd–YAG photocoagulation therapy as treatment of Barrett's oesophagus—a pilot study. *Eur J Gastroenterol Hepatol* 1996;**8**:627–30.

29. Salo JA, Salminen JT, Kiviluoto TA *et al*. Treatment of Barrett's esophagus by endoscopic laser ablation and antireflux surgery. *Ann Surg* 1998;**227**:40–4.

30. Haddad NG, Fleischer DE. Endoscopic laser therapy for esophageal cancer. *Gastrointest Endosc Clin North Am* 1994;**4**:863–74.

31. Buset M, des Marez B, Baize M *et al*. Palliative endoscopic management of obstructive esophagogastric cancer: laser or prosthesis? *Gastrointest Endosc* 1987; **33**:357–61.

32. Abdel-Wahab M, Gad-Elhak N, Denewer A *et al*. Endoscopic laser treatment of progressive dysphagia in patients with advanced esophageal carcinoma. *Hepatogastroenterology* 1998;**45**:1509–15.

33. Ertan A, Zimmerman M, Younes M. Esophageal adenocarcinoma associated with Barrett's esophagus: long-term management with laser ablation. *Am J Gastroenterol* 1995;**90**:2201–3.

34. Sharma P, Jaffe PE, Bhattacharyya A, Sampliner RE. Laser and multipolar electrocoagulation ablation of early Barrett's adenocarcinoma: long-term follow-up. *Gastrointest Endosc* 1999;**49**:442–6.

35. Wang KK. Current status of photodynamic therapy of Barrett's esophagus. *Gastrointest Endosc* 1999;**49**:S20–3.

36. Overholt BF, Panjehpour M, Haydek JM. Photodynamic therapy for Barrett's esophagus: follow-up in 100 patients. *Gastrointest Endosc* 1999;**49**:1–7.

37. Laukka MA, Wang KK. Initial results using low-dose photodynamic therapy in the treatment of Barrett's esophagus. *Gastrointest Endosc* 1995;**42**:59–63.

38. Barr H, Shepherd NA, Dix A *et al*. Eradication of high-grade dysplasia in columnar-lined (Barrett's) oesophagus by photodynamic therapy with endogenously generated protoporphyrin IX. *Lancet* 1996;**348**:584–5.

39. Harle IA, Finley RJ, Belsheim M *et al*. Management of adenocarcinoma in a columnar-lined esophagus. *Ann Thorac Surg* 1985;**40**:330–6.

40. Ackroyd R, Kelty CJ, Brown NJ *et al*. Eradication of dysplastic Barrett's oesophagus using photodynamic therapy: long-term follow-up. *Endoscopy* 2003;**35**(6): 496–501.

41. Overholt BF, Panjehpour M, Halberg DL. Photodynamic therapy for Barrett's esophagus with dyspla-

sia and/or early stage carcinoma: long-term results [see comment]. *Gastrointest Endosc* 2003;**58**(2):183–8.

42. Shaheen NJ, Inadomi JM, Overholt BF *et al*. What is the best management strategy for high grade dysplasia in Barrett's oesophagus? A cost effectiveness analysis. *Gut* 2004;**53**(12):1736–44.

43. Hur C, Nishioka NS, Gazelle GS. Cost-effectiveness of photodynamic therapy for treatment of Barrett's esophagus with high grade dysplasia. *Dig Dis Sci* 2003;**48**(7):1273–83.

44. Krishnadath K, Wang KK, Liu W *et al*. Persistent genetic abnormalities in Barrett's esophagus after photodynamic therapy. *Gastroenterology* 2000;**119**:624–30.

45. Hage M, Siersema PD, Vissers KJ *et al*. Molecular evaluation of ablative therapy of Barrett's oesophagus. *J Pathol* 2005;**205**(1):57–64.

46. Hage M, Siersema PD, van Dekken H *et al*. 5-Aminolevulinic acid photodynamic therapy versus argon plasma coagulation for ablation of Barrett's oesophagus: a randomised trial. *Gut* 2004;**53**(6): 785–90.

47. Pech O, Gossner L, May A *et al*. Long-term results of photodynamic therapy with 5-aminolevulinic acid for superficial Barrett's cancer and high-grade intraepithelial neoplasia. *Gastrointest Endosc* 2005;**62**:24–30.

48. Wang KK. Current Strategies in the management of Barrett's esophagus. *Curr Gastroenterol Rep* 2005;**7**: 196–201.

49. Wolfsen HC, Hemminger LL, Wallace MB, Devault KR. Clinical experience of patients undergoing photodynamic therapy for Barrett's dysplasia or cancer. *Aliment Pharmacol Therapeut* 2004;**20**:1125–31.

50. Etienne J, Dorme N, Bourg-Heckly G, Raimbert P, Flijou JF. Photodynamic therapy with green light and m-tetrahydroxyphenyl chlorin for intramucosal adenocarcinoma and high-grade dysplasia in Barrett's esophagus. *Gastrointest Endosc* 2004;**59**:880–9.

51. Gossner L, May A, Sroka R, Stolte M, Hahn EG, Ell C. Photodynamic destruction of high grade dysplasia and early carcinoma of the esophagus after the oral administration of 5-aminolevulinic acid. *Cancer* 1999;**86**:1921–8.

CHAPTER 21
Endoscopic Resection

Oliver Pech, Andrea May, and Christian Ell

Background

In the early 1990s, there was a marked increase in the clinical importance of Barrett's esophagus. This was mainly due to the increase in the incidence of adenocarcinoma of the esophagus and at the esophagogastric junction and a growing understanding of the pathophysiological connections between reflux disease, Barrett's metaplasia, and adenocarcinoma. Endoscopic technology (above all high-resolution video-endoscopy), the training of endoscopists, enthusiasm on the part of pathologists and gastroenterologists, and epidemiological conditions have all contributed to the current "Barrett's boom" [1].

It has been well demonstrated that acid reflux is strongly associated with the development of adenocarcinoma and that Barrett's carcinoma develops through a multistep pathway. This process is characterized by the metaplasia—intraepithelial neoplasia (low-grade intraepithelial neoplasia [LGIN]/high-grade intraepithelial neoplasia [HGIN])–adenocarcinoma sequence [2,3]. Therefore, early detection of superficial neoplasia has become important in the past several years and several techniques like chromoendoscopy, photodynamic diagnosis, optical coherence tomography, and endomicroscopy have been developed. Early detection of neoplastic lesions in Barrett's esophagus is the basis for endoscopic therapy, like photodynamic therapy (PDT) or endoscopic resection (ER) [4–6].

Radical esophageal resection has until now been the standard treatment for patients with early neoplasia in Barrett's esophagus, but it is associated with a mortality rate of at least 5% or more and a morbidity rate of at least 40%, even in experienced centers [7,8]. In patients older than 70 years, the mortality rate increases to over 10% [9], and in hospitals with a low frequency of esophageal resections, the rate can be up to 20%, even in the hands of experienced surgeons [10,11]. Therefore less invasive procedures are desirable, although they need to provide curative treatment with the same degree of certainty. ER imitates the surgical situation: The tumor is excised electrosurgically, providing the pathologist with a specimen that gives the opportunity to assess the depth of invasion, involvement of lymphatic vessels and veins, grade of differentiation, and above all in relation to the question of tumor-free margins. The aim of every ER should be the complete resection of the mucosal and submucosal layer. This can be achieved by ER with suck-and-cut technique in almost all cases.

Surgical data showed that the risk of lymph node metastases in HGIN and mucosal adenocarcinoma in Barrett's esophagus is nearly absent [7,8,12,13]. It is only when infiltration of the submucosa takes place that lymph-node metastases are encountered, in 20–25% of cases [13,14]. Thus, surgical esophageal resection is indicated in early Barrett's cancer with invasion into the submucosa. One future expansion of ER in Barrett's cancer might be infiltration in the upper third of the submucosa (T1sm1). Two recent surgical studies show that in patients with T1sm1-cancer no positive lymph nodes could be found [12,15].

History of ER

ER in the gastrointestinal tract has been used as a diagnostic and therapeutic procedure for early malignancies—in the initial period, mainly by endoscopists in Asia. In a 1984 publication, Tada *et al.* for the first time described the use of "strip-off biopsy" as a treatment option in early gastric carcinoma [16]. This was the start of the triumphant progress of ER as a therapeutic and diagnostic procedure in the upper gastrointestinal tract.

The first ER procedures for early esophageal carcinoma were carried out in the early 1990s, again by Japanese endoscopists [17,18]. It was only several years later that the first Western research groups published their preliminary experience in ER for esophageal neoplasias in a few patients [19,20]. The first larger series of ER in patients with early Barrett's neoplasia was published by our group in 2000 [6].

ER—Techniques

Strip Biopsy

In strip biopsy, a diathermy loop is introduced through the working channel of the endoscope and positioned over a polypoid lesion, which is fixed by tightening of the loop and slowly detached using electrical cutting current. This technique can especially be used in (type I) polypoid tumors, but with flat lesions it is often difficult to position the loop, and there may be a risk that the size of the removed specimen will be limited and that only piecemeal and not en bloc resection is possible in most cases.

Submucosal injection of a solution can lift flat or depressed lesions (type II) and make it easier to resect them (the "lift-and-cut" technique). In addition to extending the range of target lesions in comparison with simple strip biopsy, this procedure also has other advantages. Injection of a saline–epinephrine solution into the submucosa, for example, lifts the early carcinoma—thereby increasing the distance from the muscularis propria and potentially reducing the risk of perforation. A second advantage of the injection technique may be a reduced risk of hemorrhage, due to compression by the injected volume of liquid.

The type of injection solution has not been standardized. The solution most often used is saline with epinephrine or dextrose in various concentrations. We use generally a 1 : 100 000 epinephrine–saline solution. The advantage of the epinephrine solution, in comparison with the saline plus dextrose solution also used, is the vasoconstriction caused by the catecholamine and the resulting reduction in the risk of hemorrhage. A disadvantage of the epinephrine–saline mixture is its short dwell time (3.0 min) in comparison with a 50% dextrose solution (4.7 min) and a 1% rooster comb hyaluronic acid solution (22.1 min). These data were obtained in an experimental study in the porcine esophagus [21].

"Suck-and-Cut" Technique

The "suck-and-cut" technique is used in the esophagus more frequently than strip biopsy, due to anatomical conditions. A study by Tanabe et al. demonstrated that endoscopic suck-and-cut mucosectomy in early gastric cancer was more effective than strip biopsy with regard to the largest diameter of the resected specimen, the rate of en bloc resection, and the complication rate [22].

ER—Procedure with a Cap

In the early 1990s, Inoue and Endo developed the cap technique, thereby improving the effectiveness of ER in comparison with simple strip biopsy [23]. In the ER cap technique, a specially developed transparent plastic cap with a gutter is attached to the distal end of the endoscope. After submucosal injection under the target lesion, the lesion is sucked into the cap to create a pseudo-polyp, which can slowly be cut with the diathermy loop (Fig. 21.1). Since injecting underneath early carcinomas often makes it difficult to distinguish them, prior marking of the lesion—for example using electrocautery—is recommended. After the resected specimen is captured, for example with the cap itself or a polyp grasper, and retrieved, it should be fixed, for example on a piece of cork with needles to make it easier for the pathologist to evaluate the margins (Plate 21.1a–d; color plate section falls between pp. 148–9).

ER—Procedure with a Ligation Device

Endoscopic resection with ligation (ER-L) is another suction ER technique in which a ligation device is used. In this method, the target lesion is sucked into the ligation cylinder at the tip of the endoscope, and a polyp is created by releasing a rubber band around

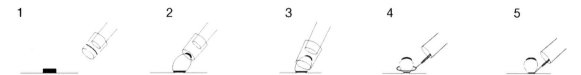

Fig. 21.1 Endoscopic resection (ER) with a ligation device. (1) Endoscope with ligation device is unserted. (2,3) Lesion is sucked into ligation device and rubber band is released to create a pseudo-polyp. (4,5) Pseudo-polyp is resected above or under the rubber band.

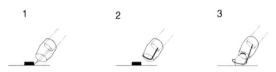

Fig. 21.2 Endoscopic resection (ER) with a transparent cap. (1) Submucosal injection under target lesion. (2) Snare is preloaded in the cap. (3) Lesion is sucked into the cap to create a pseudo-polyp. Lesion is resected with a diathermy snare.

it. The polyp is then resected at its base, either above or below the rubber band, using a diathermy loop (Fig. 21.2). This method of ER is performed in our unit without submucosal injection and therefore marking of the neoplastic margins is not necessary. In this technique, the endoscope being used for resection has to be withdrawn again and re-introduced in order to remove the ligation cylinder and introduce the loop. Ligation devices available include, in addition to single-use devices, a re-usable ligator [24], with which comparable results can be achieved at reduced cost. More recently, a multiband ligation ER device has been introduced.

Both techniques, i.e. cap and ligation, have been shown to provide equal efficacy and safety in early esophageal cancer [25]. There were no significant differences between both suck-and-cut techniques concerning the maximum diameter of the resected specimen, the resected area, and the rate of complications. Using the ligation device the endoscope had to be inserted more often (not significant), whereas using the cap a marking and submucosal injection of saline and epinephrine is necessary. Only in patients with prior mucosectomy does the ER with a ligation device seemed to be more effective than the ER using the cap (not statistically significant).

Other Resection Techniques

In addition to the suck-and-cut mucosectomy and strip-biopsy techniques, ER using a double-channel endoscope has also been described [26]. In this method, a grasping forceps is used to pull the target lesion through a diathermy loop that has been introduced through the second working channel. The lesion is then resected with the loop. Due to the large caliber of the endoscope required, double-channel procedures appear to be difficult, especially at the esophagogastric junction, and may even be almost impossible in the retroflexed position.

After ER of a neoplastic lesion, the remaining Barrett's epithelium is still at risk for malignant degradation or synchronous neoplastic areas. Seewald et al. performed circumferential resection in 12 patients with early Barrett's neoplasia with a monofilament snare without prior submucosal injection [27]. The aim of this approach was complete removal of Barrett's epithelium with early stage malignant changes. Complete removal could be performed in all patients and during a median follow-up of 9 months no recurrence of malignancy or Barrett's epithelium was observed, but the neccessary number of ER sessions per patient was very high and the procedures were acompanied by a high stricture rate (17%). Minor bleeding occurred during four of 31 ER sessions. A technique of ER associated with less stricture formation may be semicircumferential ER. Giovannini et al. reported their experience in 21 patients, in which ER of the neoplasia and semicircumferential resection of Barrett's epithelium was performed in two steps [28]. In order to prevent the formation of esophageal stenosis, the second half of the Barrett's esophagus mucosa was resected a month later. Using this technique, the authors reported no stricture formation.

In our department, to reduce the stricture rate, longitudinal resection is performed. Further longitudinal resection of neoplasia and metaplasia is usually perfomed every 6–8 weeks until HGIN or cancer is completely eradicated.

En bloc resection, where the entire tumor is removed in one piece, is often not achieved using conventional ER. Other techniques, developed in Japan, include the application of different types of knife such as the insulated-tip instrument [29]. After submucosal saline injection, circumcision and dissection of the mucosal lesions is performed with the aim of achieving *en bloc* resection. This method was first used in gastric cancer in Japan, but very limited experience in the esophagus exists in Western centers [30]. The disadvantage of this method is that *en bloc* resection with an endoscopic knife is technically very demanding, especially at the esophagogastric junction and can be associated with a high risk of bleeding and perforation. Further studies are awaited to judge the value of this method in patients with early Barrett's cancer.

Complications of ER

ER involves certain risks, and should therefore only be carried out by experienced endoscopists. The most frequent complication of ER is hemorrhage, although arterial bleeding is very rare. By contrast, oozing venous bleeding is not uncommon; it is usually not associated with a drop in hemoglobin, and can be controlled by injection therapy. Hemorrhage after ER usually occurs during the first 12–24 h. For this reason, a follow-up endoscopy may be performed 24 h following ER. The rate of bleeding after ER in the esophagus ranges from 2% to 14% in experienced centers [6,25–28].

Perforation is the most serious complication of ER. Depending on the size and location of the lesion, the figures for the frequency of perforation in the upper gastrointestinal tract range from 0.06% to 5% [31]. Localized perforations often can be treated conservatively by closing the site with metal clips and administering antibiotic treatment and parenteral nutrition. To reduce the risk of perforation, resecting large lesions in a single piece should be avoided. Invasion of the muscle layer should be ruled out by endoscopic ultrasound and good mobilization of the mucosal and submucosal layer either by suction into the ligation device or by submucosal injection is mandatory but often not sufficient in pretreated patients.

Results of ER in Early Barrett's Neoplasia

Experience in local ER treatment for early neoplasia in Barrett's esophagus is as yet very limited. In a study by Ell *et al.* of 64 patients with early Barrett's carcinoma and intraepithelial high-grade, complete remission was achieved in 82.5% of cases (97% in the low-risk group, 59% in the high-risk group) [6]. During a mean follow-up period of 12 months, recurrences or metachronous carcinomas were observed in 14% of the patients, and these lesions were again successfully treated. The rate of complications in the study was 12.5% [6].

More recent publications of our group have also confirmed the effectiveness of ER in 50 patients with early neoplasia in short segment Barrett's esophagus [33]. Twenty-eight patients received ER, 13 underwent PDT, and three were treated with argon plasma coagulation (APC). A combination of these therapies was used in six patients. Complete local remission was achieved in 98% of the patients; one patient had to undergo surgery after initial ER treatment, as there was submucosal tumor infiltration. In this study, the complication rate was again very low at 6% (bleeding, stenosis), and no major complications such as perforation or severe bleeding (hemoglobin drop > 2 g/dL) were observed. The intermediate results were similarly encouraging (average follow-up period 34 ± 10 months) in 115 patients treated using ER (n = 70), PDT (n = 32), and APC (n = 3). Multimodal therapy led to complete local remission in 98% of the patients in this group [34]. During a mean follow-up of 50 months, 37 patients (32%) had a recurrence or metachronous neoplasia, but 36 of these 37 patients could be retreated successfully by ER.

In 25 patients with lesions in Barrett's esophagus (13 adenocarcinomas, four HGIN), Nijhawan *et al.* carried out ER with a diagnostic and therapeutic intent [35]. The "lift-and-cut" technique was used in

Table 21.1 Important publications about endoscopic resection (ER) in early Barrett's neoplasia.

	No. of patients	Resection technique	Complications	5-Year follow-up
Ell *et al.* [6]	64	S & C	0% major 11% minor	—
Nijhawan & Wang [35]	17	S & C	0%	—
Buttar *et al.* [32]	17	S & C + PDT	30%	—
Seewald *et al.* [27]	12	Circumference snare resection	Stenosis 2/12 Bleeding 4/12	—
May *et al.* [34]	115	S & C 70% PDT 30%	0% major 11% minor	—
Giovannini *et al.* [28]	21	Semicircumference snare resection	0% major 19% minor	—
Behrens *et al.* [37]	44	S & C PDT	0% major 9% minor	85%*
Ell *et al.* [38]	100	S & C	0% major 10% minor	98%*
Peters *et al.* [40]	28	S & C	0% major 46% minor	—

* Deaths not tumor related.
PDT, photodynamic therapy; S & C, suck-and-cut.

the majority of cases, and the "suck-and-cut" technique with a ligation device was only used in two patients. The results were quite promising with no recurrences after a median follow-up of 9 months. In a very heterogeneous group of patients, Ahmad *et al.* carried out 101 ERs in malignant and non-malignant lesions throughout the entire gastrointestinal tract [36]. This also included 12 with lesions in Barrett's esophagus (six adenocarcinomas, six HGINs). The complication rate was 11%, and complete remission was achieved in four patients of each group.

ER was carried out in 14 patients with HGIN in Barrett's esophagus in a recently published study of our group [37]. Twenty-seven patients, in whom the HGD was not re-detectable but confirmed by reference pathologists, underwent PDT. ER and PDT were combined in three patients. Complete remission was achieved in 43 of 44 patients with HGIN (97.7%). No major complications occurred. A mean of one session was needed to achieve complete local remission and during a mean follow-up period of 36 months,

recurrent or metachronous lesions were observed in six patients (17.1%), all of whom received a second successful endoscopic treatment. A recently presented study about ER in a homogenous group of 100 patients with low-risk adenocarcinoma (macroscopic types IIa, IIb, and IIc; lesion diameter up to 20 mm; mucosal lesion without invasion into lymph vessels and veins; and histological grades G1 and G2) arising in Barrett's esophagus showed excellent short- and long-term results [36]. Complete local remission was achieved in 99 of 100 patients after 1.9 months (range 1–18 months) and a maximum of three resections. During a mean follow-up period of 36.7 months, recurrent or metachronous carcinomas were found in 11% of the patients, but successful repeat treatment with ER was possible in all cases. The calculated 5-year survival rate was 98%. Table 21.1 summarizes important studies about ER in Barrett's neoplasia.

In our own experience, involvement of the lateral margins of the resected specimens is quite frequent, especially in large or multifocal neoplastic lesions. But this fact doesn't usually mean that curative endoscopic therapy is not possible. In general, a retreatment of these patients is possible and complete remission can be achieved by further resections [6] or supportive PDT [32]. A R0 resection at the base of the neoplasia is absolutely mandatory.

Summary

In experienced hands, ER is a safe method of resecting premalignant lesions and early carcinomas in Barrett's esophagus. It has decisive advantages in comparison with other local endoscopic treatment procedures (such as thermal destruction and PDT): the opportunity for histological processing of the resected specimen provides information regarding the depth of invasion of the individual layers of the gastrointestinal tract wall, and regarding excision with healthy margins. If there is infiltration of the submucosa detected on ER, a patient with early Barrett's cancer is still able to undergo surgical resection.

Randomized and controlled studies comparing radical esophagectomy with ER are desirable, but are difficult to conduct—not least because some 5-year survival data are now available [38]. Therefore, from our point of view ER should be carried out in all patients with HGIN and mucosal cancer in Barrett's esophagus. In patients with submucosal involvement, limited esophageal resection (Merendino procedure) appears to be a good alternative with lower morbidity and mortality rate than conventional surgical resection [39]. But series with a larger cohort of patients and the results of comparative studies are awaited.

References

1. Pracht AT, MacDonald TA, Hopwood DA, Johnston DA. Increasing incidence of Barrett´s esophagus: education enthusiasm or epidemiology? *Lancet* 1997; **350**:933.

2. Cameron AJ, Carpenter HA. Barrett's esophagus, high-grade dysplasia and early adenocarcinoma: a pathological study. *Am J Gastroenterol* 1997;**92**:586–91.

3. Lagergren J, Bergstrom R, Lindgren A, Nyren O. Symptomatic gastroesophageal reflux as a risk factor for esophageal adenocarcinoma. *N Engl J Med* 1999;**340**:825–31.

4. Gossner L, Stolte M, Sroka R et al. Photodynamic ablation of high-grade dysplasia and early cancer in Barrett's esophagus by means of 5-aminolevulinic acid. *Gastroenterology* 1998;**114**:448–55.

5. Pech O, Gossner L, May A et al. Long-term results of photodynamic therapy with 5-aminolevulinic acid for superficial Barrett's cancer and high-grade intraepithelial neoplasia. *Gastrointest Endosc* 2005;**62**:24–30.

6. Ell C, May A, Gossner L et al. Endoscopic mucosal resection of early cancer and high-grade dysplasia in Barrett's esophagus. *Gastroenterology* 2000;**118**(4):670–7.

7. Heitmiller RF, Redmond M, Hamilton SR. Barrett's esophagus with high-grade dysplasia: an indication for prophylactic esophagectomy. *Ann Surg* 1996;**224**(1):66–71.

8. Hölscher AH, Bollschweiler E, Schneider PM, Siewert JR. Early adenocarcinoma in Barrett's oesophagus. *Br J Surg* 1997;**84**(10):1470–3.

9. Thomas P, Doddoli C, Neville P et al. Esophageal cancer resection in the elderly. *Eur J Cardiothorac Surg* 1996;**10**(11):941–6.

10. Birkmeyer JD, Siewers AE, Finlayson EV et al. Hospital volume and surgical mortality in the United States. *N Engl J Med* 2002;**346**:1128–37.

11. Birkmeyer JD, Stukel TA, Siewers AE et al. Surgeon volume and operative mortality in the United States. *N Engl J Med* 2003;**349**:2117–27.

12. Buskens CJ, Westerterp M, Lagarde SM et al. Prediction of appropriateness of local endoscopic treatment for high-grade dysplasia and early adenocarcinoma by EUS and histopathologic features. *Gastrointest Endosc* 2004;**60**(5):703–10.

13. Stein HJ, Feith M, Mueller J, Werner M, Siewert JR. Limited resection for early adenocarcinoma in Barrett's esophagus. *Ann Surg* 2000;**232**(6):733–42.

14. Nigro JJ, Hagen JA, DeMeester TR et al. Prevalence and location of nodal metastases in distal esophageal adenocarcinoma confined to the wall: implications for therapy. *J Thorac Cardiovasc Surg* 1999;**117**(1):16–25.

15. Stein HJ, Feith M, Bruecher BLDM, Nahrig J, Siewert JR. Early esophageal squamous cell and adenocarcinoma: Pattern of lymphatic spread and prognostic factors for long term survival after surgical resection. *Ann Surg* 2005;**242**(4):566–73.

16. Tada M, Murata M, Murakami F et al. Development of the strip-off biopsy [in Japanese]. *Gastroenterol Endosc* 1984;**26**:833–9.

17. Makuuchi H, Machimura T, Soh Y *et al*. Endoscopic mucosectomy for mucosal carcinomas in the esophagus. *Jpn J Surg Gastroenterol* 1991;**24**:2599–603.

18. Inoue H, Endo M, Takeshita K *et al*. Endoscopic resection of carcinoma *in situ* of the esophagus accompanied by esophageal varices. *Surg Endosc* 1991;**5**(4):182–4.

19. Soehendra N, Binmoeller KF, Bohnacker S *et al*. Endoscopic snare mucosectomy in the esophagus without any additional equipment: a simple technique for resection of flat early cancer. *Endoscopy* 1997;**29**:380–3.

20. Giovannini M, Bernardini D, Moutardier V *et al*. Endoscopic mucosal resection (EMR): results and prognostic factors in 21 patients. *Endoscopy* 1999;**31**:698–701.

21. Conio M, Rajan E, Sorbi D *et al*. Comparative performance in the porcine esophagus of different solutions used for submucosal injection. *Gastrointest Endosc* 2002;**56**:513–6.

22. Tanabe S, Koizumi W, Kokutou M *et al*. Usefulness of endoscopic aspiration mucosectomy as compared with strip biopsy for the treatment of gastric mucosal cancer. *Gastrointest Endosc* 1999;**50**(6):819–22.

23. Inoue H, Endo M. A new simplified technique of endoscopic esophageal mucosal resection using a cap-fitted panendoscope. *Surg Endosc* 1993;**6**:264–5.

24. Ell C, May A, Wurster H. The first reusable multiple-band ligator for endoscopic hemostasis of variceal bleeding and mucosal resection. *Endoscopy* 1999;**31**: 738–40.

25. May A, Gossner L, Behrens A, Ell C. A prospective randomized trial of two different suck-and-cut mucosectomy techniques in 100 consecutive resections in patients with early cancer of the esophagus. *Gastrointest Endosc* 2003;**58**:167–75.

26. Noda M, Kobayashi N, Kanemasa H *et al*. Endoscopic mucosal resection using a partial transparent hood for lesions located tangentially to the endoscope. *Gastrointest Endosc* 2000;**51**(3):338–43.

27. Seewald S, Akaraviputh, T, Seitz U *et al*. Circumferential EMR and complete removal of Barrett's epithelium: a new approach to management of Barrett's esophagus containing high-grade intraepithelial neoplasia and intramucosal carcinoma. *Gastrointest Endosc* 2003;**57**:854–9.

28. Giovannini M, Bories E, Pesenti C *et al*. Circumferential endoscopic mucosal resection in Barrett's esophagus with high-grade intraepithelial neoplasia or mucosal cancer. Preliminary results in 21 patients. *Endoscopy* 2004;**36**:782–7.

29. Muto M, Miyamoto S, Hosokawa A *et al*. Endoscopic mucosal resection in the stomach using the insulated-tip needle-knife. *Endoscopy* 2005;**37**:178–82.

30. Rosch T, Sarbia M, Schumacher B *et al*. Attempted endoscopic *en bloc* resection of mucosal and submucosal tumors using insulated-tip knives: a pilot series. *Endoscopy* 2004;**36**:788–801.

31. Rembacken BJ, Gotoda D, Fuji T, Axon ATR. Endoscopic mucosal resection. *Endoscopy* 2001;**33**: 709–18.

32. Buttar NS, Wang KK, Lutzke LS, Krishnadath KK, Anderson MA. Combined endoscopic mucosal resection and photodynamic therapy for esophageal neoplasia within Barrett's esophagus. *Gastrointest Endosc* 2001;**54**(6):682–8.

33. May A, Gossner L, Pech O *et al*. Intraepithelial high-grade neoplasia and early adenocarcinoma in short-segment Barrett's esophagus (SSBE): curative treatment using local endoscopic treatment techniques. *Endoscopy* 2002;**34**(8):604–10.

34. May A, Gossner L, Pech O *et al*. Local endoscopic therapy for intraepithelial high-grade neoplasia and early adenocarcinoma in Barrett's oesophagus: acute-phase and intermediate results of a new treatment approach. *Eur J Gastroenterol Hepatol* 2002;**14**(10):1085–91.

35. Nijhawan PK, Wang KK. Endoscopic mucosal resection for lesions with endoscopic features suggestive of malignancy and high-grade dysplasia within Barrett's esophagus. *Gastrointest Endosc* 2000;**52**(3):328–32.

36. Ahmad NA, Kochman ML, Long WB, Furth EE, Ginsberg GG. Efficacy, safety, and clinical outcomes of endoscopic mucosal resection: a study of 101 cases. *Gastrointest Endosc* 2002;**55**(3):390–6.

37. Behrens A, May A, Gossner L *et al*. Curative treatment for high-grade intraepithelial neoplasia in Barrett's esophagus. *Endoscopy* 2005;**37**:999–1005.

38. Ell C, May A, Pech O *et al*. Curative endoscopic resection for early esophageal adenocarcinomas (Barrett's cancer). *Gastrointest Endosc* 2006, in press.

39. Schroder W, Gutschow CA, Holscher AH. Limited resection for early esophageal cancer? *Langenbecks Arch Surg* 2003;**388**:88–94.

40. Peters FP, Kara MA, Rosmolen WD *et al*. Endoscopic treatment of high-grade dysplasia and early stage cancer in Barrett's esophagus. *Gastrointest Endosc* 2005;**61**(4):506–14.

Role of Endoscopic Ultrasound in Barrett's Esophagus and Esophageal Adenocarcinoma

Ann Marie Joyce and Gregory G. Ginsberg

Introduction

Endoscopic ultrasound (EUS) incorporates flexible endoscopy and high-frequency ultrasound to image into and through the luminal digestive tract. It enables the endosonographer to evaluate the wall layer pattern of the esophagus and to detect the presence of regional and celiac lymph nodes. EUS guided fine needle aspiration (FNA) permits directed tissue sampling of subdiaphragmatic and mediastinal lymph nodes. EUS is used for staging esophageal cancer and in the evaluation and management of Barrett's esophagus-associated dysplasia.

Endoscopic Ultrasound

EUS is available in an endoscope-based system and a catheter-based system. The endoscope-based system is divided into radial and linear array scanning. The radial echoendoscope uses a mechanically rotated transducer to generate a 360° cross-sectional image perpendicular to the long axis of the instrument. Radial scanning echoendoscopes provide imaging at 5.0, 7.5, 12.0, and 20.0 MHz.

The linear array echoendoscope has an electronically operated transducer that produces a ~270° image parallel to the long axis of the endoscope. The linear array echoendoscope permits FNA under direct EUS guidance. The linear array echoendoscope also has power Doppler capability allowing confirmation of vascular structures.

High frequency catheter ultrasound probes (CUSPs) may be passed through the accessory channel of a forward viewing endoscope allowing directed probe localization and substituting for a dedicated scope based system. The catheter-based probes may be placed directly over a small target lesion. The probes are available as 2.0, 2.4, and 2.6 mm in diameter with frequencies of 12, 15, and 20 MHz. These high frequency probes may delineate up to seven to nine layers within the esophageal wall but at the expense of a limited depth of penetration.

EUS more typically generates a five-layer wall pattern of alternating hyperechogenicity (bright) and hypoechogenicity (dark) that correlates with histology (Fig. 22.1). To improve acoustic coupling, scanning is performed with water immersion or with a water-filled balloon sheath over the probe.

EUS is used in the evaluation of regional lymph nodes. Mediastinal lymph nodes may be detected by EUS in disease and health. Lymph nodes appear as spheroid, ovoid, or pyramidal shapes. It may be difficult to differentiate between malignant and benign nodes with imaging alone. Sonographic characteristics of malignant lymph nodes include size greater than 1 cm in diameter, hypoechogenicity, and round in shape with sharp borders [1]. The introduction of FNA increases the accuracy of EUS in detecting malignant nodes [2]. The presence of malignant appearing lymph nodes in patients with Barrett's esophagus and "early" cancer, based on EUS and computed tomography (CT) scan findings, would support operative rather than endoscopic therapy.

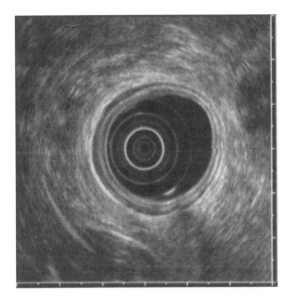

Fig. 22.1 Normal five-wall layer pattern of the esophagus as represented by endoscopic ultrasound (EUS). Innermost layer represents the interface between the probe and the wall (hyperechoic); the second layer, the superficial and deep mucosa (hypoechoic); the third layer, submucosa (hyperechoic); the fourth layer, muscularis propria (hypoechoic); and the fifth layer, adventitia (hyperechoic).

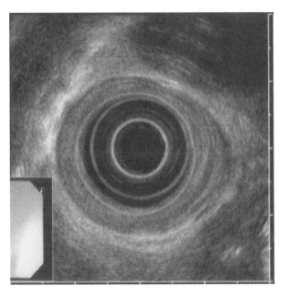

Fig. 22.2 Thickened esophageal wall may be seen with Barrett's esophagus.

EUS in Barrett's Esophagus

Barrett's esophagus is defined as metaplastic columnar epithelium replacing normal squamous mucosa in the esophagus. Gastroesophageal reflux is the major cause of Barrett's esophagus [3–5]. The relative risk of developing adenocarcinoma in Barrett's esophagus is thought to be 30–40 times higher than the general population [6]. Endoscopic surveillance is recommended in patients with Barrett's esophagus because of progression of dysplasia to carcinoma. High-grade dysplasia (HGD) in Barrett's esophagus frequently undergoes malignant transformation and can be associated with a high rate of occult malignancy [7–9].

In Barrett's esophagus, there is a thickening of the esophageal wall that can be detected by EUS (Fig. 22.2). Srivastava *et al.* compared the esophageal wall thickness of patients with Barrett's and those without using the Olympus EU-M3 (Melville, NY) at

12 MHz [10]. They studied 15 patients with Barrett's esophagus with and without dysplasia. In the control group the mean esophageal wall thickness was 2.6 mm, the non-dysplastic Barrett's esophagus group had a mean was thickness of 3.3 mm, and those with dysplasia measured 4.0 mm. The difference between the non-dysplastic measurement and the dysplastic measurement was not statistically significant. The only patients with esophageal wall thickness greater than 4 mm had dysplasia. There were two patients with a focal carcinoma with otherwise unsuspected submucosal invasion as proved on surgical pathology. Adrain *et al.* performed a similar study with high-resolution endoluminal sonographic examination using a 20 MHz ultrasound transducer [11]. In this series of patients Barrett's esophagus was identified by EUS as a second (hypoechoic) layer of the esophageal mucosa that was thicker than the first (hyperechoic) layer. All 17 patients with Barrett's esophagus were correctly identified (100% sensitivity). Ten of the 12 controls were identified as normal (specificity 86%). This study was not able to differentiate those patients with dysplasia but included only two patients with dysplasia. Kinjo *et al.* took this analysis one step further: in 39 of 56 pa-

tients with Barrett's esophagus, the esophageal wall appeared thickened as compared to controls ($P < 0.005$) [12]. Based on EUS imaging the endosonographers could not differentiate patients with non-dysplastic Barrett's esophagus, low-grade dysplasia (LGD), or HGD. There was a false positive rate of 13% in detecting cancer in patients with Barrett's esophagus and adenocarcinoma.

EUS cannot reliably differentiate between the presence and absence of dysplasia in the setting of Barrett's esophagus. Hence, EUS is not indicated for routine screening or surveillance in patients with non-dysplastic Barrett's esophagus.

EUS in Barrett's with Dysplasia

EUS may be considered in selected patients with Barrett's esophagus and HGD because co-existent adenocarcinoma may be detected in 30–47% of these patients [13–15]. The clinical evaluation of EUS in this setting has yielded conflicting results. Falk *et al.* performed preoperative EUS on nine patients with HGD and intramucosal carcinoma [16]. Four of the six patients with HGD were correctly diagnosed as T0. The two patients that were over-staged had mucosal nodularity. EUS identified tumor in only one of three patients with intramucosal carcinoma. In this small group of patients EUS did not reliably predict the presence of intramucosal carcinoma in patients with Barrett's esophagus and HGD. Conversely, a larger study by Scotiniotis *et al.* reported more promising results [17]. In 22 patients with Barrett's and HGD or intramucosal carcinoma, preoperative EUS findings were compared to surgical pathology. The emphasis in this study was the detection of locally confined versus advanced carcinoma, specifically the presence or absence of submucosal invasion or regional lymphadenopathy. EUS accurately predicted the absence of submucosal invasion as confirmed by surgical pathology in all 16 patients that were stage Tis or T1a. EUS correctly predicted submucosal invasion confirmed by histopathology in five of six patients (83% positive predictive value). There was one false positive prediction of submucosal invasion by EUS. The specificity of T stage was 94%. EUS over-staged suspected lymphadenopathy as malignant in four cases (18%) but did not under-stage any of the cases.

EUS in patients with Barrett's esophagus can change the staging that was originally predicted by esophagogastroscopy (EGD) [18]. A total of 45 patients with Barrett's esophagus with HGD had an EGD and EUS performed. Fifteen patients were suspected endoscopically with a tumor while 30 patients were thought to have just dysplasia. Thirty-six patients underwent surgical resection. The Barrett's segment staging and nodal staging were accurate in the majority of patients. Six of the 30 patients not suspected of having cancer on EGD were determined to have cancer by EUS. Five of these (83%) were found to have cancer on surgical resection. In this study, EUS helped to identify occult malignancy. These results support the use of EUS when non-operative therapy is being considered in patients with Barrett's with HGD and/or intramucosal carcinoma.

EUS is indicated in patients with Barrett's esophagus with dysphagia and/or a focal nodule or stricture as there is an increased likelihood of underlying carcinoma. Patients with a stricture or a nodule also have an increased likelihood of submucosal invasion [17]. There were 12 patients in the Scotiniotis study with a nodule and/or stricture. Five patients in this group had lesions that invaded into the submucosa, conversely there was no submucosal invasion in the group with Barrett's and no macroscopically recognizable lesions (42% vs. 0%, Fisher exact test, $P = 0.04$). All patients were on acid suppressive medications prior to the endoscopic examination which may have reduced inflammation as a contributor to false-positive staging. In an earlier study [16], the presence of nodularity in Barrett's with HGD and carcinoma resulted in over-staging of the tumor.

Accurate assessment of Barrett's esophagus by EUS in the setting of HGD enables effective stage-based therapy. Esophagectomy offers definitive treatment for patients with HGD and eliminates the need for continued rigorous surveillance programs. This may be ideal in young, fit, operative candidates. However, esophagectomy is associated with postoperative morbidity of up to 45% and a mortality rate of 2–6% [19]. Patient outcomes are best in high volume centers. Alternatives to operative resection are observation or endoluminal therapies. Emerging endoluminal eradication therapies may achieve equal efficacy to operative resection in patients with HGD and carcinoma limited to the mucosal layer [20]. This approach has particular appeal in patients deemed poor operative candidates. Resection with endoscopic mucosal resection and submucosal dissection techniques allows for further histopathological staging confirmation [21]. Ablation techniques employ photodynamic therapy and contact and non-contact thermal devices. Therefore, EUS plays an important role in patient selection.

EUS in Esophageal Carcinoma

The prognosis and treatment of esophageal carcinoma is dependent upon the stage of the disease at the time of diagnosis. The staging of esophageal carcinoma is based upon the tumor, node, and metastasis classification [22] (Table 22.1). Once the diagnosis of carcinoma is made, cross-sectional imaging should be performed to evaluate for liver and distant lymph node metastases. CT scanning is most commonly employed. Positron emission tomography (PET) scanning is gaining increasing acceptance for the detection of distant metastases as well. In the absence of distant metastases, EUS is recommended for local tumor and nodal staging when stage-based therapy is being considered. The T staging of esophageal adenocarcinoma is demonstrated in Figs 22.3–22.6.

EUS more accurately determines T stage and regional lymphadenopathy as compared to other imaging modalities [23,24]. Staging accuracy holds for both esophageal squamous cell carcinoma and adenocarcinoma. The T stage of esophageal carcinoma can also help to predict the N stage. The relationship between the T stage and N stage was studied in a retrospective review of 359 patients undergoing esophagectomy for esophageal carcinoma. The prevalence of regional lymph nodes in patients with adenocarcinoma with invasion into the lamina propria and muscularis mucosa (T1 intramucosal) was 2.8%. The prevalence of regional lymph nodes increased with the depth of tumor invasion ($P < 0.0001$) [25]. A comparison of CT scan, laparoscopic ultrasound, and EUS was made in a group of 36 patients for staging of esophagogastric carcinoma [23]. CT scan was more accurate in locally advanced

Table 22. 1 Staging: TNM classification and stage group of esophageal carcinoma.

Primary Tumor (T)

TX	Primary tumor cannot be assessed
T0	No evidence of primary tumor
Tis	Carcinoma *in situ*
T1	Tumor invades the lamina propria or submucosal
T2	Tumor invades the muscularis propria
T3	Tumor invades the adventitia
T4	Tumor invades adjacent structures

Regional Lymph Nodes (N)

NX	Regional lymph nodes cannot be assessed
N0	No regional lymph node metastases
N1	Regional lymph node metastases

Distant metastases (M)

MX	Distant metastases cannot be assessed
M0	No distant metastases
MX	Distant metastases

Tumors of the lower thoracic esophagus

M1a	Metastases of celiac lymph nodes
M1b	Other distant metastases

Tumors of the mid-thoracic esophagus

M1a	Not applicable
M1b	Non-regional lymph nodes or other distant metastases

Tumors of the upper thoracic esophagus

M1a	Metastases in cervical lymph nodes
M1b	Other distant metastases

Staging of esophageal carcinoma

Stage	T	N	M
0	Tis	N0	M0
I	T1	N0	M0
IIA	T2	N0	M0
	T3	N0	M0
IIB	T1	N1	M0
	T2	N1	M0
III	T3	N1	M0
	T4	Any N	M0
IV	Any T	Any N	M1
IVA	Any T	Any N	M1a
IVB	Any T	Any N	M1b

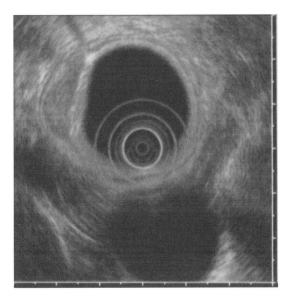

Fig. 22.3 T1 lesion of the esophagus.

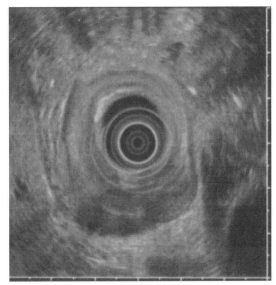

Fig. 22.5 T3 lesion of the esophagus.

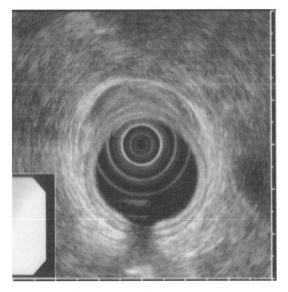

Fig. 22.4 T2 lesion of the esophagus.

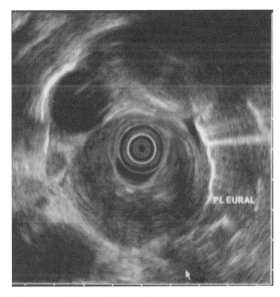

Fig. 22.6 T4 lesion of the esophagus.

tumors (T3 and T4) when compared with EUS, 95% versus 88%, respectively. EUS was the best modality for assessing early tumors and locoregional nodal involvement with accuracies of 62% and 72%, respectively. Distant metastases were more accurately detected with laparoscopic ultrasound (81%) compared with CT scan (72%). Another study performed

by Wallace *et al.* showed that combination imaging tests (i.e. PET with EUS/FNA or CT scan with EUS/FNA) proved to be more cost-effective in a decision-analysis model [26]. EUS is also superior to CT scan for detecting celiac lymph nodes. In a study of 62 patients, EUS was used to evaluate celiac lymph nodes in 95% of the patients. EUS was positive in 19 patients and CT scan was positive in two. The sensitivity and specificity of EUS were 72% and 97%, respectively, and 8% and 100%, respectively, for CT scan. EUS with FNA can identify patients with M1a disease, i.e. positive celiac lymphadenopathy, and therefore helps direct management [27]. This more accurate staging identifies patients with advanced locoregional disease who would benefit most from preoperative neoadjuvant chemoradiation therapy [28].

EUS staging has a positive clinical impact in patients with esophageal carcinoma. Hiele *et al.* analyzed the survival data of 86 patients who underwent EUS for staging of tumors of the esophagus or esophagogastric junction [29]. A surgical resection was performed in 73 patients. Survival of patients was significantly dependent upon EUS T staging ($P=0.05$), EUS N staging ($P=0.02$), and the presence of stenosis ($P = 0.02$). The worst prognosis was related to patients with celiac lymph node metastasis ($P = 0.0027$). In this study there was a decreased accuracy of T staging (59%). The majority of patients went to surgery, and only one patient had preoperative chemoradiation. Another study by Harewood and Kumar compared the outcomes of patients diagnosed with esophageal cancer in 1998 (i.e. pre-EUS) to patients diagnosed in 2000 after EUS had become available [30]. Tumor recurrence and survival were better in the EUS group. This study demonstrated that EUS more accurately identified patients who benefited from preoperative neoadjuvant therapy. A number of studies suggest that preoperative chemoradiation provides the best results for patients with stage II and III cancer, and thus it is important to identify these patients so that they receive the most appropriate care. EUS can provide more accurate staging and therefore improve patient outcome.

EUS staging in esophageal cancer also contributes to improved cost-effectiveness. Shumaker *et al.* performed a retrospective review of the CORI (Clinical Outcomes Research Initiative) database to identify patients who had a preoperative EUS for esophageal carcinoma [31]. Cost analysis was done on 188 procedures. It was assumed that patients with stage I disease would go directly to surgery while patients with stage IV disease would not have combined modality therapy. In this study group, 26% of patients were spared the combined modality therapy and that resulted in a cost savings. A prospective case series by Chang *et al.* demonstrated similar findings [32]. In this study, there was decreased cost of care by $12 340 per patient by reducing the number of thoracotomies because of improved staging. Harewood *et al.* used a computer model to determine the cost of EUS in the staging of esophageal cancer [33]. In this study, EUS FNA provided the least costly approach to patients with celiac lymph node involvement as compared with CT FNA and surgery. These data were dependent upon the prevalence of celiac lymph nodes of 16%. These three studies show that there are cost savings for patients that undergo EUS as appropriate treatment can be provided due to more accurate staging.

Cancer with Stenosis

In up to 30% of cases of adenocarcinoma of the esophagus concurrent luminal stenosis does not permit the echoendoscope to traverse the tumor without dilation. This is important to allow complete staging to include inspection for celiac adenopathy. When tumor stenosis is encountered several options are available including dilation to allow passage of the echoendoscope, use of miniprobes, or abort the procedure with limited staging information. Since the risk of perforation accompanies dilation of malignant strictures, these options should be individualized. In an early experience, Van Dam *et al.* reported a complication rate of 24% [34]. In this study the strictures were dilated up to 18 mm to accommodate larger diameter, more primitive echoendoscopes which may have contributed to the high complication rate. A later study performed by Pfau *et al.* included 81 patients that required dilation to allow passage of the Olympus GF-UM20 echoendoscope [35]. The dilations were performed in a stepwise fashion with Savary–Guilliard wire-guided dilators or through-the-scope dilating hydrostatic balloons (Microvasive, Natick, MA) to about 14 mm. The majority of dilations were performed in one session. Immediately following dilation, the echoendoscope was able to traverse the stricture in 85.2% of patients. There were no complications. Similar results were obtained by Kallimanis *et al.* [36]. Given these findings, and with the further reduction in the diameter of echoendoscopes, stepwise dilation can generally be safely performed to allow complete tumor and nodal staging with EUS in patients with esophageal cancer and malignant stenosis.

The use of catheter ultrasound miniprobes is another means of tumor staging in patients with a tight esophageal stricture related to the tumor. The miniprobes can be passed through the accessory channel of the endoscope and across the stricture under fluoroscopic guidance. A study was carried out by Menzel *et al.* to compare the results using an echoendoscope (GF-UM3, Olympus, Melville, NY), versus the miniprobe (MH-908, Olympus) [37]. The overall T staging was more accurate with the miniprobe as compared with the echoendoscope 80% versus 57%. The miniprobe was also more accurate with regards to the presence or absence of periesophageal lymph nodes. There were no complications reported with the use of the miniprobes. However, these results have not been validated and most authorities perceive that high frequency miniprobes do not provide an adequate depth of imaging to satisfy tumor and lymph node assessment in large tumors.

Re-Staging after Neoadjuvant Therapy

EUS may also be used in re-staging esophageal carcinoma after chemoradiation. This is employed to determine response to the treatment and candidacy for operative resection. However, studies evaluating this performance have yielded varying results. When the TNM classification is used in re-staging the tumor, the majority of tumors are over-staged. Kalha *et al.* showed that T classification was assessed correctly by EUS in only 22 patients (29%) [38]. In evaluating the N classification, the sensitivity was 48% for N0 disease and 52% for N1 disease. In a pilot study, EUS with FNA was performed on enlarged lymph nodes and the accuracy of identifying malignant cells was 87.5% [39,40]. One promising method is to measure the size and cross-sectional area of the tumor. Isenberg *et al.* demonstrated that the measurement of the maximal cross-sectional area of the tumor was more useful than the TNM classification. In a small group of patients, there was a statistically significant decrease in this measure-

ment in patients that responded to chemotherapy. Larger studies are needed to further evaluate the impact that the maximal cross-sectional area of the tumor has on patient survival.

Limitations of EUS in Barrett's Esophagus and Esophageal Cancer

EUS is highly operator dependent. The training and experience of the endosonographer impacts the accuracy of EUS. In a study performed to compare the findings on EUS by inexperienced and experienced endosonographers [41], interobserver agreement amongst the experienced endosonographers was excellent for all T stages except for T2. In the inexperienced group of endosonographers, the agreement for T staging was poor but was better for the detection of lymph nodes.

EUS artifacts can be created by oblique scanning and balloon compression of the esophageal wall. These artifacts may result in over-staging of the tumor. Ideally, the echoendoscope should be placed perpendicular to the tissue being examined. The balloon should be inflated so as not to compress the esophageal wall and thereby distort the imaging. The anatomic configuration at the esophagogastric junction may not permit ideal transducer positioning for staging lesions in this region. The tubular esophagus does not lend itself to water-filling and so circumstances are encountered in which acoustic coupling cannot be ideally achieved.

Conclusions

EUS has a substantive role in the evaluation and management of patients with esophageal carcinoma and in patients with dysplastic Barrett's esophagus. It is effectively used in patients with Barrett's esophagus and HGD to detect otherwise unrecognizable invasive carcinoma and thus the consideration of operative versus non-operative therapies. For established carcinoma of the esophagus, EUS is the most accurate tool for tumor and nodal staging. Accurate TNM staging directs stage-based therapy.

References

1. Catalano MF, Sivak MV, Jr, Rice T. Endoscopic features

predictive of lymph node metastasis. *Gastrointest Endosc* 1994;**40**(4):442–6.

2. Vazquez-Sequeiros E, Wiersema MJ, Clain JE *et al.* Impact of lymph node staging on therapy of esophageal carcinoma. *Gastroenterology* 2003;**125**(6):1626–33.

3. Mann NS, Tsai MF, Nair PK. Barrett's esophagus in patients with symptomatic reflux esophagitis. *Am J Gastroenterol* 1989;**84**:1494–6.

4. Winters C, Jr, Spurling TJ, Chobanian SJ *et al.* Barrett's esophagus. A prevalent occult complication of gastroesophageal reflux disease. *Gastroenterology* 1987;**92**:118–24.

5. Lieberman DA, Oehlke M, Helfand M. Risk factors for Barrett's esophagus in community-based practice. *Am J Gastroenterol* 1997;**92**:1293–7.

6. Eckardt VF, Kanzler G, Bernhard G. Life expectancy and cancer risk in patients with Barrett's esophagus: a prospective controlled investigation. *Am J Med* 2001;**111**:33–7.

7. Falk GW, Rice TW, Goldblum JR *et al.* Jumbo biopsy forceps protocol still misses unsuspected cancer in Barrett's esophagus with high-grade dysplasia. *Gastrointest Endosc* 1999;**49**:170–6.

8. Reid BJ, Blount PL, Feng Z *et al.* Optimizing endoscopic biopsy detection of early cancers in Barrett's high-grade dysplasia. *Am J Gastroenterol* 2000;**95**:3089–96.

9. Heitmiller RF, Redmond M, Hamilton SR. Barrett's esophagus with high-grade dysplasia. An indication for prophylactic esophagectomy. *Ann Surg* 1996;**224**: 66–71.

10. Srivastava AK, Vanagunas A, Kamel P *et al.* Endoscopic ultrasound in the evaluation of Barrett's esophagus: a preliminary report. *Am J Gastroenterol* 1994;**89**(12): 2192–5.

11. Adrain AL, Ter HC, Cassidy MJ *et al.* High-resolution endoluminal sonography is a sensitive modality for the identification of Barrett's metaplasia. *Gastrointest Endosc* 1997;**46**(2):147–51.

12. Kinjo M, Maringhini A, Wang KK *et al.* Is endoscopic ultrasound (EUS) cost effective to screen for cancer in patients with Barrett's esophagus? *Gastrointest Endosc* 1994;**40**:205A.

13. Altorki NK, Sunagawa M, Little AG *et al.* High-grade dysplasia in the columnar-lined esophagus. *Am J Surg* 1991;**26**:1–32.

14. Cameron AJ, Carpenter HA. Barrett's esophagus, high-grade dysplasia, and early adenocarcinoma; a pathological study. *Am J Gastroenterol* 1997;**92**: 586–91.

15. Ferguson MK, Naunheim KS. Resection for Barrett's mucosa with high-grade dysplasia: implications for prophylactic photodynamic therapy. *J Thorac Cardiovasc Surg* 1997;**114**:824–9.

16. Falk GW, Catalano MF, Sivak MV, Jr *et al.* Endosonography in the evaluation of patients with Barrett's esophagus and high-grade dysplasia. *Gastrointest Endosc* 1994;**40**(2):207–12.

17. Scotiniotis IA, Kochman ML, Lewis JD *et al.* Accuracy of EUS in the evaluation of Barrett's esophagus and high grade dysplasia or intramucosal carcinoma. *Gastrointest Endosc* 2001;**54**:689–96.

18. Wang KK, Norbash A, Geller A *et al.* Endoscopic ultrasonography in the assessment of Barrett's esophagus with high grade dysplasia or carcinoma. *Gastroenterology* 1996;**110**(4):A611.

19. Ruol A, Zaninotto G, Costantini M *et al.* Barrett's esophagus: management of high-grade dysplasia and cancer. *J Surg Res* 2004;**117**:44–51.

20. Pacifico RJ, Wang KK, Wongkeesong LM *et al.* Combined endoscopic mucosal resection and photodynamic therapy versus esophagectomy for management of early adenocarcinoma in Barrett's esophagus. *Clin Gastroenterol Hepatol* 2003;**1**(4):252–7.

21. Nijhawan PK, Wang KK. Endoscopic mucosal resection for lesions with endoscopic features suggestive of malignancy and high-grade dysplasia within Barrett's esophagus. *Gastrointest Endosc* 2000;**52**(3):328–32.

22. Greene FL, Page DL, Fleming ID *et al.*, eds. *American Joint Committee on Cancer. Cancer Staging Manual*, 6th edn. New York: Springer, 2002: 91–8.

23. Wakelin SJ, Deans C, Crofts TJ *et al.* A comparison of computerized tomography, laparoscopic ultrasound and endoscopic ultrasound in the preoperative staging of oesophago-gastric carcinoma. *Eur J Radiol* 2002; **41**(2):161–7.

24. Reed CE, Mishra G, Sahai AV *et al.* Esophageal cancer staging: improved accuracy by endoscopic ultrasound of celiac lymph nodes. *Ann Thoracic Surg* 1999;**67**(2): 319–21.

25. Rice TW, Zuccaro G, Jr, Adelstein DJ *et al.* Esophageal carcinoma: depth of tumor invasion is predictive of regional lymph nodes status. *Ann Thorac Surg* 1998;**65**:787–92.

26. Wallace MB, Nietert PJ, Earle C *et al.* An analysis of multiple staging management strategies for carcinoma of the esophagus: computed tomography, endoscopic ultrasound, positron emission tomography, and thoracoscopy/laparoscopy. *Ann Thorac Surg* 2002;**74**: 1026–32.

27. Parmar KS, Zwischenberger JB, Reeves AL *et al.* Clinical impact of endoscopic ultrasound-guided fine needle aspiration of celiac axis lymph nodes

(M1a disease) in esophageal cancer. *Ann Thorac Surg* 2002;**73**(3):916–20.

28. Lerut T, Coosemans W, De Leyn P *et al.* Optimizing treatment of carcinoma of the esophagus and gastroesophageal junction. *Surg Oncol Clin N Am* 2001;**10**:863–4,x.

29. Hiele M, De Leyn P, Schurmans P *et al.* Relation between endoscopic ultrasound findings and outcome of patients with tumors of the esophagus or esophagogastric junction. *Gastrointest Endosc* 1997;**45**(5): 381–6.

30. Harewood GC, Kumar KS. Assessment of clinical impact of endoscopic ultrasound on esophageal cancer. *J Gastroenterol Hepatol* 2004;**19**:433–9.

31. Shumaker DA, de Garmo P, Faigel DO. Potential impact of preoperative EUS on esophageal cancer management and cost. *Gastrointest Endosc* 2002;**56**:391–6.

32. Chang KJ, Soetikno RM, Bastas D *et al.* Impact of endoscopic ultrasound combined with fine-needle aspiration biopsy in the management of esophageal cancer. *Endoscopy* 2003;**35**(11):962–6.

33. Harewood GC, Wiersema MJ. A cost analysis of endoscopic ultrasound in the evaluation of esophageal cancer. *Am J Gastroenterol* 2002;**97**(2):452–8.

34. Van Dam J, Rice TW, Catalano MF *et al.* High-grade malignant stricture is predictive of esophageal tumor stage. *Cancer* 1993;**71**:2910–7.

35. Pfau PR, Ginsberg GG, Lew RJ *et al.* Esophageal dilation for endosonographic evaluation of malignant esophageal strictures is safe and effective. *Am J Gastroenterol* 2000;**95**(10):2813–5.

36. Kallimanis GE, Gupta PK, al-Kawas FH *et al.* Endoscopic ultrasound for staging of esophageal cancer, with or without dilation, is clinically important and safe. *Gastrointest Endosc* 1995;**41**(6):613–5.

37. Menzel J, Hoepffner N, Nottberg H *et al.* Preoperative staging of esophageal carcinoma: miniprobe sonography versus conventional endoscopic ultrasound in a prospective histopathology verified study. *Endoscopy* 1999;**31**(4):291–7.

38. Kalha I, Kaw M, Fukami N *et al.* The accuracy of endoscopic ultrasound for restaging esophageal carcinoma after chemoradiation therapy. *Cancer* 2004;**101**:940–7.

39. Agarwal B, Swisher S, Ajani J *et al.* Endoscopic ultrasound after preoperative chemoradiation can help identify patients who benefit maximally after surgical esophageal resection. *Am J Gastroenterol* 2004; **99**(7):1258–66.

40. Isenberg G, Chak A, Canto MI *et al.* Endoscopic ultrasound in restaging of esophageal cancer after neoadjuvant chemoradiation. *Gastrointest Endosc* 1998;**48**(2):158–63.

41. Burtin P, Napoleon B, Palazzo L. Interobserver agreement in endoscopic ultrasonography staging of esophageal and cardia cancer. *Gastrointest Endosc* 1996;**43**(1):20–4.

CHAPTER 23

Surgical Therapy of Barrett's Esophagus and Cancer

Dave R. Lal and Brant K. Oelschlager

Introduction

Barrett's esophagus is an acquired abnormality that is best defined as the displacement of the squamo-columnar junction proximal to the gastroesophageal junction with the presence of esophageal intestinal metaplasia found on biopsy. Risk factors for Barrett's esophagus include severe and long-standing gastroesophageal reflux disease (GERD), obesity, the presence of a hiatal hernia, male gender, and Caucasian ethnicity [1]. The incidence of Barrett's esophagus has increased dramatically in the last 20 years [2]. Concomitant to this had been a 10-fold increase in the incidence of esophageal adenocarcinoma over the past decade strongly supporting a link between the two [3].

Treatment for Barrett's esophagus, before it has progressed to high-grade dysplasia (HGD) or cancer, should seek to accomplish three goals: (i) to provide long-term control of reflux symptoms; (ii) provide a durable gastroesophageal barrier to acid and bile; and (iii) promote the regression or reduce the progression of Barrett's esophagus thus decreasing the risk of adenocarcinoma. Treatment of HGD or Barrett's associated adenocarcinoma shifts towards eradication of disease with the least amount of morbidity.

Surgical therapy plays an important role in Barrett's esophagus and cancer. We will review the role of surgery with regard to these goals and in relation to other available therapies.

Symptom Control

Medical Therapy

Antisecretory therapy with proton pump inhibitors (PPIs) for GERD is very effective in patients with uncomplicated reflux disease. In patients with Barrett's, however, conventional doses are less likely to control symptoms completely, and usually require larger doses to provide relief. Still, in most patients symptoms can be controlled with medical therapy. Interestingly, and almost paradoxically, some patients have relatively minor symptom complaints for the quantitative amounts of reflux that is occurring. This "diminished esophageal sensitivity" may be a result of the injury and mucosal change that accompanies intestinal metaplasia. Nevertheless, Barrett's esophagus is usually synonymous with severe GERD, thus patients are more likely to be poorly controlled and seek other solutions.

Surgical Therapy

Surgical antireflux procedures are now almost exclusively performed via the laparoscopic approach. In experienced hands, an equal and perhaps better fundoplication can be constructed as compared to open (because of superior exposure and visualization of the hiatus), with the benefits of less morbidity and faster recovery. Long-term outcomes after laparoscopic antireflux surgery (LARS) for Barrett's esophagus are sparse due to the relatively short existence of laparoscopy. Still, the control of GERD-related symptoms with LARS is excellent. Although several studies have reported that achievement of symptom control is not as great in patients without Barrett's esophagus [4,5], Farrell *et al.* reported ex-

Table 23.1 Comparison of pre and postoperative symptoms in 106 patients with Barrett's esophagus who underwent paparoscopic antireflux surgery. Reprinted with permission from Oelschlager *et al.* [14]. Copyright Lippincott, Williams & Wilkins.

Symptom	Preoperative incidence n (%)	Resolution n (%)	Improvement n (%)	No improvement n (%)
Heartburn	98 (92%)	69 (70%)	25 (26%)	4 (4%)
Regurgitation	69 (65%)	52 (75%)	6 (9%)	11 (16%)
Dysphagia	33 (31%)	21 (64%)	6 (18%)	6 (18%)
Cough	31 (29%)	22 (71%)	2 (6%)	7 (23%)
Chest pain	30 (28%)	20 (67%)	6 (20%)	4 (13%)
Hoarseness	25 (24%)	21 (84%)	1 (4%)	3 (12%)

cellent short-term results in patients with Barrett's esophagus undergoing LARS that did not deteriorate with extended follow-up (2–5 years) [6]. Similarly, Parrilla *et al.* published a prospective randomized trial comparing medical versus surgical therapy of Barrett's esophagus [7]. With a median follow-up of 5 years, they reported excellent or good symptom control in 91% of patients undergoing antireflux surgery.

We have found that with long-term follow-up (mean 43 months) after LARS, 95% of our Barrett's esophagus patients continued to report improvement of their preoperative heartburn and regurgitation. These results are identical to patients without Barrett's esophagus [8]. Furthermore, dysphagia, which was associated with impaired motility in many of the patients, improved in more than 80% of patients who presented with it. Other symptoms of GERD also diminished or resolved and remained so several years after the repair (Table 23.1). Collectively, these studies demonstrate that durable control of GERD can be achieved with surgery.

Reflux Control

Medical Therapy

Control of reflux related symptoms is not synonymous with control of acid reflux as detected by pH probe monitoring. In fact, many patients with Barrett's esophagus have adequate control of their symptoms with a markedly abnormal acid exposure by 24-h pH monitoring. Katzka and Castell reported that 80% of patients with Barrett's who reported

control of their reflux symptoms had abnormal esophageal acid exposure when tested. Moreover, two studies that were specifically designed to medically (high-dose PPI therapy) normalize esophageal acid exposure in Barrett's esophagus patients failed in 16% of patients [9,10].

Esophageal acid exposure is not the only contributor to Barrett's esophagus; bile reflux also plays an intimate role. Several authors have shown that the incidence of duodenogastric reflux in patients with Barrett's esophagus is markedly elevated. Medical therapy, aimed at reducing acid production, has a limited ability to treat or prevent bile reflux. Measurements of esophageal bile exposure by spectrophotometer have shown an exponential relationship between bile reflux and GERD severity [11]. Fifty-four percent of patients with Barrett's esophagus have been reported to have elevated esophageal bile acid exposure with levels equivalent to those seen after partial gastrectomy [11,12]. Therefore, although medical therapy may control or reduce symptoms in patients with Barrett's esophagus, it is unlikely to completely control acid and bile reflux.

Surgical Therapy

Fundamental to antireflux surgery is the correction of the anatomy of the cardia and creating a barrier to reflux. If successful, surgery should intuitively be more successful than medical therapy at controlling acid and bile reflux and in fact this has been demonstrated. Hofstetter *et al.* reported normal pH monitoring in 81% of patients after fundoplication [13]. In the randomized control trial of medical versus surgical treatment of Barrett's esophagus, fundoplication was much more successful in attaining nominalization of esophageal acid exposure as compared to PPI therapy (85% vs. 25%, respectively) [7]. Likewise, Bilitec monitoring showed normal esophageal exposure to duodenogastric reflux after surgical intervention in 92% versus 25% of the medical treated group.

It has been our experience that although a vast majority of patients have decreased esophageal acid exposure after LARS, approximately one-quarter of patients with Barrett's esophagus do not achieve normal DeMeester or esophageal acid exposure measurements [14]. Reasons for this are likely related to the high incidence of associated complicating factors in those with Barrett's esophagus, making failure or ineffective operations more likely. In our series, factors that contributed to inferior results in patients included; a high incidence of re-operations, paraesophageal hernia repair, ineffective esophageal motility requiring partial fundoplication, peptic stricture, and foreshortened esophagus. However, the failure to achieve normalization of acid exposure in our study (and presumably others) may be an overestimation of the true incidence, since all patients who returned with symptoms underwent pH monitoring as part of their evaluation, whereas a minority (<40%) of the totally asymptomatic patients agreed to this test postoperatively. The findings of this study underscore the impact that associated anatomic abnormalities have on the results of surgery in patients with Barrett's esophagus and suggest that earlier referral to surgical therapy (i.e. before complications develop) may be important to improve the chances of a successful outcome.

Barrett's Regression

The third goal of therapy, and perhaps the most important in patients with Barrett's esophagus, is halting the progression and possibly even causing regression of Barrett's epithelium. Since Barrett's esophagus carries with it a risk of progressing to adenocarcinoma, the most effective form of therapy would be directed at decreasing this risk while providing symptom relief. However, this is not currently included as a priority of treatment by most practitioners. In fact, the Practice Parameters Committee of the American College of Gastroenterology states that the goal of treatment for Barrett's esophagus should be "the control of the symptoms of GERD" [15]. In contrast to medical treatment, surgical therapy, by reducing refluxate that contributes to ongoing esophageal injury, may be able to control symptoms and induce a complete regression of Barrett's esophagus.

Medical Therapy

Whether the natural history of Barrett's esophagus can be affected by intervention is still a matter of debate, but one thing that is clear is the inability of medical therapy to effect the complete regression of intestinal metaplasia. Almost all studies of Barrett's esophagus and medical therapy have as an endpoint either relief of symptoms or "normalization" of esophageal acid exposure. Regression of intestinal metaplasia is rarely reported and thus not a common endpoint [16–18]. In one of the most rigorous longitudinal follow-up studies involving 309 patients with Barrett's esophagus for an average of 3.8 years, no cases of complete Barrett's regression were found [19]. Similarly, in a recent retrospective study by El-Serag et al., which reviewed 236 veterans over a 20-year period, PPI usage resulted in reduced incidence of dysplasia but not regression of Barrett's [20].

Surgical Therapy

Conversely, the literature is replete with evidence for regression after surgical therapy. In 1980, Brand et al. were the first to report regression of Barrett's esophagus after surgery in four of 10 patients [21]. Since that time, many series have reported modest rates (10–38%) of complete regression after antireflux surgery [22–25]. Gurski et al. reported on 77 consecutive patients undergoing antireflux surgery and found that low-grade dysplasia (LGD) regressed to non-dysplastic Barrett's in 68% and intestinal metaplasia to cardiac mucosa in 21% [25]. Similarly, Hofstetter et al. found 44% of patients having complete resolution of their preoperative LGD and 14% regressed from intestinal metaplasia to cardiac mucosa, after antireflux surgery [13]. The implications of these results deserve further consideration as they are far superior to any published studies utilizing medical treatment.

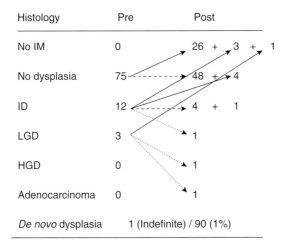

Histology	Pre	Post
No IM	0	26 + 3 + 1
No dysplasia	75	48 + 4
ID	12	4 + 1
LGD	3	1
HGD	0	1
Adenocarcinoma	0	1
De novo dysplasia	1 (Indefinite) / 90 (1%)	

Fig. 23.1 Fate of the Barrett's epithelium after laparoscopic antireflux surgery (LARS) in patients with endoscopic follow-up; includes all patients in series. Key: No IM: no evidence of intestinal metaplasia by endoscopy or histology; No dysplasia: intestinal metaplasia without dysplasia on biopsy; ID: indefinite for dysplasia; LGD: low-grade dysplasia; HGD: high-grade dysplasia; (—) regression; (– –) stable; (···) progression. HGD, high-grade dysplasia; ID, indefinite for dysplasia; LGD, low-grade dysplasia; No dysplasia, intestinal metaplasia without dysplasia on biopsy; No IM, no evidence of intestinal metaplasia by endoscopy or histology; —, regression; – –, stable; ···, progression. Reproduced with permission from Oelschlager *et al.* [14]. Copyright Lippincott, Williams & Wilkins.

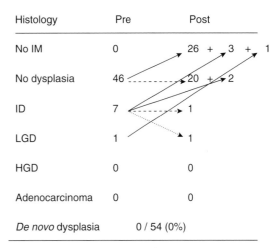

Histology	Pre	Post
No IM	0	26 + 3 + 1
No dysplasia	46	20 + 2
ID	7	1
LGD	1	1
HGD	0	0
Adenocarcinoma	0	0
De novo dysplasia	0 / 54 (0%)	

Fig 23.2 Fate of the Barrett's epithelium after laparoscopic antireflux surgery (LARS) in patients with endoscopic follow-up; includes patients with short segment only (<3 cm). Key: No IM: no evidence of intestinal metaplasia by endoscopy or histology; No dysplasia: intestinal metaplasia without dysplasia on biopsy; ID: indefinite for dysplasia; LGD: low-grade dysplasia; HGD: high-grade dysplasia; (—) regression; (– –) stable; (···) progression. HGD, high-grade dysplasia; ID, indefinite for dysplasia; LGD, low-grade dysplasia; No dysplasia, intestinal metaplasia without dysplasia on biopsy; No IM, no evidence of intestinal metaplasia by endoscopy or histology; —, regression; – –, stable; ···, progression. Reproduced with permission from Oelschlager *et al.* [14]. Copyright Lippincott, Williams & Wilkins.

We recently reported the results of 106 patients with Barrett's esophagus after LARS [14]. After a median follow-up of 40 months, 33% of patients had complete regression of intestinal metaplasia (Fig. 23.1). All of the patients with complete regression had short segments of Barrett's esophagus (<3 cm) before the operation, and in this group the regression rate was 55% (Fig. 23.2). The fact that complete regression was observed exclusively in patients with short segment Barrett's esophagus is not surprising. Gurski *et al.* reported regression of Barrett's esophagus was significantly more common in short segment than long segment Barrett's esophagus after antireflux surgery (58% vs. 20%, respectively, *P* = 0.0016) [25]. Similarly, DeMeester *et al.* found that 73% of patients with Barrett's esophagus confined to the gastroesophageal junction had complete regression after surgery [5]. If, as some recent studies on the pathogenesis of Barrett's esophagus suggest,

the disease is initially localized and then becomes progressively longer, the results of the preceding studies would strongly suggest that earlier referral for antireflux surgery in patients with Barrett's esophagus may yield the best chance for complete regression.

Progression to Cancer

The demonstration that any form of therapy reduces the risk of developing adenocarcinoma, among patients with Barrett's esophagus, is difficult due to the low rate of progression. Rudolph *et al.* reported a 3.4%/year chance of progression to cancer in a group of 309 patients followed for a mean of 3.8 years [19]. However, if patients presenting with HGD were excluded the rate decreased to 0.8%/year. Most studies examining the incidence of progression from Barrett's esophagus to cancer involve patients receiving medical therapy; thus, the true rate of progression without any treatment is unknown.

Medical versus Surgical Therapy

Multiple studies have concluded that there is no difference in progression to cancer between those treated medically or surgically, although there are no comparative trials with enough patients to show a difference even if one exists. For example, the most recent randomized clinical trial in the USA concluded the risk was the same, yet two patients in the medical arm developed esophageal cancer with none in the surgical arm [26].

Whether medical or surgical therapies can ultimately affect the progression from Barrett's esophagus to cancer remains highly controversial. Corey *et al.* performed a meta-analysis to examine if ARS was associated with a reduction in the incidence of esophageal adenocarcinoma when compared to medically treated patients [27]. They reported that patients treated with ARS had a rate of 3.8 cancers/1000 patient years compared to 5.3 cancers in the medical group. This did not reach significance ($P = 0.29$). A large retrospective cohort study from Sweden also reported no decrease in the rate of progression to cancer after antireflux surgery [28].

Still, many have shown a difference in cohorts of patients where significantly more medically treated patients developed dysplasia and cancer than surgical patients. Katz *et al.* for example, found the 9-year dysplasia- and cancer-free survival was 100% in patients treated surgically, and only 50% in those receiving medical therapy [29].

Data from our center support the premise that an effective antireflux barrier reduces the progression of Barrett's esophagus. None of our patients without dysplasia before operation progressed to HGD or cancer. Only one of our patients with long segment intestinal metaplasia and LGD was found to have adenocarcinoma, but this occurred within a year of operation. Given the short period, it is likely that this focus was either missed prior to the operation, or the dysplasia–carcinoma sequence was irreversible at the time of operation. In fact, in most studies of the natural history of Barrett's esophagus, patients who develop a cancer within 6 months to a year are ex-

cluded because they are thought to have harbored the disease when first seen [30]. McDonald *et al.* have shown that most cancers after antireflux surgery present in the first year postoperatively, suggesting that in these patients, the dysplastic process has entered an irreversible phase before the operation [31]. They also found that very few patients develop HGD or cancer when followed for longer periods. Even so, including our patient equates to one cancer in 274 patient-years of follow-up (incidence, 0.3%/year). If the three largest published series of LARS for Barrett's esophagus are compiled; only one cancer has developed in 1021 patient-years of follow-up (incidence, 0.09%/year).

In contrast to McDonalds study, Csendes *et al.* reported a 4.1% progression from Barrett's esophagus to adenocarcinoma from 4–18 years after antireflux surgery [32]. This group also had an unusually high rate of recurrent GERD, more so than other centers. This is important because the development of adenocarcinoma was related to recurrence of reflux symptoms and failure of the antireflux surgery. What is clear from this study is that patients with Barrett's esophagus undergoing antireflux surgery need to be followed long-term and those with recurrent pathologic reflux are at increased risk for adenocarcinoma.

In our study, most patients (10 of 15) with preoperative evidence of dysplasia had regression to non-dysplastic metaplasia or to normal (no Barrett's) after LARS. This supports the findings from other groups, which have demonstrated up to a 70% chance of regression of dysplasia after successful antireflux surgery [5,6,23]. Thus, it appears that if the integrity of the antireflux mechanism is restored and remains intact over several years, preventing the continued injury from acid and bile reflux, patients with Barrett's esophagus have a good chance of disease regression and limited risk of progression.

The evidence to date strongly suggests that LARS, while not perfect, is currently the most effective treatment for patients with Barrett's esophagus. In comparison to medical therapy, surgery has been shown to effectively control patient symptoms, provide a durable barrier to gastroesophageal reflux, stimulate the regression of Barrett's esophagus, and reduce the risk of adenocarcinoma.

High-Grade Dysplasia

Treatment of HGD remains controversial. HGD is an intermediary between metaplasia and adenocarcinoma. Estimated rates of progression from HGD to cancer have been reported as high as 59% 5-year cumulative incidence [33]. Options for patients found to have HGD include surveillance, prophylactic esophagectomy, and endoscopic ablative techniques (endoscopic mucosal resection [EMR] and photodynamic therapy [PDT]).

The goal of surveillance is to detect the transformation of HGD to adenocarcinoma at an early stage allowing for surgical resection. In order for surveillance to be successful there must not be significant survival difference in patients opting for surveillance as opposed to esophagectomy or ablative therapies. The main limitation of surveillance is its ability to detect the progression to adenocarcinoma at its earliest point, which is influenced by sampling error and/or understaging by pathologists. Standard endoscopy and biopsy forceps have a rate as high as 38% of missed invasive adenocarcinoma in patients diagnosed with HGD who subsequently underwent prophylactic esophagectomy [34]. In an effort to diminish this false negative rate, jumbo biopsies taken in four quadrants every 2 cm was advocated. Falk *et al.* found that even with this technique 33% of patients undergoing esophagectomy were found to have invasive adenocarcinoma [34]. Further efforts have sought to increase the area sampled thus diminishing sampling error. Reid *et al.* showed that a biopsy protocol utilizing jumbo biopsies every 1 cm in four quadrants was more efficacious and missed fewer cancers than when performed every 2 cm [35]. This protocol also relied on an experienced gastrointestinal pathologist. Still, even with their more rigorous sampling protocol, one of 32 (3%) patients in their series progressed to metastatic esophageal cancer despite surveillance.

The benefit of surveillance depends upon both the skill of the endoscopist and pathologist, as well as the mortality associated with esophageal resection, since mortality varies between 2–20% depending on surgeon and institution experience.

Because of the high rate of progression and morbidity and mortality of resection, less morbid methods of eliminating the dysplastic epithelium have been investigated. In an effort to ablate the dysplastic mucosal tissue responsible for progression to cancer with low morbidity, PDT and EMR have been utilized. Studies have reported the success of PDT in ablating HGD. Overholt *et al.* recently reported on 83 patients undergoing follow-up of over 50 months after PDT [36]. They found 94% of patients had sustained resolution of their HGD. However, this was associated with a 30% stricture rate and 4.6% progression to adenocarcinoma. EMR allows the histologic evaluation of resected tissue to determine extent and depth of dysplasia/adenocarcinoma and ensure adequate margins. Resection of HGD has been reported with success of up to 98%. [37] This rate has not been uniformly achieved and authors have reported recurrence of HGD and progression to invasive cancer after successful EMR [37,38]. Both therapies should be limited to very controlled, high volume centers.

Prophylactic esophagectomy after the diagnosis of HGD eradicates cells at risk of degeneration to cancer and should serve as the standard that all other treatment modalities are compared with. Due to sampling error and difficulties in differentiating HGD from cancer, 38–56% of patients diagnosed with HGD have been found to have invasive adenocarcinoma after esophagectomy with 3% having metastatic disease [39–42]. This high rate of undiagnosed invasive cancer in the background of HGD has lead many authors to advocate esophagectomy for any patient diagnosed with HGD. The advantage of complete eradication of dysplastic cells must be weighed against the morbidity and mortality associated with esophagectomy. Large meta-analysis looking at the mortality after esophagectomy have reported declining rates from 13% in the 1980s to a current rate of 3–6%, at high volume centers.

In the end, no perfect treatment is available for HGD. With vigilant surveillance and numerous frequent biopsies, cancer has been missed with progressing to metastatic disease. Ablative techniques remain relatively new with few long-term follow-up studies. These techniques are likely to improve with time and prolonged follow-up, making them an attractive alternative to esophagectomy. Esophagectomy, although completely removing the organ at risk, has varying degrees of associated morbidity and mortality. These rates vary greatly depending on the experience and operative volume of the surgeon and medical center. Thus, physicians caring for patients with HGD must weigh the risk of cancer progression (patient age, surveillance compliance, healthcare access) with the morbidity and mortality of esophagectomy and unknown efficacy of evolving endoscopic ablative techniques.

Esophageal Cancer

Esophageal cancer progresses insidiously, thus often presenting at a late stage with a poor prognosis. There are two main types, squamous cell and adenocarcinoma. In the last 20 years, esophageal cancer in the USA and Western countries has undergone a transformation from predominantly squamous cell carcinoma to adenocarcinoma. Largely responsible for this shift is the identification of Barrett's esophagus as a precursor to esophageal adenocarcinoma. Due to accepted screening and surveillance methods for Barrett's, esophageal adenocarcinoma is being detected more commonly at an earlier stage, before symptoms develop, and at a more curable stage.

At present, surgical resection is an integral component of treatment for cure. In these cases the surgical diagnosis, work-up, and treatment are key to the management of this disease. While there is overlap, we will concentrate on the management of patients with Barrett's associated adenocarcinoma.

Presentation

The classic presentation of a patient with esophageal cancer is that of progressive dysphagia initially to solids and with time liquids. Patients typically describe a change in their eating habits from solids to soft foods and eventually to liquids. Weight loss is common. Esophageal luminal compromise can also lead to odynophagia, regurgitation, and emesis. As mentioned, increased screening and surveillance have led to a greater proportion of patients detected at earlier stages. Still, complications like recurrent aspirations from tracheoesophageal fistula and vocal hoarseness from encasement of the recurrent laryngeal nerve or invasion of the vocal cords can occur. Rarely, patients present with massive hematemesis

after local invasion into the aorta, though most of these are associated with squamous cell carcinoma.

Diagnosis

The most economical and easily accessible screening test for patients suspected of harboring an esophageal malignancy is an esophagram. Esophageal anatomy, size and location of mucosal abnormalities and masses, as well as fistulas can be visualized. If not the initial diagnostic test, esophagoscopy is the next logical choice. Esophagoscopy allows visual characterization of the lesion with concomitant biopsy. If clinical and gross appearances of esophageal lesions are consistent with malignancy, a negative biopsy should initiate repeat biopsy.

Staging

Once the diagnosis of esophageal cancer has been made, staging becomes paramount. In addition to providing prognostic information, the TNM-based staging system developed by the American Joint Committee on Cancer, allows for the stratification of patients who will benefit from surgery. Operative resection is essential for long-term survival. Patients with unresectable or metastatic disease are offered palliative care. Early esophageal lesions are treated with sole surgical resection. Locally advanced disease can either be approached immediately with operative intervention or surgical resection after neoadjuvant therapies.

Computed tomography (CT) scanning of the chest and abdomen is necessary to evaluate for distant metastasis and local tumor invasion or extension. Though it does give information on lymphadenopathy, CT is notoriously poor in its accuracy of detecting malignant lymph nodes (approximately 55%). Size criteria (>1 cm) is not definitive for nodal disease as enlarged benign reactive lymph nodes are common in patients with esophageal cancer. CT scan is more accurate in the evaluation of metastatic disease to the liver and lung as well as ruling out tumor invasion into surrounding organs.

Endoscopic ultrasound (EUS) has become the modality of choice in the evaluation of tumor depth and regional nodal involvement. EUS allows for the most accurate assessment of T (85–90%) and N stage

(70–90%) and allows for fine needle aspiration of suspicious lymph nodes (>90% accuracy).

Positron emission tomography (PET) can be a useful adjunct for patients suspected of metastatic disease or equivocal findings on imaging studies. PET localizes areas of high cellular metabolic demand as is common with malignancy. The results of PET can occasionally be misleading, negatively influencing treatment decisions. Therefore, further confirmation of metastatic disease either detected by diagnostic imaging or physical exam, should be confirmed with tissue diagnosis via fine needle aspiration, percutaneous, thorascopic, laparoscopic, or open biopsy.

Neoadjuvant Therapy

In efforts to prolong survival and reduce local recurrence, neoadjuvant chemotherapy and radiation have been advocated. Definitive studies demonstrating the efficacy of this therapy are few and thus it remains controversial. There is one randomized clinical trial demonstrating a survival benefit of this approach compared with surgery alone [43]. Still, other trials have shown no significant benefit [44–46]. There are no trials demonstrating a benefit of adjuvant therapy. Patients with locally advanced tumor (stage IIB, III), i.e. node-positive disease or those in whom negative microscopic margins are unlikely to be achieved, may benefit from neoadjuvant therapy. The utility of this is twofold. First, if successful, it allows reduction in tumor size and stage thus making complete surgical resection possible (RO resection) and in a subset of patient (20–25%) resulting in complete pathologic response. Second, it provides for immediate treatment of micrometastatic disease which is otherwise delayed until after surgery and recovery. Once neoadjuvant therapy is complete, patients undergo restaging. As long as the patients have not progressed to metastatic disease, esophagectomy is performed 4–6 weeks after completion of neoadjuvant therapy.

Preoperative Assessment

Overall, operative mortality after esophagectomy has steadily declined since its first published review by Ochsner and DeBakey [47] in 1941 with a 72% mortality rate to 29% in the 1960s–1970s [48], 13%

in the 1980s [49], and 3–6% currently [50]. A portion of the improvement in patient survival is likely attributable to advances in patient selection and preoperative care.

Patients presenting with esophageal cancer commonly have significant comorbidities increasing the risk of perioperative morbidity and mortality. Different comorbidities have been found to be associated with esophageal adenocarcinoma and squamous cell carcinoma, thus helping to guide preoperative workup. Patients with esophageal adenocarcinoma, a disease of Western countries, have a high prevalence of obesity, increased cardiovascular disease, and renal impairment. The reported prevalence has been as high as 50% with obesity, 28% with cardiac impairment, and 17% with renal insufficiency [51]. Patients with esophageal squamous cell cancer are more likely to have sequela of tobacco and alcohol abuse, specifically impaired hepatic and pulmonary function.

Patients being evaluated for esophagectomy should undergo a detailed history and physical exam specifically focusing on cardiovascular, pulmonary, and nutritional parameters. Cardiopulmonary complications after esophagectomy are responsible for up to 70% of perioperative mortality. During esophagectomy significant strain is placed on the myocardium with intravascular fluid shifts and operative maneuvers including mediastinal dissection and single lung ventilation. Routine preoperative pulmonary and cardiac function testing should be performed on patients thought to be at increased risk. Cardiac evaluation should include an electrocardiogram and chest X-ray. Abnormalities identified should be further investigated with selective use of a stress test (either exercise or chemical), echocardiography, myocardial perfusion imaging, or angiography, in collaboration with a cardiologist.

Pulmonary complications have been reported to be directly responsible for a 4.5-fold increase in mortality. Utilizing prospective data on 228 patients undergoing esophagectomy, major pulmonary complications were significantly associated with smoking history ($P = 0.03$) and abnormal preoperative spirometry ($P = 0.002$) [52]. In efforts to decrease this, preventative efforts have focused on preoperative smoking cessation, risk stratification with spirometry, and aggressive pulmonary physiotherapy, incentive spirometry and ambulation postoperative. Two large studies have shown the forced expiratory volume in 1 s (FEV_1) to be predictive of postoperative pulmonary complications. Law *et al.* retrospectively looked at 523 patients undergoing esophagectomy and found patients with an FEV_1 less than 81% predicted had significant pulmonary morbidity [53]. Likewise, Ferguson and Durkin reported that on multivariate analysis of 292 patients, abnormal FEV_1 was an independent predictor of pulmonary complications [54]. Although multiple studies have looked at the predictive value of other individual measured pulmonary function tests, none have consistently been shown to predict postoperative morbidity or mortality.

In summary, most patients with esophageal cancer are greater than 65 years and often have significant comorbidities. The intervention (esophagectomy) is substantial, thus careful attention to the patients overall health and physiologic status is very important. While most patients should be operated on in a timely manner (4–6 weeks), there is usually time for a thorough work-up.

Operative Techniques
Open Approach

Many different operative approaches are utilized in resection of the esophagus, each with their proponents. In the USA, esophageal resection is most commonly performed using one of the following approaches: transhiatal esophagectomy (THE), transthoracic (Ivor–Lewis esophagectomy), multi-incision esophagectomy, and left thoracoabdominal esophagectomy. Each has theoretically advantages and disadvantages, and currently none is widely accepted as the approach of choice.

THE involves both a midline laparotomy and a left cervical incision. The short gastric and left gastric arteries are ligated, while the right gastric artery and right gastroepiploic arcade are carefully preserved. The main advantages of THE include a cervical gastroesophageal anastamosis and avoidance of a thoracic incision. If anastomotic leaks do occur, they are usually contained in the neck and rarely evolve into empyema or mediastinitis. Treatment, therefore, consists of simply opening and draining the neck incision and allowing healing via secondary intention. The morbidity and mortality of a cervical leak is nearly 10-fold less than for a thoracic leak. With THE, the thoracic cavity and pleura is not typically violated, therefore pulmonary complications are less likely. Although perioperative morbidity and mortality is decreased in most studies, critics contend that since the thoracic esophagus is mobilized blindly, lymph nodes can be left behind which could negatively impact long-term survival and local control.

Transthoracic esophagectomy (TTE) or the Ivor–Lewis esophagectomy also requires two incisions, a midline laparotomy, and a right posterolateral thoracotomy. *En bloc* resection is performed from the hiatus to the apex of the chest. Hilar, subcarinal, and periesophageal nodes can be carefully resected with the esophagus. A gastroesophageal anastamosis is performed in the right chest and chest tubes are placed for drainage. TTE allows for the direct visualization and resection of the intrathoracic esophagus and complete lymphadenectomy. As a result, this is the approach of choice for locally advanced mid-esophageal tumors (mostly squamous cell cancers) that potentially involve surrounding mediastinal organs, such as the trachea, bronchus, thoracic duct, azygous vein, and recurrent laryngeal nerve. The improved exposure afforded by TTE comes at the price of increased postoperative complications related to the thoracotomy incision. Division of the accessory muscles of respiration leads to the impairment of pulmonary mechanics. Additionally, pain from the incision and necessary chest tube leads to splinting, atelectasis, and decreased respiratory reserve. Pivotal in the reduction of pulmonary complications after TTE has been the thoracic epidural. Watson and Allen [55] compared patients undergoing esophagectomy with and without epidural anesthesia. They found that epidural anesthesia was associated with fewer respiratory failure events (13% vs. 30%), respiratory related deaths (0% vs. 5%), and 30-day hospital mortality (6% vs. 9%). Similarly, Whooley *et al.* examined their institutions decline in operative mortality and pulmonary complications in 710 patients undergoing primarily TTE over a 17-year period [56]. They found that during this time operative mortality decreased from 16% to 3% and pulmonary complication declined from 15% to 6%. Concomitant with this improvement was the introduction and standard use of epidural anesthetic. Utilizing a logistical regression analysis, epidural anesthesia was shown to significantly contribute to the reduction in postoperative mortality ($P < 0.0001$).

Multi-incision esophagectomy is performed less often and requires three incisions: midline laparotomy, thoracotomy, and a cervical incision. This is more commonly performed for upper or middle esophageal squamous cell carcinomas and allows the addition of cervical lymphadenectomy. A left thoracoabdominal esophagectomy involves one incision extended across the abdomen and posterolateral chest. Regardless of the incisional approach, the same operative procedure is performed, i.e. esophagogastrectomy with regional lymph node resection.

The two most common approaches utilized for distal esophageal adenocarcinoma are the transhiatal and transthoracic (TT) esophagectomy. Controversy exist as to whether the lower perioperative morbidity and mortality with THE is outweighed by the TTE's more radical lymphadenectomy. Multiple studies have sought to answer this dilemma. Four randomized controlled trials have been published. Three have suffered from small sample sizes and have thus been criticized as suffering from a type II error. The first from France randomized 32 patients to THE and 35 to TTE [57]. They reported no difference in operative blood loss, morbidity, pulmonary complications, intensive care unit and hospital stay, or long-term survival. They did find a significant difference in median operative duration with THE being shorter (4 vs. 6 h). A smaller German study randomized 16 patients each to THE and TTE [58]. A significant decrease in mean operative length (190 vs. 330 min, $P = 0.005$), mean operative blood loss (1000 vs. 2270 mL, $P = 0.003$), and pulmonary complications (four vs. eight events) were found in the THE group. There was no difference between groups in 30-day hospital mortality or survival at 1 year. A study of distal third squamous cell cancers from Hong Kong enrolled 20 patients into the THE cohort and 19 into the TTE group [59]. No difference was found in operative blood loss although intraoperative hypotension was significantly more frequent in the THE group ($P = 0.001$). THE was completed with a shorter mean operative length (174 vs. 210 min, $P = 0.001$). Two patients in the TTE group underwent

re-exploration (persistent air leak and fundal necrosis) with none in the THE group. No difference existed in pulmonary complications, hospital length, or median survival.

Hulscher *et al.* conducted the largest randomized controlled trial comparing THE to TTE [60]. One hundred and six patients were assigned to the THE group and 114 to the TTE group, virtually all with adenocarcinoma. These groups were evenly matched for age, American Society of Anesthesiologists class, and tumor stage. Operative time and blood loss in the THE group were almost half of that in the TTE group (3.5 h vs. 6.0 h, $P < 0.001$ and 1.0 vs. 1.9 L, $P < 0.001$ respectively). As predicted, specimens from the TTE group had significantly more lymph nodes identified in the pathologic specimen (mean, 31 vs. 16, $P < 0.001$). Perioperative morbidity was lower in the THE group, specifically, pulmonary complications (27% vs. 57%, $P < 0.001$) and development of chylous leak (2% vs. 10%, $P = 0.02$). Although no significant difference existed in anastamotic leak rate, two leaks in the TTE required re-operation with none in the THE group. Increased perioperative morbidity in the TTE group contributed to the groups overall increase in intensive care unit and hospital stay ($P < 0.001$ for both) as well as a 56% higher overall cost. Hospital mortality between groups was not significant and low at 3%. With a median follow-up of 4.7 years (range 2.5–8.3), no difference existed in local–regional recurrence or distant recurrence with 70% of patients dying in the THE group and 60% in the TTE group ($P = 0.12$). Although no difference in overall survival or disease-free survival occurred at the time of median follow-up, if projected out to 5 years both trended toward increased survival in the TTE group.

Despite four randomized controlled trials, controversy continues as to which operative approach is superior. Some of the differences in findings may be related to the variance in cancer subtype between studies (adenocarcinoma vs. squamous cell carcinoma), geographical differences in patient populations (Europe vs. Asia), and perioperative care. What is clear is that all four studies reported no statistical difference in cancer survival between patients undergoing THE and TTE. Therefore, extended lymphadenectomy for esophageal cancer remains an unproven method of improving survival and both

Table 23.2 Reported results of minimally invasive esophagectomy (MIE).

Author	N	Conversion (%)	OR time (min)*	Major complications (%)	Anastomotic leak rate (%)	Hospital stay (days)†	Mortality (%)
Nguyen *et al.* [63]	46	2.2	350	17.4	8.7	8	4.3
Luketich *et al.* [62]	222	7.2	NR	32	11.7	7	1.4

* Reported as mean.
† Reported as median.
NR, not reported; OR time, operative time.

THE and TTE are effective operations for distal esophageal cancer.

Esophagectomy whether performed transhiatal or transthoracic, results in prolonged convalescence. De Boer *et al.* examined the long-term effect THE and TTE had on quality of life assessed via two validated quality-of-life (QOL) questionnaires (Rotterdam Symptom Checklist and Medical Outcomes Studies Short Form-20) [61]. Patients in both groups reported a decline in physical and psychological symptoms as well as activity level immediately after surgery with a gradual return to preoperative levels within a year after surgery. Interestingly, global QOL measurements initially declined then re-bounded too and remained above preoperative results 8 months after surgery. Comparing THE to TTE at 5 weeks postoperative, pain was significantly less in the THE group. Likewise at 3 months, the THE group reported significant increases in energy level, physical and mental functioning as compared to patients undergoing TTE. However with continued follow-up the recovery of the TTE group met the THE group and at 1 year no statistical difference existed in QOL scores between groups. With sustained follow-up of over 3 years, QOL remained similar between groups.

Minimally Invasive Approach

In efforts to decrease operative morbidity, hospital stays, and postoperative convalescence, surgeons began reporting on the feasibility of minimally invasive esophagectomy (MIE) in 1992. Similar to the open approach, multiple variations exist in technique; thorascopic, laparoscopic, and a combination there of. Two large studies have reported on the combined laparoscopic and thorascopic approach to esophagectomy and results are displayed in Table 23.2 [62,63]. Both studies demonstrate the technical feasibility of MIE with a low conversion rate, hospital stay, and mortality rate. Mean operative times were 350 min, equivalent to those reported by Hulscher *et al.* with open TTE (360 min) [60]. Major complications, anastomotic leak rate, and cumulative survival, based on TNM stage, were comparable to outcomes after open surgery. An admitted shortcoming of MIE is the loss of tactile sensation which can make discerning the extent of tumor difficult, thus possible jeopardizing attainment of negative margins. By utilizing intraoperative endoscopy to delineate proximal and distal extension of the malignancy, Nguyen *et al.* obtained negative margins in all patients [63]. Other theoretical concerns include port site recurrences, which have not been reported in either study with mean follow-up of 26 months.

Although technically challenging, MIE can be performed with equivalent operative morbidity, mortality, and cancer survival as reported with open surgery. A few studies have reported decreased cardiopulmonary complications and faster recovery with MIE. Still more experience, longer follow-up, and ideally a randomized control trial is needed to determine if MIE protracts any advantage over open esophagectomy.

References

1. Gerson LB, Shetler K, Triadafilopoulos G. Prevalence of Barrett's esophagus in asymptomatic individuals. *Gastroenterology* 2002;**123**(2):461–7.

2. Conio M, Cameron AJ, Romero Y *et al.* Secular trends in the epidemiology and outcome of Barrett's oesophagus in Olmsted County, Minnesota. *Gut* 2001;**48**(3):304–9.

3. Pera M, Cameron AJ, Trastek VF, Carpenter HA, Zinsmeister AR. Increasing incidence of adenocarcinoma of the esophagus and esophagogastric junction. *Gastroenterology* 1993;**104**(2):510–3.

4. Williamson WA, Ellis FH, Jr, Gibb SP, Shahian DM, Aretz HT. Effect of antireflux operation on Barrett's mucosa. *Ann Thorac Surg* 1990;**49**(4):537–41; discussion 541–32.

5. DeMeester SR, Campos GM, DeMeester TR *et al.* The impact of an antireflux procedure on intestinal metaplasia of the cardia. *Ann Surg* 1998;**228**(4):547–56.

6. Farrell TM, Smith CD, Metreveli RE *et al.* Fundoplication provides effective and durable symptom relief in patients with Barrett's esophagus. *Am J Surg* 1999;**178**(1):18–21.

7. Parrilla P, Martinez de Haro LF, Ortiz A *et al.* Long-term results of a randomized prospective study comparing medical and surgical treatment of Barrett's esophagus. *Ann Surg* 2003;**237**(3):291–8.

8. Eubanks TR, Omelanczuk P, Richards C, Pohl D, Pellegrini CA. Outcomes of laparoscopic antireflux procedures. *Am J Surg* 2000;**179**(5):391–5.

9. Fass R, Sampliner RE, Malagon IB *et al.* Failure of oesophageal acid control in candidates for Barrett's oesophagus reversal on a very high dose of proton pump inhibitor. *Aliment Pharmacol Ther* 2000;**14**(5):597–602.

10. Ortiz A, Martinez de Haro LF, Parrilla P *et al.* Twenty-four hour pH monitoring is necessary to assess acid reflux suppression in patients with Barrett's oesophagus undergoing treatment with proton pump inhibitors. *Br J Surg* 1999;**86**(11):1472–4.

11. Stein HJ, Kauer WK, Feussner H, Siewert JR. Bile reflux in benign and malignant Barrett's esophagus: effect of medical acid suppression and nissen fundoplication. *J Gastrointest Surg* 1998;**2**(4):333–41.

12. Champion G, Richter JE, Vaezi MF, Singh S, Alexander R. Duodenogastroesophageal reflux: relationship to pH and importance in Barrett's esophagus. *Gastroenterology* 1994;**107**(3):747–54.

13. Hofstetter WL, Peters JH, DeMeester TR *et al.* Long-term outcome of antireflux surgery in patients with Barrett's esophagus. *Ann Surg* 2001;**234**(4):532–8; discussion 538–9.

14. Oelschlager BK, Barreca M, Chang L, Oleynikov D, Pellegrini CA. Clinical and pathologic response of Barrett's esophagus to laparoscopic antireflux surgery. *Ann Surg* 2003;**238**(4):458–64; discussion 464–56.

15. Sampliner RE. Practice guidelines on the diagnosis, surveillance, and therapy of Barrett's esophagus. The Practice Parameters Committee of the American College of Gastroenterology. *Am J Gastroenterol* 1998;**93**(7):1028–32.

16. Sharma P, Sampliner RE, Camargo E. Normalization of esophageal pH with high-dose proton pump inhibitor therapy does not result in regression of Barrett's esophagus. *Am J Gastroenterol* 1997;**92**(4):582–5.

17. Malesci A, Savarino V, Zentilin P *et al.* Partial regression of Barrett's esophagus by long-term therapy with high-dose omeprazole. *Gastrointest Endosc* 1996; **44**(6):700–5.

18. Peters FT, Ganesh S, Kuipers EJ *et al.* Endoscopic regression of Barrett's oesophagus during omeprazole treatment; a randomised double blind study. *Gut* 1999;**45**(4):489–94.

19. Rudolph RE, Vaughan TL, Storer BE *et al.* Effect of segment length on risk for neoplastic progression in patients with Barrett esophagus. *Ann Intern Med* 2000;**132**(8):612–20.

20. El-Serag HB, Aguirre TV, Davis S *et al.* Proton pump inhibitors are associated with reduced incidence of dysplasia in Barrett's esophagus. *Am J Gastroenterol* 2004;**99**(10):1877–83.

21. Brand DL, Ylvisaker JT, Gelfand M, Pope CE, II. Regression of columnar esophageal (Barrett's) epithelium after anti-reflux surgery. *N Engl J Med* 1980; **302**(15):844–8.

22. Attwood SE, Barlow AP, Norris TL, Watson A. Barrett's oesophagus: effect of antireflux surgery on symptom control and development of complications. *Br J Surg* 1992;**79**(10):1050–3.

23. Low DE, Levine DS, Dail DH, Kozarek RA. Histological and anatomic changes in Barrett's esophagus after antireflux surgery. *Am J Gastroenterol* 1999;**94**(1): 80–5.

24. O'Riordan JM, Byrne PJ, Ravi N, Keeling PW, Reynolds JV. Long-term clinical and pathologic response of Barrett's esophagus after antireflux surgery. *Am J Surg* 2004;**188**(1):27–33.

25. Gurski RR, Peters JH, Hagen JA *et al.* Barrett's esophagus can and does regress after antireflux surgery: a study of prevalence and predictive features. *J Am Coll Surg* 2003;**196**(5):706–12; discussion 712–3.

26. Spechler SJ, Lee E, Ahnen D *et al.* Long-term outcome of medical and surgical therapies for gastroesophageal reflux disease: follow-up of a randomized controlled trial. *JAMA* 2001;**285**(18):2331–8.

27. Corey KE, Schmitz SM, Shaheen NJ. Does a surgical antireflux procedure decrease the incidence of

esophageal adenocarcinoma in Barrett's esophagus? A meta-analysis. *Am J Gastroenterol* 2003;**98**(11):2390–4.

28. Ye W, Chow WH, Lagergren J, Yin L, Nyren O. Risk of adenocarcinomas of the esophagus and gastric cardia in patients with gastroesophageal reflux diseases and after antireflux surgery. *Gastroenterology* 2001; **121**(6):1286–93.

29. Katz D, Rothstein R, Schned A *et al.* The development of dysplasia and adenocarcinoma during endoscopic surveillance of Barrett's esophagus. *Am J Gastroenterol* 1998;**93**(4):536–41.

30. Schnell TG, Sontag SJ, Chejfec G *et al.* Long-term nonsurgical management of Barrett's esophagus with high-grade dysplasia. *Gastroenterology* 2001; **120**(7):1607–19.

31. McDonald ML, Trastek VF, Allen MS, Deschamps C, Pairolero PC. Barretts's esophagus: does an antireflux procedure reduce the need for endoscopic surveillance? *J Thorac Cardiovasc Surg* 1996;**111**(6):1135–8; discussion 1139–40.

32. Csendes A, Burdiles P, Braghetto I, Korn O. Adenocarcinoma appearing very late after antireflux surgery for Barrett's esophagus: long-term follow-up, review of the literature, and addition of six patients. *J Gastrointest Surg* 2004;**8**(4):434–41.

33. Reid BJ, Levine DS, Longton G, Blount PL, Rabinovitch PS. Predictors of progression to cancer in Barrett's esophagus: baseline histology and flow cytometry identify low- and high-risk patient subsets. *Am J Gastroenterol* 2000;**95**(7):1669–76.

34. Falk GW, Rice TW, Goldblum JR, Richter JE. Jumbo biopsy forceps protocol still misses unsuspected cancer in Barrett's esophagus with high-grade dysplasia. *Gastrointest Endosc* 1999;**49**(2):170–6.

35. Reid BJ, Blount PL, Feng Z, Levine DS. Optimizing endoscopic biopsy detection of early cancers in Barrett's high-grade dysplasia. *Am J Gastroenterol* 2000;**95**(11):3089–96.

36. Overholt BF, Panjehpour M, Halberg DL. Photodynamic therapy for Barrett's esophagus with dysplasia and/or early stage carcinoma: long-term results. *Gastrointest Endosc* 2003;**58**(2):183–8.

37. May A, Gossner L, Pech O *et al.* Local endoscopic therapy for intraepithelial high-grade neoplasia and early adenocarcinoma in Barrett's oesophagus: acute-phase and intermediate results of a new treatment approach. *Eur J Gastroenterol Hepatol* 2002;**14**(10):1085–91.

38. van Hillegersberg R, Haringsma J, ten Kate FJ, Tytgat GN, van Lanschot JJ. Invasive carcinoma after endoscopic ablative therapy for high-grade dysplasia in Barrett's oesophagus. *Dig Surg* 2003;**20**(5):440–4.

39. Peters JH, Clark GW, Ireland AP *et al.* Outcome of adenocarcinoma arising in Barrett's esophagus in endoscopically surveyed and nonsurveyed patients. *J Thorac Cardiovasc Surg* 1994;**108**(5):813–21; discussion 821–12.

40. Pera M, Trastek VF, Carpenter HA *et al.* Barrett's esophagus with high-grade dysplasia: an indication for esophagectomy? *Ann Thorac Surg* 1992;**54**(2):199–204.

41. Altorki NK, Sunagawa M, Little AG, Skinner DB. High-grade dysplasia in the columnar-lined esophagus. *Am J Surg* 1991;**161**(1):97–99; discussion 99–100.

42. Heitmiller RF, Redmond M, Hamilton SR. Barrett's esophagus with high-grade dysplasia. An indication for prophylactic esophagectomy. *Ann Surg* 1996; **224**(1):66–71.

43. Walsh TN, Noonan N, Hollywood D *et al.* A comparison of multimodal therapy and surgery for esophageal adenocarcinoma. *N Engl J Med* 1996;**335**(7):462–7.

44. Urba SG, Orringer MB, Turrisi A *et al.* Randomized trial of preoperative chemoradiation versus surgery alone in patients with locoregional esophageal carcinoma. *J Clin Oncol* 2001;**19**(2):305–13.

45. Apinop C, Puttisak P, Preecha N. A prospective study of combined therapy in esophageal cancer. *Hepatogastroenterology* 1994;**41**(4):391–3.

46. Bosset JF, Gignoux M, Triboulet JP *et al.* Chemoradiotherapy followed by surgery compared with surgery alone in squamous-cell cancer of the esophagus. *N Engl J Med* 1997;**337**(3):161–7.

47. Ochsner A, DeBakey M. Surgical aspects of carcinoma of the esophagus: review of the literature and report of four cases. *J Thorac Surg* 1941;**10**:401–45.

48. Earlam R, Cunha-Melo JR. Oesophageal squamous cell carcinoma: I. A critical review of surgery. *Br J Surg* 1980;**67**(6):381–90.

49. Muller JM, Erasmi H, Stelzner M, Zieren U, Pichlmaier H. Surgical therapy of oesophageal carcinoma. *Br J Surg* 1990;**77**(8):845–57.

50. Jamieson GG, Mathew G, Ludemann R *et al.* Postoperative mortality following oesophagectomy and problems in reporting its rate. *Br J Surg* 2004;**91**(8): 943–7.

51. Bollschweiler E, Schroder W, Holscher AH, Siewert JR. Preoperative risk analysis in patients with adenocarcinoma or squamous cell carcinoma of the oesophagus. *Br J Surg* 2000;**87**(8):1106–10.

52. Griffin SM, Shaw IH, Dresner SM. Early complications after Ivor Lewis subtotal esophagectomy with two-field lymphadenectomy: risk factors and management. *J Am Coll Surg* 2002;**194**(3):285–97.

53. Law SY, Fok M, Wong J. Risk analysis in resection of squamous cell carcinoma of the esophagus. *World J Surg* 1994;**18**(3):339–46.

54. Ferguson MK, Durkin AE. Preoperative prediction of the risk of pulmonary complications after esophagectomy for cancer. *J Thorac Cardiovasc Surg* 2002;**123**(4):661–9.

55. Watson A, Allen PR. Influence of thoracic epidural analgesia on outcome after resection for esophageal cancer. *Surgery* 1994;**115**(4):429–32.

56. Whooley BP, Law S, Murthy SC, Alexandrou A, Wong J. Analysis of reduced death and complication rates after esophageal resection. *Ann Surg* 2001; **233**(3):338–44.

57. Goldminc M, Maddern G, Le Prise E *et al.* Oesophagectomy by a transhiatal approach or thoracotomy: a prospective randomized trial. *Br J Surg* 1993; **80**(3):367–70.

58. Jacobi CA, Zieren HU, Muller JM, Pichlmaier H. Surgical therapy of esophageal carcinoma: the influence of surgical approach and esophageal resection on cardiopulmonary function. *Eur J Cardiothorac Surg* 1997;**11**(1):32–7.

59. Chu KM, Law SY, Fok M, Wong J. A prospective randomized comparison of transhiatal and transthoracic resection for lower-third esophageal carcinoma. *Am J Surg* 1997;**174**(3):320–4.

60. Hulscher JB, van Sandick JW, de Boer AG *et al.* Extended transthoracic resection compared with limited transhiatal resection for adenocarcinoma of the esophagus. *N Engl J Med* 2002;**347**(21):1662–9.

61. de Boer AG, van Lanschot JJ, van Sandick JW *et al.* Quality of life after transhiatal compared with extended transthoracic resection for adenocarcinoma of the esophagus. *J Clin Oncol* 2004;**22**(20):4202–8.

62. Luketich JD, Alvelo-Rivera M, Buenaventura PO *et al.* Minimally invasive esophagectomy: outcomes in 222 patients. *Ann Surg* 2003;**238**(4):486–94; discussion 494–85.

63. Nguyen NT, Roberts P, Follette DM, Rivers R, Wolfe BM. Thoracoscopic and laparoscopic esophagectomy for benign and malignant disease: lessons learned from 46 consecutive procedures. *J Am Coll Surg* 2003; **197**(6):902–13.

CHAPTER 24

Chemoprevention for Barrett's Esophagus

Janusz Jankowski and Edyta Zagorowicz

Abstract

The esophageal adenocarcinoma (EAC) incidence has been increasing for the last few decades at an alarming rate and its burden in the UK is higher than in other Western countries. The prognosis for advanced EAC is poor. A majority of those cancers arise from Barrett's esophagus in the course of a well-established metaplasia–dysplasia–carcinoma sequence. Endoscopic surveillance for dysplasia and early carcinoma detects cancer in less advanced stages but has not proven to diminish cancer incidence or improve general outcomes. Neither has antireflux surgery been shown to protect against EAC development. Currently different available endoscopic ablative techniques for Barrett's mucosa are limited to high-risk patients groups with dysplasia. Therefore other strategies that would inhibit carcinogenesis process are needed. Chemoprevention is a specific medical treatment of carcinogenesis that stops the process in the early phases before an advanced cancer develops. There is evidence that proton pump inhibitor (PPI) treatment of Barrett's esophagus increases cell differentiation and apoptosis, reduces cyclooxygenase-2 (COX-2) level and proliferation and possibly reduces the length of Barrett's epithelium and dysplasia incidence. Epidemiological studies show that use of aspirin and other non-steroidal anti-inflammatory drugs (NSAIDs), probably due to inhibition of COX-2 and other non-COX-2 inflammatory pathways, correlates with a lower incidence of esophageal cancer. Chemoprevention with aspirin in patients with Barrett's esophagus may be cost-effective, at least in populations with high cancer incidence. A large randomized trial (ASpirin Esomeprazole Chemoprevention Trial—ASPECT) in Barrett's esophagus has begun to study if intervention with aspirin and high-dose PPIs can decrease mortality or conversion from Barrett's metaplasia to adenocarcinoma or high-grade dysplasia (HGD).

Introduction

Epidemiology

Gastroesophageal reflux disease (GERD) affects 7–10% of the general population and the development of esophageal adenocarcinoma (EAC) is its most serious complication. For the last three decades the incidence of esophageal carcinoma, which has become a dominant form of esophageal cancer in Westernized countries, has been rapidly increasing. The UK has one of the highest rates of 12–16/100 000 compared with 3–5/100 000 in the USA [1,2], with a peak incidence at the age of 55–69 years. Despite recent developments in diagnostics and treatment modalities the prognosis remains poor with an overall 5 year survival rate of 10%. Only early detection of stage 1 tumors carries substantial improved outcomes.

Although some studies suggest that chronic reflux symptoms predispose to the carcinoma itself, Barrett's esophagus is detected before or at the diagnosis of adenocarcinoma in almost two-thirds of patients [3]. Barrett's metaplasia is present in up to 12% patients with symptomatic GERD. In addition autopsy studies showed that in the general population its prevalence is about 1% [4]. A vast majority of cases remains unidentified. More recent studies on populations of American subjects who underwent upper endoscopy in addition to screening sigmoidoscopy or colonoscopy, report the prevalence of 6.8% to as much as 25% [5,6].

The other recognized demographic and clinical characteristics that correlate with the higher cancer incidence include Caucasian ethnicity, male sex, obesity, smoking, reflux duration, frequency and severity, the length of Barrett's esophagus; high-grade dysplasia (HGD), a positive Barrett's esophagus or EAC family history, possibly the absence of *Helicobacter pylori* infection, and increased hiatal hernia size [3,7,8]. Non-steroidal anti-inflammatory drugs (NSAIDs), aspirin, and perhaps proton pump inhibitor (PPI) use shows a negative correlation with the EAC occurrence [9–11].

Although it is generally accepted that the majority of Barrett's esophagus and EAC are sporadic, familial aggregation of both conditions (familial Barrett's esophagus) has been repeatedly reported. In a hospital-based epidemiological series, Chak *et al.* showed that up to 20% of all Barrett's esophagus presentations were familial and therefore might have a small and undetermined genetic component [7,12]. Autosomal dominant transmission pattern was observed in most series but a causative gene has yet to be identified [7,12]. In a recent study, screening endoscopy identified Barrett's esophagus and EAC in a substantial proportion of first-degree relatives of affected members of families [13].

The strongest predictor of the adenocarcinoma risk in Barrett's esophagus is HGD. Its presence determines 30–60% cumulative risk of cancer development within 5 years and in some patients occult cancer is already present at the time of dysplasia detection. It is estimated that in the UK the cancer incidence rate in Barrett's esophagus is 1%/year and it appears to be higher when compared with other Western European countries and the USA [14,15]. The evaluation of the exact conversion rate into dysplasia and cancer is hampered by false positive Barrett's esophagus diagnoses and this limitation might be particularly true for large population studies [16,17]. The diagnosis of columnar esophagus with no intestinal metaplasia may result from hiatal hernia biopsying and intestinal metaplasia may be found in biopsies from the gastroesophageal junction.

EAC prevention

Once Barrett's esophagus, and so the increased cancer risk, has been recognized, some measures need to be taken to detect cancer at an early stage to lower or prevent the adenocarcinoma incidence. Given a 0.5–1.0% annual risk of cancer with Barrett's esophagus, the majority of those patients will not develop EAC and only 5% of them will die with this disease. Any current preventive strategy will benefit only one in 20 patients and so the economic burden of an intervention is of particular importance. One approach to this problem is better identification within Barrett's esophagus population those patients who are particularly at risk so that a preventive intervention might be limited to them. Presently, however, only dysplasia is taken into account in the clinical algorithm that stratifies the cancer risk and adjusts the preventive management accordingly. Dysplasia is a late cancer risk marker but it is preceded by specific molecular alterations that might provide surrogate markers of the increased risk. Some intensively studied parameters being validated in prospective studies are inactivation of *p16* and *p53*, which are tumor supressor genes, and overexpression of cyclin D, which acts in opposition to *p16* and stimulates cell proliferation by promoting cell cycle transition from G1 to S [18]. The most advanced and promising data concerns DNA aneuploidy and tetraploidy detected in flow cytometry that were already shown to predict progression to EAC [19,20], but those data have not yet been widely reproduced in other centers and in randomized controlled trials. The selection of prognostic molecular markers will be of critical importance for timing of preventive interventions and for targeted designs for future studies.

Diet and Lifestyle

Obese subjects with a body mass index (BMI) > 30 may have up to a 16-fold increase of the EAC risk compared with those with a BMI < 22 [3]. Unfortunately, although clinical trials have shown that combined low-calorie diet, increased physical activity, and behavioral therapy result in a substantial weight reduction, when the therapeutic intervention is stopped the majority of subjects will progressively regain lost kilograms and reach the same weight as before the treatment or even higher. The same is true for pharmacological weight reduction strategies, and the safety of long-term therapy has not been established.

The association between dietary factors and the risk of EAC is not fully understood. Studies that analyzed dietary patterns in cancer patients suggest that a greater intake of nutrients from plant sources, particularly from fruit, vegetables, and whole-grains, as well as fish and diary products may be associated with a lower risk. [21-23]. These foods contain α-tocopherol, vitamin C, vitamin B_6, β-carotene, folate, and dietary fiber that have been shown to be inversely associated with the EAC risk. More recently, serum selenium levels were found to be inversely correlated with the incidence of markers of neoplastic progression in Barrett's esophagus patients [24]. Greater intake of meat, dietary fat, and cholesterol show a positive relation with the cancer incidence.

Smoking is a major risk factor for EAC and the increase in smoking prevalence observed in the last century may partly explain the rising incidence of these tumors in the past decades [25]. The recent decrease in smoking may not yet have had an impact. The same authors found that also poor educational levels and low socioeconomic status seem to be associated with the increased EAC incidence. Excessive alcohol use is probably another related factor [26,27].

These data more precisely define target populations for preventive interventions and suggest that general education on healthy nutrition and healthy lifestyle may be of value for EAC prevention. In addition some deficient nutrients supplementation might potentially have a chemopreventive effect.

Helicobacter pylori

Infection with *H. pylori* and particularly *cag*A+ strains is inversely associated with the risk of EAC (odds ratio [OR], 0.4; 95% confidence interval [CI], 0.2–0.8) [28]. Chronic *H. pylori* infection may lead to atrophic gastritis and can lower gastric acidity, which might have a protective effect against the complications of acid reflux including EAC. It has been suggested that the rising EAC incidence may reflect the decreasing *H. pylori* infection prevalence. This problem, and the balance between benefits and risks of

eradication therapy, especially in GERD patients, needs further studies.

Pharmacological Treatment

Currently there is no medical treatment proven to protect from EAC. Antacids and H2-receptor antagonists (H2RAs) were the most widely used drug classes in GERD patients before the appearance of PPIs. It has been suggested that these drugs may allow reflux to continue without symptoms and that uncontrolled reflux may lead to increased esophageal damage. This hypothesis was partly based on results of some case controlled studies which showed that subjects who developed EAC reported the use of H2RAs and antacids more often than the general population [29], and those who died of EAC were more likely to use H2RAs than subjects who died from cardiovascular disorders [30]. These results, however, should be interpreted with caution since the increased drug consumption may only reflect the severity of reflux. The comparison to non-reflux populations does not allow for separating the influence of pathologic mechanisms present in GERD, from the drug effect. Direct evidence that effective acid suppressant therapy with PPI modifies cancer risk is lacking [31]. There is data from experimental and epidemiological studies that acid and inflammation control may significantly influence transition process from metaplasia to dysplasia and carcinoma. These issues are discussed in more detail in the next sections.

Surgery

Antireflux surgery in a population with GERD and in patients with Barrett's esophagus does not seem to lower the cancer incidence and this is thought to be due to incomplete acid reflux control, even when symptoms are reduced [32,33].

Endoscopic Screening and Surveillance

According to current American College of Gastroentenology recommendations, regular surveillance endoscopy with histological examination of metaplastic tissue for dysplasia is performed more frequently when low-grade dysplasia (LGD) is detected, while HGD is treated with esophagectomy or endoscopic ablation. Endoscopic screening and repeated surveillance procedures needs to be accepted by a patient and requires expert endo-scopists and pathologists, given the major interpretation problems with dysplasia. It results in the detection of cancers at an earlier stage and prognosis of these patients is better compared with those with symptomatic tumors. However there is no direct evidence from randomized studies that this improves overall survival compared to the general population [34]. Cost-effectiveness analyses indicate that highly sensitive surveillance endoscopy can only be justified in subpopulations with the highest risk; the lower the adenocarcinoma incidence, the longer interval between endoscopies is worthwhile [35]. In the USA, a population with an estimated 0.4% cancer incidence per year, the cost-effective management includes a surveillance procedure every 5 years with an incremental cost-effectiveness ratio (ICER) of $98 000/quality-adjusted life-years (QALY) (see later). Although debatable, a one-time endoscopic screening for Barrett's esophagus in 50-year-old GERD patients might be a cost-effective strategy compared with no screening with an ICER of $24 700/QALY, and even an alternative to surveillance if effective measures in patients at risk could be taken [36,37].

Endoscopic Ablation Therapies

Endoscopic mucosal ablation therapies (photodynamic therapy, argon plasma coagulation, and mucosal resection) are increasingly used in specialized centers for treatment of HGD. These methods, combined with medically or surgically achieved acid control may lead to partial regression of Barrett's esophagus mucosa and squamous re-epithelialization, but there is no direct evidence that this reduces the EAC incidence. Moreover, dysplasia or cancer may develop in the residual metaplastic epithelium and also under the squamous re-epithelialization layer [38], thereby making detection even more difficult.

Chemoprevention – General Information

Definitions

Cancer chemoprevention was first defined by Sporn in 1976 as a use of natural, synthetic, or biologic chemical agents to reverse, suppress, or prevent carcinogenic progression, and his definition included a model of field carcinogenesis and multistep carcinogenesis [39]. According to this hypothesis, due to chronic exposure of a surface epithelium to environmental carcinogens, epithelial cells may undergo gradual genetic changes that predispose them to multifocal development of dysplasia and cancer. The original conception has been expanded and it was shown that genetic and epigenetic changes in oncogenes and tumor supressor genes, along with growth factors, imbalances, and enzyme dysregulation in some cytoplasmic and nuclear signal pathways, lead to accumulation of changes in a single clone of cells. Progression from normal tissue to dysplasia and then to cancer occurs usually over decades. Multifocal occurrence of this evolution implies that not all changed cells in a given tissue will develop the same genetic lesions. Chemoprevention can also be defined as the treatment of carcinogenesis, i.e. intervention in the disease process at earlier stages before it reaches its terminal invasive and metastatic phase.

Primary anticancer chemoprevention strategy is aimed to prevent the development of malignancies in a healthy population that may be characterized by high risk, such as specific genetic mutations that predispose to cancer (e.g. prevention of colorectal carcinoma in patients with familial adenomatous polyposis (FAP) or prevention of breast cancer in women with known *BRCA* mutation). Secondary preventive intervention includes patients with established premalignant lesions (i.e. colon adenomas, Barrett's esophagus) to prevent their progression to cancers. Tertiary prevention is employed to prevent the development of second primary tumors (SPTs) in patients cured of initial cancer or premalignant lesion, like women with a history of breast cancer or patients definitely treated for oral leukoplakia [40].

Chemopreventive Agents Development

Possible mechanisms of action of chemopreventive agents were originally described by Kelloff *et al.* and include carcinogen blocking activities, antioxidant activities, and antiproliferation activities [41]. The list of potential agents is long and still expanding, but the most intensively studied molecules include nutrients, particularly retinoids, and NSAIDs for different organs, estrogen receptor modulators (tamoxifen and raloxifene) for breast cancer, and finasteride for prostate cancer. Similar to the new drug evaluation process, based on epidemiological and experimental studies candidate agents are selected in a scrutinized preclinical evaluation of its preventive effect, metabolism, kinetics, and toxic effects including potential carcinogenicity. If the agent has promising organ-specific activity, is safe, tolerable, with a mathematically proven cost-effectiveness in a population at risk, subsequent phases of clinical trials are conducted. Phase I trials may be omitted in case of nutrients or drugs already approved for use in humans. Phase II studies are short-term trials conducted in a premalignant phase of a disease perhaps using surrogate markers. Long-term phase III studies are best based on hard endpoints such as the cancer incidence. Typically in the latter phase a reduced cancer incidence or mortality is required to show the chemopreventive efficacy. Such trials are usually at least 5–10 years duration and involve large groups of patients. For economic reasons, few academic centers and pharmaceutical manufacturers can undertake them and that substantially limits the number of candidate agents that can be developed using rigorous protocols.

Another novel strategy to advance chemoprevention trials is not to depend on the cancer as the endpoint, but on inhibition of earlier phases in the carcinogenesis process basing on surrogate (intermediate) endpoints for evaluation of its efficacy. This approach may allow chemoprevention efficacy to be demonstrated in a shorter duration. The potential surrogate endpoints for cancer incidence are both phenotypic and genotypic and their identification and validation is the subject of many ongoing studies. The primary phenotypic surrogate endpoint used in present chemopreventive trials is histological modulation of significant precancerous lesions, specifically intraepithelial neoplasia (IEN) in epithelial tissues [41,42]. IEN is a non-invasive lesion that has genetic abnormalities, loss of cellular control functions, and some phenotypic characteristics of invasive cancer and is a strong predictor of invasive cancer. An established IEN (dysplasia in Barrett's esophagus, colorectal adenoma, prostatic IEN, cervi-

cal IEN) is currently an indication to invasive surgical intervention or increased surveillance, but it may also be a goal for medical intervention to reduce the cancer risk and also morbidity associated with surgery. Another potential advantage of pharmacological intervention over surgery is that its effect is not limited to the established IEN but is exerted on the whole epithelial field involved. It means that, apart from inhibiting progression of a precancerous lesion to cancer, an effective agent might lower the risk of development of similar lesions in the surrounding tissue. When the mechanism of action of a new drug is well understood and the treatment benefits only a subset of patients, their accurate identification and targeted design may dramatically reduce the number of patients required for the study [43], such as estrogen antagonists in breast cancer or epidermal growth factor inhibitors in EAC.

Chemoprevention Cost-Effectiveness

Unger *et al.* [44] developed a method of assessing the potential impacts of new cancer therapies on the mortality of the US population and compared it with successful cancer prevention using the example of the prostate cancer prevention with finasteride [45]. The absolute impact of a new treatment on survival can be measured as the extension of life, that is the potential number of person-years saved (PYS) in a defined population as a result of the treatment. Person-years lived (PYL) is the product of the number of patients treated and the average number of years lived by those patients. PYS is the difference between PYL on the experimental arm and PYL on the standard arm:

PYS = PYL experimental — PYL standard.

First the authors analyzed eight phase III therapeutic trials in oncology in which the experimental therapy showed significantly better survival. For each study they constructed 5-year survival curves for standard and experimental groups and calculated PYS for each new therapy as a percentage of the number of PYL with standard therapy. Then, based on cancer population data from the SEER (Surveillance, Epidemiology and End Results) registry, they referred it to the whole US population.

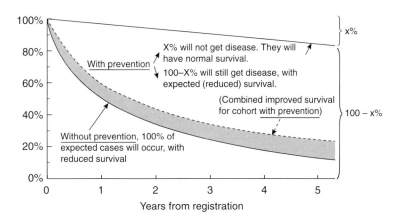

Fig. 24.1 Estimating person-years saved (PYS) in the prevention setting. Adapted from Unger *et al.* [44].

In the prevention-setting, PYS is the difference between PYL in the cohort that received prevention regimen and PYL in the cohort without prevention. In a cohort without prevention, where 100% expected cancers will occur, the estimated survival will be reduced. In a cohort with prevention, some subjects will not get the disease and they will have similar survival as normal people and some will still get the disease and will have survival as the cohort without prevention. Combining the component prevented from getting the disease with the component not prevented from getting the disease will result in improved overall survival for the cohort with prevention (Fig. 24.1).

The authors were able to show that the potential number of PYS as a result of chemoprevention of the prostate cancer in the US population within the first 5 years is similar to the number of person-years that would have been saved due to the new therapies for advanced cancer from eight recent positive phase III therapeutic trials in oncology.

Cost-effectiveness is one more requirement that has to be fulfilled for a new intervention approval. The average cost-effectiveness ratio (CER) is the average costs for a particular intervention, divided by the years of life saved (PYS) as a result of that management:

CER = costs/PYS

The incremental cost-effectiveness ratio (ICER) is the additional or incremental costs and benefits compared with an alternative practice. Instead of PYS, quality-adjusted life-years (QALYs) are usually used in the denominator, a measure that adjusts life expectancy by the quality of life associated with it:

ICER = the difference in costs/QALYs

The ICER provides the critical information because it compares the cost and benefits of one strategy with another and shows what the additional benefit is in a robust way. For a preventive strategy, like endoscopic surveillance in Barrett's esophagus, ICER is the costs of regular surveillance endoscopy minus the costs of no surveillance (the costs of cancer treatment) divided by the life expectancy of patients with surveillance minus the life expectancy of patients without surveillance [35,46]. The suggested ICER for prevention strategies is $40 000/life-year saved, but some well-accepted practices, like cervical cancer screening, are much more costly.

Landmark Chemopreventive Studies

Breast Cancer Prevention Trial results were the landmark achievement in this field that made the US Food and Drug Administration (FDA) approve tamoxifen for primary prevention of breast cancer in healthy high-risk women (40–50% reduction of incidence) [47]. Waiting for approval is finasteride with strong supportive evidence for its protective effect against prostate cancer development [45].

Agents for Chemoprevention in Barrett's Esophagus

The progression to cancer in patients with Barrett's

esophagus is thought to be driven by the reflux of acid and bile, and the resulting mucosal damage is accompanied by an inflammatory cell infiltrate. Precise molecular mechanisms responsible for the malignant transformation and the relative contribution of specific insults are still poorly understood. Despite symptomatic improvement with PPI treatment the majority of Barrett's esophagus patients may not achieve adequate acid control [48]. After a pulse but not continuous exposure to acid *in vitro*, metaplastic cells show an increase in proliferation and expression of cyclooxygenase-2 (COX-2) antiapoptotic protein [49]. In Barrett's mucosa exposed to acid *in vivo* the activation of mitogen activated protein kinase (MAPK) pathways is observed that transmit growth-regulating signals to effector genes in the nucleus [50]. The rise in COX-2-expression in Barrett's mucosa specimens was also seen in response to bile acid exposure [49]. Bile acids are mostly toxic in combination with acid but they are not likely to be important as a single agent, as gastric surgery does not increase EAC risk [51]. The acidified bile acid *in vitro* upregulate the expression of oncogene c-*myc* in esophageal cells [52]. The inflammatory infiltration may contribute to DNA damage by generation of free radicals and induction of cytokines and growth factors expression that are responsible for epithelial proliferation, resistance to apoptosis, and cell migration [53,54]. It is speculated that the nuclear transcription factor kappa B (NFκB) activation may have a cancer promoting effect and provides an important mechanism linking inflammation and numerous cytokine abnormalities to esophageal carcinogenesis [55,56]. Overall, this data suggests it is biologically plausible that some pharmacological interventions might have a chemopreventive effect for Barrett's esophagus. Since no preventive intervention in Barrett's esophagus is currently recommended to lower the cancer risk until high-risk tissue abnormalities develop, finding effective agents that stop this process would be highly desirable.

Non-Steroidal Anti-Inflammatory Drugs
Chemopreventive Properties of NSAIDs

The chronic use of NSAIDs has been associated with a decreased incidence of several types of gastrointestinal neoplasia including EAC. The strongest data, coming from animal studies, human observational studies, and also clinical trials in FAP patients and populations with colorectal adenomas, concern colorectal cancer.

The principal mechanism of action of NSAIDs is the inhibition of both identified isoforms of cyclooxygenase (COX) that are rate-limiting enzymes for the production of prostaglandins from arachidonic acid. COX-1 is constitutively expressed in the majority of tissues; it regulates blood flow and platelet function and also protects gastrointestinal mucosa. COX-2 is normally found in the kidney and brain but in other tissues its expression is inducible and rises during inflammation, wound healing, and neoplastic growth in response to inteleukins, cytokines, hormones, growth factors, and tumor promoters. COX-2 and derived prostaglandin E_2 (PGE2) occur to be implicated in carcinogenesis because they prolong the survival of abnormal cells that favors accumulation of genetic changes. They reduce apoptosis and cell adhesion, increase cell proliferation, promote angiogenesis and invasion, and make cancer cells resistant to the host immune response [57].

NSAIDs vary in their abilities to inhibit COX-1 and COX-2 at different concentrations and different tissues, and coxibs selectively inhibit COX-2. The recent rofecoxib, and to a degree celecoxib, withdrawn from the market due to promotion of thrombosis and the increased incidence of coronary events during long-term treatment, which seems to be a class effect, is likely to result in a greater interest in the classic NSAIDs chemopreventive role. NSAIDs work mainly by restoration of apoptosis and inhibition of angiogenesis. This had been mainly attributed to the inhibition of COX but now a large body of evidence exists that the chemopreventive activity of NSAIDs depends also on COX-independent mechanisms. Compounds that do not inhibit COX activity, such as sulindac sulphone, also stimulate apoptosis in experimental settings. The chemopreventive effect of aspirin was shown in COX-2-negative neoplastic cells [58] and also in humans when a low dose of 81 mg was given that has an antiplatelet but not a COX-2 inhibitory effect [59].

Aspirin promotes cell apoptosis through a number of mechanisms including activation of *p53* signaling and inhibition of NFκB, MAPK, wnt signaling pathway, and downregulation of antiapoptotic protein Bcl-2 (Table 24.1). Inhibitory effects of aspirin on β-catenin signaling pathway are presented in Table 24.2. Activation of β-catenin signaling via enriching its free cytosolic pool has been recently proposed as one of the important mechanisms linking inflamma-

tion and cancer. Once stabilized in the cytoplasm, β-catenin translocates into the nucleus and interacting with T-cell factor (TCF) enhances transcription of variety of genes involved in cell cycle regulation, adhesion, and development, including c-*myc*, cyclin D and *COX-2* genes. The contributory role of aberrant β-catenin signaling has been documented in various

Table 24.1 Cyclooxygenase (COX)-dependent and COX-independent mechanisms of aspirin antineoplastic action.

Pathway	Mechanism	Refs
Inhibition of COX-2 and prostaglandin E$_2$	Induction of apoptosis Inhibition of proliferation and angiogenesis	[57]
Inhibition of wingless-type (Wnt) signaling and β-catenin/T-cell transcription factor signaling	Inhibition of clonal epithelial cell proliferation	[81]
Activation of *p53*	Induction of apoptosis	[82,83]
Reduction of Bcl-2 protein expression	Induction of apoptosis	[58,84]
Inhibition of nuclear transcription factor kappa B (NFκB) pathway	Inhibition of proliferation	[85,86]
Mitogen-activated protein kinase (MAPK) activation	Inhibition of NFκB activation and induction of apoptosis	[87]
Increase in mismatch repair proteins (MMR) expression	Reduction of microsatellite instability and induction of apoptosis	[88]

Table 24.2 The documented effects of aspirin and related compounds on β-catenin signaling pathway.

Compound	Effect	Cells	Refs
Aspirin	Reduced cyclin D$_1$ expression	SW948, SW480, HCT226, and LoVo colorectal cancer lines	[81]
Aspirin	Increased phosphorylation and subsequent degradation of β-catenin Reduced β-catenin-dependent TCF transcriptional activity	SW948 and SW480 colorectal cancer lines	[89]
NO-donating aspirin	Disrupted nuclear β-catenin-TCF-4 association Reduced β-catenin- dependent TCF-4 transcriptional activity Reduced cyclin D$_1$ expression	SW480 colorectal cancer line	[90]
Sodium salicylate	Increased degradation of β-catenin	HCT116 colorectal cancer line	[91]

NO, nitric oxide.

cancers development and abnormal cytoplasmatic β-catenin distribution in Barrett's esophagus has also been shown [60].

COX-2 Expression in Barrett's Esophagus and EAC

COX-2 is expressed in the normal esophagus but its expression was found to be significantly increased in Barrett's esophagus and even more in HGD and EAC [49,61,62]. Some authors speculated that COX-2 expression might be of prognostic value in EAC as the COX-2 immunoreactivity study in cancer tissues showed that patients with high COX-2 expression were more likely to develop distant metastases and local recurrence and had significantly reduced survival rates when compared to those with low expression [63].

Epidemiological Data on NSAIDs and EAC Incidence

In addition to physiologic and experimental data, cumulative results of observational epidemiological studies support attempts of chemoprotective intervention with NSAIDs against EAC in patients at risk. Based on two cohort and seven case control studies containing 1813 esophageal cancer cases, a recent meta-analysis performed by Corley *et al.* provided the most conclusive retrospective data on the association of aspirin/NSAIDs use and esophageal cancer [9]. It showed that both intermittent and frequent medication usage was protective against adenocarcinoma and squamous cell carcinoma. NSAIDs were associated with 25% reduction in the odds of developing esophageal carcinoma with a borderline statistical significance while aspirin was associated with the significant 50% reduction. The highest level of protection was seen in subjects with most frequent aspirin/NSAIDs use. More recently a Canadian study analyzed the association between NSAIDs or coxibs use and the incidence of esophageal cancer in a cohort of 86 895 patients who underwent esophageal imaging. The authors found that chronic intake of selective COX-2 inhibitors was related to significant reduction in the cancer risk but the effect of NSAIDs was even stronger (OR 0.63 and 0.47, respectively) [64]. These studies seem to further confirm the role

of COX-2 independent mechanisms in chemopreventive effect of NSAIDs.

Clinical Studies with NSAIDs

Clinical data on NSAIDs role in EAC chemoprevention from randomized trails are not yet available. A short-term study with rofecoxib 25 mg orally given for 10 days was conducted in 12 Barrett's esophagus patients on PPI therapy. Biopsies obtained before the treatment were compared with biopsies taken at the completion of the study and rofecoxib decreased COX-2 expression in Barrett's esophagus by 77%, PGE2 content by 59%, and PCNA (proliferating cell nuclear antigen which is a marker of proliferation) expression by 62.5% [65]. A randomized phase IIb trial with celecoxib in patients with Barrett's HGD or LGD has been started [66]. The study's primary objective is to evaluate the change in dysplasia occurrence after 12 months of celecoxib treatment in 200 patients.

Timing and Cost-Effectiveness of Aspirin Chemoprevention in Barrett's Esophagus

The optimal timing of chemoprevention is not known. It seems logical that the earlier phase of molecular transformation the intervention starts, the greater effect might be expected. It is possible that aspirin primarily prevents subjects from developing Barrett's esophagus rather than preventing Barrett's metaplasia from progressing into cancer, but in patients with a history of colorectal adenomas the beneficial effect of aspirin against new adenomas development was seen already after 2 years [59]. Barrett's esophagus patients also have higher than average incidence of ischaemic heart disease or cardiac deaths and this itself provides a reason for which aspirin prevention might decrease the overall mortality in this group. A significant cardio protective effect of aspirin in primary prevention is observed within the first few years of treatment [67]. These considerations encourage intervening with aspirin even in the older subgroup of Barrett's esophagus population. A recently published cost-effectiveness analysis of aspirin chemoprevention for Barrett's esophagus was performed using modified Markov decision model that presumed 50% reduction in the incidence of EAC in aspirin users (325 mg/day) and included known complications related to the therapy. It showed that aspirin either in addition to no therapy or to endoscopic surveillance is a dominant strategy. The aspirin therapy was more effective and less costly than no therapy. Additional analyses on the timing of prevention with aspirin revealed that aspirin alone was better than no therapy at all ages. The analysis did not include additional potential benefits of aspirin usage regarding cardiovascular system and chemoprevention of other cancers [68].

Proton Pump Inhibitors

Data on the role of acid suppression with PPI therapy in patients with Barrett's esophagus are controversial. Lansoprazole treatment for 6 months decreased proliferation (PCNA) and increased differentiation (villin expression) in Barrett's esophagus biopsy specimens [69], but prognostic value of those markers is unsure. The length of Barrett's esophagus is an independent cancer risk factor and the important question is whether regression of Barrett's epithelium occurs in response to PPI therapy. Although in some studies profound suppression of acid secretion resulted in the appearance of squamous islands within previous metaplastic area, that effect was not consistently observed and complete regression is rare [70,71]. Notably, there is no evidence that the reduction of Barrett's metaplasia length or surface lowers the risk of EAC.

Two more recent retrospective studies in Barrett's esophagus patients addressed the influence of PPI on hard endpoints, namely dysplasia incidence and progression. In an Australian study 350 Barrett's esophagus patients were analyzed who underwent endoscopic surveillance with median follow-up of 4–7 years. The patients in whom PPI therapy commenced 2 years or more after the diagnosis of Barrett's esophagus had five to six times the risk of LGD was compared with patients who started PPI in the first year. Similar results were seen for HGD and adenocarcinoma [10]. Further evidence that PPI may reduce the risk of developing dysplasia in Barrett's esophagus comes from an American cohort [11]. A retrospective analysis of data for 236 patients with Barrett's esophagus followed-up for 1170 patient-years showed that 56 developed dysplasia (annual incidence rate 4.7%) and 14 of them had HGD.

Cumulative incidence of dysplasia was significantly lower among patients who received PPI after Barrett's esophagus diagnosis than in those with no therapy or H2RA treatment and the hazard ratio in PPI users was 0.25. Similar findings were observed when only cases with HGD were analyzed and, as in the previous study, the longer duration of therapy was associated with less frequent occurrence of dysplasia.

The importance of the timing of acid suppressive therapy was earlier shown in a study of Carlson *et al.* who found that during acid suppression therapy progression in dysplasia and DNA ploidy status is more likely in patients with initial *p53* overexpression in biopsies [72].

One of concerns related to PPI is the increase in GERD and EAC incidence following the widespread use of this drug class, but there is no evidence that this coincidence reflects causality relation. PPI treatment may induce marked hypergastrinemia and gastrin has an important role in the regulation and proliferation of epithelial cells in the GI tract. It has been recently shown that gastrin induces COX-2 and PGE2 expression and cell proliferation via the CCK2 receptor in Barrett's mucosa [73,74]. The mitogenic effect of gastrin was reversed by COX-2 inhibitor suggesting that proliferation occurred as a result of COX-2 induction. It was also found that Barrett's epithelium expressed more amounts of endogenous gastrin mRNA compared with other tissues, which suggests an importance of autocrine or paracrine way of gastrin signaling in this setting. Another important downstream effect of CCK2 activation is phosphorylation/activation of protein kinase B (PKB/Akt) which is a potent antiapoptotic factor. It was recently shown that gastrin activates PKB/Akt in various esophageal cell lines. Thereby it may reduce cell death in metaplastic Barrett's esophagus and promote malignant progression [75].

Prospective randomized trails with PPI treatment for Barrett's esophagus are urgently needed to verify retrospective clinical data and hypotheses arisen from experimental studies. Summarized rationale for NSAIDs/aspirin and PPIs use in chemoprevention for Barrett's esophagus is shown in Table 24.3.

Table 24.3 Summarized rationale for non-steroidal anti-inflammatory drugs (NSAIDs)/aspirin and proton pump inhibitors (PPIs) use in chemoprevention for Barrett's esophagus.

Candidate agent	NSAIDs	Aspirin	PPIs
Effects of potential anticancer properties	COX-2 inhibition Decreased cell proliferation Decreased angiogenesis Increased apoptosis Increased cell adhesion Reduced development of esophageal adenocarcinoma in animal models [92]		Increased cell differentiation and decreased proliferation Decreased COX-2 expression Reduced bile exposure
Clinical data	Inverse association between aspirin/NSAIDs intake and esophageal adenocarcinoma: Better protection with more frequent use Significant effect of aspirin and borderline of NSAIDs		Reduced cell proliferation in Barrett's esophagus Partial regression of metaplastic epithelium in Barrett's esophagus* Reduced dysplasia occurrence in Barrett's esophagus
Additional benefits		Possible protection against numerous other malignancies Reduced cardiovascular disease incidence and mortality	GERD symptoms control
Major concerns	GI toxicity Increased risk of cardiovascular/thromboembolic incidents in selective NSAIDs users	GI toxicity† Aspirin resistance	Rise in EAC incidence parallel to PPIs introduction Potential procancerogenic activity of gastrin increased increased in response to acid suppression

* This effect was not consistently found in all studies.
† Cost-effectiveness in Barrett's esophagus population shown in a decision model analysis.
COX-2, cyclooxygenase-2; EAC, esophageal adenocarcinoma; GI, gastrointestinal.

Other Potential Chemopreventive Agents for Use in Barrett's Esophagus

Epidemiological and clinical data suggest that the other potential chemopreventive agents for use in EAC may include other acid suppression agents (antacids, H2RAs), bile-reducing agents, some nutrients (vitamins A–E, folic acid), and also general dietary manipulations like vegetables and fruits-rich low-calorie low-fat diets) [76].

Four nutrient combinations: retinol and zinc; riboflavin and niacin; vitamin C and molybdenum; and β-carotene, α-tocopherol, and selenium were evaluated in two randomized nutrition intervention trials conducted in Linxian in China. This region has some of the world's highest rates of esophageal and stomach cancer and a population with chronic deficiency of several nutrients. One of these four combinations was given to 29 584 adults for 5.25 years and small but significant reductions in total (relative risk [RR] = 0.91) and cancer (RR = 0.87) mortality was observed in subjects receiving β-carotene, α-tocopherol, and selenium but not the other nutrients. The second trial provided daily multiple vitamin and mineral supplementation or placebo to 3318 persons with esophageal dysplasia. After 6 years insignificant reductions in total and cancer mortality were observed [77].

Current studies focus on a strictly pharmacologic approach to the problem of carcinogenesis and its prevention. One of the numerous enzymes upregulated in esophageal carcinogenesis is inducible nitric oxide synthase (iNOS) that is thought to be involved in the *p53* mutation process [61]. The expression of iNOS and nitrate scavenger thioproline that neutralises reactive nitrogen species (RNS) was recently evaluated in rats with gastroduodenal reflux. Animals belonging to the control group ($n = 18$) were given normal diet and the intervention group of 13 rats was administered food with 0.5% thioproline. EAC developed in seven rats in the control group but in none in the therapeutic group. The authors suggest that iNOS overexpression and RNS as nitric oxide play an important role in the development of EAC [78]. Another agent of potentially chemopreventive properties evaluated in EAC cell lines include telomerase inhibitor [79] and leukotriene B$_4$ inhibitor bestatin that interferes with abnormal arachidonic acid metabolism [80]. Ongoing molecular studies continue to provide new putative targets for specific pharmacologic interventions such as MAPK, NFκB and PPARγ (peroxisome proliferator-activated receptor gamma) (Fig. 24.2).

ASPECT Study

The ASPECT study, a phase IIIb, randomized study of Aspirin and Esomeprazole Chemoprevention in Barrett's metaplasia, started in April 2004 in the UK. It is organized by the National Cancer Research Institute (NCRI) and funded mainly by Cancer Research UK. This is a national, multicenter, randomized, controlled 2×2 factorial trial of low- or high-dose esomeprazole with or without low-dose aspirin for 8 years. The expected number of subjects is 5000–9000. Patients receive either continuous PPI 20 mg/day or continuous PPI 80 mg/day with or without aspirin 300 mg/day (Table 24.4). It is aimed to study if intervention with aspirin can result in a decreased mortality or conversion rate from Barrett's metaplasia to adenocarcinoma or HGD and if high-dose PPI therapy can decrease the cancer risk further. Secondary objectives are identification of clinical and molecular risk factors than can be identified in Barrett's metaplasia for the development of Barrett's adenocarcinoma and the evaluation of cost-effectiveness of aspirin and/or PPI treatment in the prevention of Barrett's adenocarcinoma. The population studied are men between 40–75 years with circumferential at least 2 cm above the gastroesophageal junction (histologically proven by intestinal metaplasia be at least one sample).

Patients will be endoscoped at baseline and thereafter at 2-yearly intervals. Each time any macro-

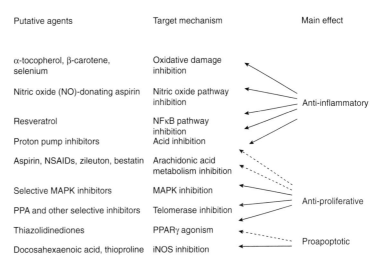

Fig. 24.2 Target mechanisms for chemoprevention in Barrett's esophagus identified in molecular studies and putative agents. iNOS, inducible nitric oxide synthase; MAPK, mitogen activated protein kinase; NFκB, nuclear transcription factor kappa B; NSAIDs, non-steroidal anti-inflammatory drugs; PPA, piperidino-propionamido-anthracenedione; PPARγ, peroxisome proliferator-activated receptor gamma.

Table 24.4 The ASPECT (ASpirin Esomeprazole Chemoprevention Trial) study design summary.

Arm A: 20 mg PPI Symptomatic treatment only = standard therapy control ARM	Arm B: 80 mg PPI Strong acid suppression ARM	No aspirin (A + B)
Arm C: 20 mg PPI Symptomatic treatment and low-dose aspirin ARM	Arm D: 80 mg PPI Strong acid suppression and low-dose aspirin ARM	Aspirin (C + D)
Low-dose PPI (A + C)	High-dose PPI (B + D)	

PPI, proton pump inhibitor.

scopic abnormality of the Barrett's metaplasia will be biopsied and systematic quadrantic biopsies taken using from the lower, middle, and upper levels of the Barrett's zone for formalin fixation and histological assessment for dysplasia. DNA and RNA will be extracted for single nucleotide polymorphism (SNP) analysis and micro-array analysis. Every 2 years blood samples will also be taken for cardiovascular risk factors and the remainder stored for analysis of circulating genetic mutations as and when reliable assays become available. Questionnaires dealing with demographics, family history, drug history, smoking, cardiac disease, alcohol, diet, and quality-of-life measures will be also assessed at 2-yearly intervals such as ASPECT now recruiting.

Conclusion

Neither the existing endoscopic strategies, including surveillance and mucosal ablation, nor antireflux surgery have proved to reduce mortality from EAC. Therefore, alternative interventions are needed and chemoprevention appears to be a promising approach that requires evaluation in a randomized, controlled fashion. There is little data to justify dietary interventions in large randomized controlled trials such as ASPECT now recruiting.

The challenging task for future studies is to better identify cohorts of Barrett's esophagus patients with the highest risk, find most precise phenotypic and genotypic surrogate endpoints and new targets of drug activity for development of new potential chemopreventive agents. Probably combinatory chemoprevention would be most promising with agents of different mechanisms of action that may have synergistic or additive effects.

References

1. Devesa SS, Blot WJ, Fraumeni JF, Jr. Changing patterns in the incidence of esophageal and gastric carcinoma in the United States. *Cancer* 1998;**83**:2049–53.
2. Jankowski J. *CRC Cancerstats: Esophageal Cancer*. London: Cancer Research Campaign Press, 2005 (updated edition).
3. Lagergren J, Bergstrom R, Lindgren A, Nyren O. Symptomatic gastroesophaeal reflux as a risk factor for esophageal adenocarcinoma. *N Engl J Med* 1999;**340**:823–31.
4. Cameron AJ, Zinsmeister AR, Ballard DJ, Carney JA. Prevalence of columnar-lined (Barrett's) esophagus. Comparison of population based clinical and autopsy findings. *Gastroenterology* 1990;**99**:918–22.
5. Gerson LB, Shetler K, Triadafilopoulos G. Prevalence of Barrett's esophagus in asymptomatic individuals. *Gastroenterology* 2002;**123**:461–7.
6. Rex DK, Cummings OW, Shaw M *et al*. Screening for Barrett's esophagus in colonoscopy patients with and without heartburn. *Gastroenterology* 2003;**125**:1670–7.
7. Chak A, Lee T, Kinnard MF *et al*. Caucasian adults oesophagogastric junctional adenocarcinoma in oesophageal adenocarcinoma and familial aggregation of Barrett's esophagus. *Gut* 2002;**51**:323–8.
8. Weston AP, Sharma P, Mathur S *et al*. Risk stratification of Barrett's esophagus: updated prospective multivariate analysis. *Am J Gastroenterol* 2004;**99**:1557–66.
9. Corley DA, Kerlikowske K, Verma R, Buffler P. Protective association of aspirin/NSAIDs and esophageal cancer: a systematic review and meta-analysis. *Gastroenterology* 2003;**124**:47–56.
10. Hillman LC, Chiragakis L, Shadbolt B, Kaye GL, Clarke AC. Proton-pump inhibitor therapy and the development dysplasia in patients with Barrett's esophagus. *Med J Aus* 2004;**180**(8):387–91.
11. El-Serag HB, Aguirre TV, Davis S *et al*. Proton pump inhibitors are associated with reduced incidence of

dysplasia in Barrett's esophagus. *Am J Gastroenterol* 2004;**99**:1877–83.

12. Drovdlic CM, Goddard KAB, Chak A *et al*. Demographic and phenotypic features of 70 families segregating Barrett's oesophagus and oesophageal adenocarcinoma. *J Med Genet* 2003;**40**:651–6.

13. Chak A, Faulx A, Kinnard M *et al*. Identification of Barrett's esophagus in relatives by endoscopic screening. *Am J Gastroenterol* 2004;**99**(11):2107–14.

14. Shaheen NJ, Crosby MA, Bozymski EM, Sandler RS. Is there publication bias in the reporting of cancer risk in Barrett's esophagus? *Gastroenterology* 2000;**119**:333–8.

15. Jankowski J, Provenzale D, Moayyedi P. Esophageal adenocarcinoma arising from Barrett's metaplasia has regional variations in the West. *Gastroenterology* 2002;**122**:588–9.

16. Murray L, Watson P, Johnston B *et al*. Risk of adenocarcinoma in Barrett's esophagus: population based study. *BMJ* 2003;**327**(7414):534–5.

17. Solaymani-Dodaran M, Logan RF, West J, Card T, Coupland C. Risk of esophageal cancer in Barrett's esophagus and gastro-esophageal reflux. *Gut* 2004; **53**(8):1070–4.

18. Reid BJ, Blount PL, Rabinowitch PS. Biomarkers in Barrett's esophagus. *Gastrointest Endosc Clin N Am* 2003;**13**:369–97.

19. Reid BJ, Levine DS, Longton G, Blount PL, Rabinovitch PS. Predictors of progression to cancer in Barrett's esophagus: baseline histology and flow cytometry identify low- and high-risk patient subsets. *Am J Gastroenterol* 2000;**95**:1669–76.

20. Rabinowitch PS, Longton G, Blount PL, Levine DS, Reid BJ. Predictors of progression in Barrett's esophagus III: baseline flow cytometric variables. *Am J Gastroenterol* 2001;**96**:3071–83.

21. Mayne ST, Risch HA, Dubrow R *et al*. Nutrient intake and risk of subtypes of esophageal and gastric cancer. *Cancer Epidemiol Biomarkers Prev* 2001;**10**(10):1055–62.

22. Terry P, Lagergren J, Ye W, Nyren O, Wolk A. Antioxidants and cancers of the esophagus and gastric cardia. *Int J Cancer* 2000;**87**(5):750–4.

23. Chen H, Ward MH, Graubard BI *et al*. Dietary patters and adenocarcinoma of the esophagus and distal stomach. *Am J Clin Nutr* 2002;**75**:137–44.

24. Rudolph RE, Vaughan TL, Kristal AR *et al*. Serum selenium levels in relation to markers of neoplastic progression among persons with Barrett's esophagus. *J Natl Cancer Inst* 2003;**95**(10):750–7.

25. Gammon MD, Schoenberg JB, Ahsan H *et al*. Tobacco, alcohol, and socioeconomic status and adeno-carcinoma of the esophagus and gastric cardia. *J Natl Cancer Inst* 1999;**89**(17):1247–9.

26. Vaughan TL, Davis S, Kristal A, Thomas DB. Obesity, alcohol, and tobacco as risk factors for cancers of the esophagus and gastric cardia: adenocarcinoma versus squamous cell carcinoma. *Cancer Epidemiol Biomarks Prev* 1995;**4**:85–92.

27. Zeka A, Gore R, Kriebel D. Effects of alcohol and tobacco on aerodigestive cancer risks: a metaregression analysis. *Cancer Causes Control* 2003;**14**(9): 897–906.

28. Chow WH, Blaser MJ, Blot WJ *et al*. An inverse relation between *cag*A$^+$ strains of *Helicobacter pylori* infection and risk of esophageal and gastric cardia adenocarcinoma. *Cancer Res* 1998;**58**:588–90.

29. Farrow DC, Vaughan TL, Sweeney C *et al*. Gastroesophageal reflux disease, use of H2 receptor antagonists, and risk of esophageal and gastric cancer. *Cancer Causes Control* 2000;**11**(3):231–8.

30. Suleiman UL, Harrison M, Britton A, McPherson K, Bates T. H2-receptor antagonists may increase the risk of cardio-esophageal adenocarcinoma: a case-control study. *Eur J Cancer Prev* 2000;**9**(3):185–91.

31. Sharma P, McQuaid K, Dent J *et al*. A critical review of the diagnosis and management of Barrett's esophagus: the AGA Chicago workshop. *Gastroenterology* 2004; **127**:310–30.

32. Ye W, Chow WH, Lagergren J, Yin L, Nyren O. Risk of adenocarcinomas in the esophagus and gastric cardia in patients with gastroesophageal reflux disease and after antireflux surgery. *Gastroenterology* 2001;**121**: 1286–93.

33. Corey KE, Schmitz SM, Shaheen NJ. Does a surgical anti-reflux procedure decrease the incidence of esophageal adenocarcinoma in Barrett's esophagus? A meta-analysis. *Am J Gastroenterol* 2003;**98**:2390–4.

34. Corley DA, Levin TR, Habel LA. Surveillance and survival in Barrett's adenocarcinomas: a population-based study. *Gastroenterology* 2002;**122**:633–40.

35. Provenzale D, Schmitt C, Wong JB. Barrett's esophagus: a new look at surveillance based on emerging estimates of cancer risk. *Am J Gastroenterol* 1999;**94**: 2043–53.

36. Soni A, Sampliner RE, Sonnenberg A. Screening for high-grade dysplasia in gastro-oesophageal reflux disease: is it cost-effective? *Am J Gastroenterol* 2000; **95**:2086–93.

37. Inadomi JM, Sampliner R, Lagergren J *et al*. Screening and surveillance for Barrett's esophagus in high-risk groups: a cost-utility analysis. *Ann Intern Med* 2003; **138**:176–86.

38. Van Laethem JL, Peny MO, Salmon I, Cremer M, Deviere J. Intramucosal adenocarcinoma arising under squamous re-epithalisation of Barrett's esophagus. *Gut* 2000;**46**:574–7.

39. Sporn MB. Approaches to prevention of epithelial cancer during the preneoplastic period. *Cancer Res* 1976;**36**:2699–702.

40. Tsao AE, Kim SK, Hong WK. Chemoprevention of cancer. *CA Cancer J Clin* 2004;**54**:150–80.

41. Kelloff GJ, Sigman CC, Johnson KM *et al*. Perspectives on surrogate end points in the development of drugs that reduce the risk of cancer. *Cancer Epidemiol Biomarks Prev* 2000;**9**:127–37.

42. O'Shauhgnessy JA, Kellof GJ, Gordon GB *et al*. Treatment and prevention of intraepithelial neoplasia: an important target for accelerated new agent development. *Clin Cancer Res* 2002;**8**:3114–346.

43. Simon R, Maitournam A. Evaluating the efficiency of targeted designs for randomised clinical trials. *Clin Cancer Res* 2004;**10**:6759–63.

44. Unger JM, LeBlanc M, Crowley JJ *et al*. Estimating the impact of new clinical trial proven cancer therapy and cancer chemoprevention on population mortality: the Karnofsky memorial lecture. *J Clin Oncol* 2003;**21**:246–52.

45. Thompson IM, Goodman PJ, Tangen CM *et al*. The influence of finasteride on the development of prostate cancer. *N Eng J Med* 2003;**349**:215–24.

46. Provenzale D. The cost-effectiveness of aspirin for chemoprevention of colorectal cancer. *Gastroenterology* 2002;**122**:230–3.

47. Dunn BK, Ford LG. Breast cancer prevention: results of the national surgical adjuvant breast and bowel project (NSABP) breast cancer prevention trial (NSABP P-1: BCPT). *Eur J Cancer* 2000;**36**(suppl 4):S49–50.

48. Gerson LB, Boopari V, Ullah N, Triadafilopoulos G. Esophageal and gastric pH in patients with gastro-oesophageal reflux disease and Barrett's esophagus treated with proton pump inhibitors [abstract]. *Gastroenterology* 2004;**126**(suppl 2):A57.

49. Shirvani VN, Ouatu-Lascar R, Kaur BS, Omary MB, Triadafilopoulos G. Cyclooxygenase-2 expression in Barrett's esophagus and adenocarcinoma: *ex vivo* induction by bile salts and acid exposure. *Gastroenterology* 2000;**118**:487–96.

50. Souza RF, Shewmake K, Terada LS, Spechler SJ. Acid exposure activates the mitogen-activated protein kinase pathways in Barrett's esophagus. *Gastroenterology* 2002;**122**:299–307.

51. Avidan B, Sonnenberg A, Schnell TG, Sontag SJ. Gastric surgery is not a risk for Barrett's esophagus or

esophageal adenocarcinoma. *Gastroenterology* 2001; **1221**:1502–6.

52. Tselepis C, Morris CD, Wakelin D *et al*. Upregulation of the oncogene c-*myc* in Barrett's adenocarcinoma: induction of c-*myc* by acidified bile acid *in vitro*. *Gut* 2003;**52**(2):174–80.

53. Jankowski J, Harrison RF, Perry I, Balkwill F, Tselepis C. Seminar: Barrett's metaplasia. *Lancet* 2000;**356**:2079–85.

54. Jankowski JA, Wright NA, Meltzer SJ *et al*. Molecular evolution of the metaplasia–dysplasia–adenocarcinoma sequence in the esophagus. *Am J Pathol* 1999; **154**:965–73

55. Jenkins GJ, Harries K, Doak SH *et al*. The bile acid deoxycholic acid (DCA) at neutral pH activates NF-κB and induces IL-8 expression in esophageal cells *in vitro*. *Carcinogenesis* 2004;**25**(3):317–23.

56. Konturek PC, Nikiforuk A, Kania J *et al*. Activation of NFκB represents the central event in the neoplastic progression associated with Barrett's esophagus: a possible link to the inflammation and overexpression of COX-2, PPARγ and growth factors. *Dig Dis Sci* 2004;**49**(7–8):1075–83.

57. Thun MJ, Henely SJ, Patrono C. Non-steroidal anti-inflammatory drugs as anticancer agents: mechanistic, pharmacologic and clinical issues. *J Natl Cancer Inst* 2002;**94**:252–66.

58. Yu HG, Huang JA, Yang YN *et al*. The effects of acetylsalicylic acid on proliferation, apoptosis, and invasion of cyclooxygenase-2 negative colon cancer cells. *Eur J Clin Invest* 2002;**32**(11):838–46.

59. Baron JA, Cole BF, Sandler RS *et al*. A randomized trial of aspirin to prevent colorectal adenomas. *N Eng J Med* 2003;**348**(10):891–9.

60. Seery JP, Syrigos KN, Karayiannakis AJ, Valizadeh A, Pignatelli M. Abnormal expression of the E-cadherin–catenin complex in dysplastic Barrett's esophagus. *Acta Oncol* 1999;**38**(7):945–8.

61. Wilson KT, Fu S, Ramanujam KS, Meltzer SJ. Increased expression of inducible nitric oxide synthase and cyclooxygenase-2 in Barrett's esophagus and associated carcinomas. *Cancer Res* 1998;**58**: 2929–34.

62. Morris CD, Armstrong GR, Bigley G, Green H, Attwood SE. Cyclooxygenase-2 expression in the Barrett's metaplasia–dysplasia–adenocarcinoma sequence. *Am J Gastroenterol* 2001;**96**(4):990–6.

63. Buskens CJ, van Rees BP, Sivula A *et al*. Prognostic significance of elevated cyclooxygenase expression in patients with adenocarcinoma of the esophagus. *Gastroenterology* 2002;**122**(7):1808–7.

64. Bardou M, Barkun AN, Ghosn J, Hudson M, Rahme E. Effect of chronic intake of NSAIDs and cyclooxygenase 2-selective inhibitors on esophageal cancer incidence. *Clin Gastroenterol Hepatol* 2004;**2**(10): 880–7.

65. Kaur BS, Khamnehei N, Iravani M *et al*. Rofecoxib inhibits cyclooxygenase 2 expression and activity and reduces cell proliferation in Barrett's esophagus. *Gastroenterology* 2002;**123**(1):60–7.

66. Heath EI, Canto MI, Wu TT *et al*. Chemoprevention for Barrett's esophagus trial. Design and outcome measures. *Dis Esophagus* 2003;**16**(3):177–86.

67. Collaborative Group of the Primary Prevention Project (PPP). Low-dose aspirin and vitamin E in people at cardiovascular risk: a randomised trial in general practice. *Lancet* 2001;**357**:89–95.

68. Hur C, Nishioka NS, Gazelle GS. Cost-effectiveness of aspirin chemoprevention for Barrett's esophagus. *J Natl Cancer Inst* 2004;**96**(4):316–25.

69. Ouatu-Lascar R, Fitzgerald RC, Triadafilopoulos G. Differentiation and proliferation in Barrett's esophagus and the effects of acid suppression. *Gastroenterology* 1999;**117**:325–7.

70. Sharma P, Sampliner RE, Camargo E. Normalization of esophageal pH with high dose proton pump inhibitor therapy does not result in regression of Barrett's esophagus. *Am J Gastroenterol* 1997;**92**:582–5.

71. Peters FT, Ganesh S, Kuipers EJ *et al*. Endoscopic regression of Barrett's esophagus during omeprazole treatment; a randomized double blind study. *Gut* 1999;**45**:489–94.

72. Carlson N, Lechago J, Richter J *et al*. Acid suppression therapy may not alter malignant progression in Barrett's metaplasia showing p53 protein accumulation. *Am J Gastroenterol* 2002;**97**:1340–5.

73. Haigh CR, Attwood SE, Thompson DG *et al*. Gastrin induces proliferation in Barrett's metaplasia through activation of the CCK2 receptor. *Gastroenterology* 2003;**124**:615–25.

74. Abdalla SI, Lao-Sirieix P, Novelli MR *et al*. Gastrin-induced cyclooxygenase-2 expression in Barrett's carcinogenesis. *Clin Can Res* 2004;**10**:4784–92.

75. Harris JC, Clarke PA, Awan A, Jankowski J, Watson S. An antiapoptotic role for gastrin and the gastrin/CCK-2 receptor in Barrett's esophagus. *Can Res* 2004;**64**: 1915–9.

76. Jankowski J, Anderson M. Review article: management of esophageal adenocarcinoma—control of acid, bile and inflammation in intervention strategies for Barrett's esophagus. *Aliment Pharmacol Ther* 2004; **20**(suppl 5):71–80.

77. Wang GQ, Dawsey SM, Li JY *et al*. Effects of vitamin/mineral supplementation on the prevalence of histological dysplasia and early cancer of the esophagus and stomach: results from the general population trial in Linxian, China. *Cancer Epidemiol Biomarkers Prev* 1994;**3**(2):161–6.

78. Kumagai H, Mukaisho K, Sugihara H *et al*. Thioproline inhibits development of esophageal adenocarcinoma induced by gastroduodenal reflux in rats. *Carcinogenesis* 2004;**25**(5):723–7.

79. Shammas MA, Koley H, Beer DG *et al*. Growth arrest, apoptosis, and telomere shortening of Barrett's-associated adenocarcinoma cells by a telomerase inhibitor. *Gastroenterology* 2004;**126**(5):1337–46.

80. Chen X, Li N, Wang S *et al*. Aberrant arachidonic acid metabolism in esophageal adenocarcinogenesis, and the effects of sulindac, nordihydroguaiaretic acid, and α-difluoromethylornithine on tumorigenesis in a rat surgical model. *Carcinogenesis* 2002;**23**(12):2095–102.

81. Dihlmann S, Siermann A, von Knebel Doeberitz M. The non-steroidal anti-inflammatory drugs aspirin and inomethacin attenuate β catenin/TCF-4 signalling. *Oncogene* 2001;**20**:645–53.

82. Shao J, Fujiwara T, Kadowaki Y *et al*. Overexpression of the wild-type *p53* gene inhibits NF-κB activity and synergizes with aspirin to induce apoptosis in human colon cancer cells. *Oncogene* 2000;**19**(6):726–36.

83. Ho CC, Yang XW, Lee TL *et al*. Activation of *p53* signalling in acetylsalicylic acid-induced apoptosis in OC2 human oral cancer cells. *Eur J Clin Invest* 2003;**33**(10):875–82.

84. Sheng H, Shao J, Morrow JD, Beauchamp RD, DuBois RN. Modulation of apoptosis and *Bcl-2* expression by prostaglandin E$_2$ in human colon cancer cells. *Cancer Res* 1998;**58**(2):362–6.

85. Kopp E, Ghosh S. Inhibition of NF-κB by sodium salicylate and aspirin. *Science* 1994;**265**(5174):956–9.

86. Stark LA, Din FV, Zwacka RM, Dunlop MG. Aspirin-induced activation of the NF-κB signaling pathway: a novel mechanism for aspirin-mediated apoptosis in colon cancer cells. *FASEB J* 2001;**15**:1273–5.

87. Schwenger P, Alpert D, Skolnik EY, Vilcek J. Activation of *p38* mitogen-activated protein kinase by sodium salicylate leads to inhibition of tumor necrosis factor-induced IκB phosphorylation and degradation. *Mol Cell Biol* 1998;**18**(1):78–84.

88. Goel A, Chang DK, Ricciardiello L, Gasche C, Boland CR. A novel mechanism for aspirin-mediated growth inhibition of human colon cancer cells. *Clin Cancer Res* 2003;**9**:383–90.

89. Dihlmann S, Klein S, Doeberitz Mv MK. Reduction of β-catenin/T-cell transcription factor signaling by aspirin and indomethacin is caused by an increased stabilization of phosphorylated β-catenin. *Mol Cancer Ther* 2003;**2**(6):509–16.

90. Nath N, Kashfi K, Chen J, Rigas B. Nitric oxide-donating aspirin inhibits β-catenin/T cell factor (TCF) signaling in SW480 colon cancer cells by disrupting the nuclear β-catenin–TCF association. *Proc Natl Acad Sci U S A* 2003;**100**(22):12 584–9.

91. Lee EJ, Park HG, Kang HS. Sodium salicylate induces apoptosis in HCT116 colorectal cancer cells through activation of p38^{MAPK}. *Int J Oncol* 2003;**23**(2):503–8.

92. Buttar NS, Wang KK, Leontovich O *et al.* Chemoprevention of esophageal adenocarcinoma by COX-2 inhibitors in an animal model of Barrett's esophagus. *Gastroenterology* 2002;**122**(4):1101–12.

CHAPTER 25

Management of High-Grade Intraepithelial Neoplasia in Barrett's Esophagus

Jacques J. G. H. M. Bergman and Paul Fockens

Introduction

Barrett's esophagus is a condition in which the normal squamous lining of the distal esophagus has been replaced by columnar epithelium with intestinal metaplasia. Barrett's esophagus is considered to be a premalignant condition that predisposes to esophageal adenocarcinoma [1]. Malignant degeneration of Barrett's esophagus is thought to be a multistep process in which intestinal metaplasia progresses through low-grade and high-grade dysplasia into intramucosal and invasive carcinoma [2,3]. Endoscopic surveillance with random biopsies is currently the monitoring technique of choice in patients with Barrett's esophagus. Endoscopic surveillance aims at identifying patients with early and curable malignancy [4]. Whereas most centers recommend treatment in patients with histologically manifest early cancer, there is much controversy regarding the management of high-grade intraepithelial neoplasia (HGIN). In these patients, management alternatives include endoscopic follow-up, application of endoscopic treatment modalities such as endoscopic mucosal resection (EMR) and/or photodynamic therapy (PDT), or surgical resection [5–7]. In this chapter we will discuss the management options in HGIN. Up-to-date reviews on the different management alternatives are given in separate chapters in this book; therefore, we will discuss the different approaches from a patient's care perspective without describing the underlying studies in too much detail.

Since the diagnosis of HGIN in Barrett's esophagus is not a straightforward task, we will first discuss the controversies regarding making the *histological* diagnosis, followed by discussing the importance of endoscopic imaging for making the *clinical* diagnosis of HGIN. We will then discuss the pros and cons of the different management options and give practical advice concerning their optimal use.

Histological Diagnosis of HGIN

Histological Diagnosis of Dysplasia: "East versus West"

Histopathological diagnosis is of paramount importance for clinical decision making in the evaluation of patients with Barrett's esophagus. The presence and the degree of dysplasia determine whether treatment or follow-up will be advised. The histological diagnosis by itself is not without controversies. Classically, there have been major differences between the Western and Eastern histological classification of gastrointestinal epithelial neoplasia, including those of the esophagus [8]. For Eastern pathologists the focus lies more on cellular and nuclear characteristics, whereas their Western colleagues pay more attention to the coherence of the histological architecture. Lesions, which would be high-grade dysplasia according to the conventional European classification, will often be diagnosed as carcinoma by Japanese pathologists. Schlemper *et al.* have reviewed these differences together with the results of international consensus meetings in Padova and

Diagnosis	Clinical management
1 Negative for neoplasia	Optional follow-up
2 Indefinite for neoplasia	Follow-up
3 Non-invasive low-grade neoplasia	Endoscopic resection or follow-up
4 Non-invasive high-grade neoplasia	
4.1 High-grade dysplasia	
4.2 Non-invasive carcinoma (CIS)	
4.3 Suspicious for invasive carcinoma	
5 Invasive carcinoma	
5.1 Intramucosal carcinoma	Endoscopic or surgical resection
5.2 Submucosal carcinoma and beyond	Surgical resection

Table 25.1 Histological categories with corresponding clinical management in the revised Vienna classification for gastrointestinal (GI) epithelial neoplasias.

CIS, carcinoma *in situ*.

Vienna, where attempts were made to reach a common worldwide classification system and terminology for gastrointestinal epithelial neoplasia [8]. The so-called "revised Vienna classification" led to the highest agreement and lowest interobserver variability. This classification not only reduces inter and intraobserver variability but also produces categories that are clinically meaningful and useful in terms of natural history and clinical management [9] (Table 25.1). It is important to note that in the aforementioned consensus meetings mainly squamous lesions were used and that few Barrett's lesions were included.

In the year 2000, the World Health Organization (WHO) classification recommended not to use the term "dysplasia" anymore since this term carries different meanings in different countries [10]. In the revised Vienna classification the term dysplasia is therefore not used and, according to the WHO advice, the term "high-grade intraepithelial neoplasia" (HGIN) replaces the diagnoses high-grade dysplasia and carcinoma *in situ*.

Histological Diagnosis of HGIN: Questions Concerning the Interpretation of the Histological Findings

One of the limitations of surveillance of Barrett's esophagus is the interobserver variation in the histological diagnosis of biopsies. Studies have shown that this is most pronounced for the categories indefinite for dysplasia and low-grade intraepithelial neoplasia

(LGIN) and less for HGIN [11]. When faced with the histological diagnosis of HGIN in biopsies obtained at a surveillance endoscopy, the clinician should ask him or herself (and the pathologist!) the following questions concerning the interpretation of the histological findings:

1 How extensive are the histological abnormalities? Is their presence restricted to just a limited number of crypts in a single biopsy; i.e. "focal HGIN," [12] or can they be shown in multiple biospies obtained at different levels in the Barrett's segment? Extensive HGIN at multiple levels may be more relevant than focal HGIN from a prognostic standpoint but may also increase the credibility of the histological findings.

2 What was the worst prior histological diagnosis in this patient? If the patient has been diagnosed with LGIN at earlier surveillance endoscopies, a diagnosis of HGIN may be a less surprising finding than when the patient has had multiple endoscopies showing no evidence of dysplasia [13].

3 Were the neoplastic abnormalities accompanied with extensive inflammatory changes or did they occur against the "normal" background of mild chronic inflammation? This holds especially for biopsies obtained at the squamocolumnar junction where reactive inflammatory changes are most prominent. For dubious cases additional immunohistochemical (IHC) staining may be useful. For instance, the presence of positive Ki67-staining (marking the proliferation in the epithelium) in the upper part of the villi is suggestive of neoplastic changes whereas in reactive changes the proliferative compartment remains restricted to the crypts. In addition, the presence of positive p53 staining may be considered an extra argument for the neoplastic character of the abnormalities [14]. These tests should be performed at experienced centers.

4 How experienced is the pathologist in diagnosing early neoplasia in Barrett's esophagus? Most pathologists will not encounter HGIN at a regular basis and one may speculate that their interpretation may be less reliable than those coming from units with a high-case volume where biopsies are discussed in multidisciplinary meetings. Montgomery *et al.* found only a moderate and fair interobserver reproducibility for HGIN and LGIN, respectively, when a group of 12 pathologists independently reviewed a set of 125 slides with Barrett's pathology [11]. The corresponding kappa values were 0.40 and 0.23 for HGIN and LGIN, respectively. Skacel *et al.* found a higher risk of progression to HGIN or adenocarcinoma when there was a consensus between at least two pathologists on the diagnosis of LGIN [13] and one may speculate that the same will hold for diagnosing HGIN. We therefore recommend review of biopsies by a gastrointestinal pathologist with experience in this field before deciding on the management of patients with HGIN [15].

Clinical Diagnosis of HGIN

Quality of the Endoscopic Work-Up

In addition to the uncertainty and the controversies in the *histological diagnosis* of HGIN in Barrett's esophagus, the quality of the endoscopic procedure during which biopsies were taken also plays a substantial part in the accuracy of the diagnosis. Important aspects include the endoscopic appearance of the Barrett's segment, the experience of the endoscopist, the quality and type of endoscopic equipment, and the biopsy protocol employed.

When faced with a histological diagnosis of HGIN in biopsies obtained from a Barrett's esophagus, the clinician should ask the following questions concerning the quality of the endoscopic work-up:

1 Were the biopsies with HGIN obtained from visible abnormalities (i.e. targeted biopsies) or were no suspicious lesions seen? The relevance of this is best illustrated by an example: Plate 25.1a–d (color plate section falls between pp. 148–9) shows an endoscopic image of a Barrett's carcinoma. This patient was referred for endosonographic staging of this lesion. At the referring hospital, a diagnosis of HGIN was made after three biopsies were obtained from the lesion for histological analysis. The patient underwent esophagectomy and the surgical specimen showed a moderately differentiated adenocarcinoma with invasion of the muscularis propria, and three of 14 positive lymph nodes. Although this patient had a preoperative *histological* diagnosis of HGIN, he was operated under the *clinical* diagnosis of esophageal cancer based on the endoscopic aspect of his Barrett's segment. The combination of the histological diagnosis of HGIN and the presence of visible abnormalities at endoscopy strengthens the likelihood that the patient has a true neoplastic lesion and should make the clinician aware that the histological diagnosis of HGIN may in fact underestimate the correct diagnosis.

2 Were there signs of active reflux esophagitis or inflammatory changes within the Barrett's segment (Plate 25.2a,b; color plate section falls between pp. 148–9)? Under these circumstances the clinician should be aware that the histological diagnosis of HGIN may be an overestimation of the patient's true condition, since microscopically, inflammatory, and reactive changes may resemble neoplastic transformation. Most guidelines, therefore, advise against biopsies in the presence of reflux esophagitis and to repeat the endoscopy after the patient has been treated with acid suppressive therapy for 6–8 weeks [1]. Such a policy may be too conservative in patients who endoscopically only show minor reflux changes (e.g. grade A or B reflux esophagitis according to the Los Angeles (LA) classification) but stresses the importance of correlating the diagnosis of intraepithelial neo-plasia with endoscopic and/or histological signs of inflammation.

3 In the absence of visible abnormalities at endoscopy: Who performed the procedure and with what equipment? Is it possible that a more advanced lesion was overlooked? HGIN and early cancer in Barrett's esophagus may be difficult to detect during

routine endoscopy. Most endoscopists will not encounter these lesions on a regular basis and their detection rate may be less than that of endoscopists
working at high-volume centers. Apart from the experience of the endoscopist, the endoscopic equipment is also important in this respect. Fiber-optic
endoscopes provide inferior quality images of the
Barrett's mucosa and should not be used in the work-
up of patients with HGIN (Plate 25.3a,b; color plate
section falls between pp. 148–9). High-resolution
endoscopes with high-quality CCD-chips (>850 000
pixels) and a variable focal distance are now
commercially available. These devices allow endoscopists to magnify parts of the mucosa optically, i.e.
by means of an adjustable focal distance. The image
quality of these endoscopes is clearly superior to that
of standard video- and fiber-optic endoscopes (see
Plate 25.3a,b; color plate section falls between pp.
148–9). Recent studies have shown that the vast majority of early neoplastic lesions in Barrett's esophagus can be detected with high-resolution endoscopy
only, and this technique should be considered the
imaging technique of choice in the surveillance of
Barrett's patients [16,17].

4 Was the Barrett's segment carefully inspected, and
were random biopsies obtained? Many early neoplastic lesions in Barrett's esophagus occur at the distal end of the Barrett's segment, where they can be
easily overlooked if inspection is performed with the
endoscope only in the antegrade position. Adequate
imaging of a Barrett's esophagus, therefore, also
requires an inspection in the retroflexed position
(Plate 25.4; color plate section falls between pp.
148–9). The endoscopist should carefully withdraw
the retroflexed instrument into the hiatal hernia and
inspect the distal portion of the Barrett's segment
while inflating air.

The current ACG guidelines recommend that in
the absence of visible abnormalities four-quadrant
random biopsies be obtained every 2 cm of the Barrett's segment, starting at the upper end of the gastric
folds [18]. Studies, however, suggest that in daily
practice a lower number of biopsies are obtained, resulting in sampling error and thus underestimation
of the patient's true condition. Furthermore, data
from Reid *et al.* indicate that the four-quadrant 2 cm
biopsy protocol may not be sensitive enough to de-

tect invasive cancer in patients with HGIN: the detection of invasive cancer was increased by 50% when
random biopsies were obtained every centimeter of
Barrett's mucosa [19].

HGIN: a Clinical Diagnosis

In our opinion, for the *clinical* diagnosis HGIN, the
following should be considered: (i) a prior histological diagnosis of HGIN; (ii) review of biopsies by
an independent expert pathologist; (iii) repeat
endoscopic imaging in a specialized center; (iv) using
a 1-cm four-quadrant biopsy protocol for sampling;
and (v) absence of endoscopic lesions suspicious for
malignancy.

The importance of a strict definition of the clinical
diagnosis HGIN is best illustrated by discussing the
risk of synchronous cancers in patients with HGIN.

Risk of Synchronous Cancers in HGIN

In the literature there are many series that describe
the existence of cancer in Barrett's segments resected
with the preoperative histological diagnosis of HGIN
[20–40]. In a meta-analysis by Collard *et al.* the percentage of "missed carcinomas" in these studies
varied between 11% and 73% [41]. These striking
figures raise the important question: how adequate
was the preoperative work-up in these patients? Was
the preoperative histological and endoscopic work-
up adequately performed to support the presump-
tive *clinical* diagnosis of HGIN? One may argue that, if
the histological HGIN by itself is considered sufficient
to justify surgical resection (as it was in most centers
in the recent past) it is irrelevant to diagnose a carcinoma preoperatively, since this would not alter the
indication for esophagectomy (see Plate 25.1a–d;
color plate section falls between pp. 148–9). However, some investigators use the rate of carcinomas
found in specimens resected for "HGIN" as an argument to recommend surgical resection in all patients
with HGIN and to discourage endoscopic follow-up
and/or treatment [41]. The data from these studies
should be carefully interpreted when deciding on
the current management of patients with HGIN. We
have evaluated the preoperative work-up in 21 studies published in the English literature that reported
variable percentages of adenocarcinoma in patients
who underwent esophagectomy under the pre-

sumptive diagnosis of HGIN in Barrett's esophagus [20]. Most studies were performed in an era when mainly fiber-optic endoscopes were used and no study used repeat endoscopy, high-resolution endoscopy, chromoendoscopy, EMR, or other advanced imaging techniques for diagnosis. Some studies had described endoscopic abnormalities, but in spite of that the endoscopy was not repeated before proceeding to surgery, and it was not reported whether the presence of endoscopic abnormalities were associated with carcinoma in the resected specimen. Moreover, many studies did not describe the biopsy protocol, which makes it difficult to estimate the chance of their results being affected by sampling error. Finally, in several studies there was no review of the histological diagnosis by an expert gastrointestinal pathologist, which is essential for making the diagnosis HGIN. This means that for virtually none of these studies, the aforementioned requirements for the *clinical* diagnosis of HGIN were met.

Management of HGIN

Endoscopic Surveillance

Few studies have reported the results of endoscopic follow-up for HGIN in Barrett's esophagus. The aim of endoscopic follow-up is careful continued surveillance of patients with HGIN; esophageal resection being reserved only for patients who progress to invasive cancer. Table 25.2 shows a summary of these studies [5,12,18,42]. Weston *et al.* surveyed patients with unifocal HGIN (defined as HGIN found in a single Barrett's mucosal segment or biopsy specimen) [42]. Four out of 15 patients (27%) progressed to adenocarcinoma during a follow-up duration of 17–35 months. Reid *et al.* reported that a 4-quadrant 1-cm interval biopsy protocol was superior to the widely used 2-cm interval protocol [19]. During a mean follow-up of 23 months in 110 patients with HGIN they diagnosed 32 cases of cancer (29%). They calculated that a 2 cm protocol would have missed 50% of these cancers. Buttar *et al.* investigated the correlation between the extent of HGIN and progression to adenocarcinoma [12]. Four of 24 patients (17%) with focal HGIN (defined as HGIN in <5 crypts in a single biopsy) developed cancer during follow-up (median duration 36.6 months). In the same study, 28 of 42 patients (67%) with diffuse HGIN (defined as HGIN in >5 crypts or in more than one biopsy specimen) developed cancer during follow-up (median duration 19.5 months). They concluded that diffuse HGIN carried a higher risk of progression to adenocarcinoma than focal HGIN. The relatively high rates of cancer occurrence in these series was contrasted by a study of Schnell *et al.* who concluded that endoscopic surveillance was a safe follow-up strategy in patients with HGIN [5]. In their study, during a median follow-up period of 7.3 years, cancer was detected in only 12 of 75 patients (16%). Most of the cancers were in an early and curable stage.

The follow-up studies failed to report a uniform long-term outcome of surveillance endoscopy for HGIN in Barrett's esophagus. Each study had a different objective and design, which makes it difficult to compare the results of these studies. In some reports, there were a significant number of patients in whom no further HGIN was seen during follow-up [5,42]. Although some authors attribute this to an apparent regression of HGIN to a lesser degree of dysplasia [5], this raises the question whether the original diagnosis of HGIN was correct, and whether the apparent regression of HGIN during follow-up was not "pseudoregression" due to an initial over-diagnosis of HGIN. For example, in the study by Schnell *et al.* all patients with HGIN were diagnosed by a single study pathologist, and there was no review of histology by an independent pathologist. In this study, the surveillance population consisted of 1099 patients with Barrett's esophagus and the diagnosis LGIN was made at least on one occasion in 67% of these patients [5]. This percentage is considerably higher than the 3.5–12.0% reported in other surveillance populations [2,43]. This may suggest that there was a low threshold for classifying patients as having LGIN, and consequently for HGIN since their percentage HGIN (7%) was also considerably higher than reported in previous studies (0–2%) [2,43]. This raises the possibility that HGIN may have been over-diagnosed in this study. This is also illustrated by the high rate of (pseudo) regression in this study: only 32% of patients with an initial diagnosis of HGIN were detected with HGIN during follow-up endoscopies [5].

Table 25.2 Summary of studies that investigated endoscopic follow-up of high-grade intraepithelial neoplasia (HGIN) in Barrett's esophagus.

Author and year of publication	No. of patients with HGIN	No. of cancers detected	No. detected during first year	Follow-up duration	Follow-up interval	Independent review of histology?	Biopsy protocol	Endoscopic findings and no. of patients	Cancer stage or no. of cured cancers
Weston et al. [42] 2000	15	4	0	17–35 months	3–6 months	Yes	Lesions + 4 Q, 1 cm interval	1 had esophigitis grade 2, 1 had a Barrett's ulcer	2 intramucosal, 1 submucosal, 1 T2 Nx tumor
Reid et al. [19] 2000	110	32	12	Mean 22.8 months	1st follow-up 1–3 months, 2nd 3–6 months, every 6 months afterwards	N/R	Lesions + 4 Q, 1 cm interval	15 cancers diagnosed from targeted biopsies	96% intramucosal, 2 submucosal, 1 regional metastasis
Schnell et al. [5] 2001	75	12	None due to the "1-year hunting for cancer" (4 detected, not included)	7.3 years	Year 1 quarterly, year 2 every 6 months, then every 12 months	Single pathologist	Lesions + 4 Q, 2 cm interval	7/12 had flat mucosa, 5 had either nodules, elevations or mass	11/12 cured, the 12th patient was non-compliant
Buttar et al. [12] 2001 Focal HGIN	24	4	2	Mean 41 months	3 months	2 experienced blinded GI pathologists	4 Q, 1 cm interval	2 patients had nodularity	N/R for all patients, 1 patient had celiac metastasis
Buttar et al. [12] 2001 Diffuse HGIN	42	28	17	Mean 23 months	3 months	2 experienced blinded GI pathologists	4 Q, 1 cm interval	5 patients had nodularity	N/R

GI, gastrointestinal; N/R, not reported; 4 Q, four quadrants.

Apart from the "HGIN-over-diagnosis dilemma" in the follow-up studies, another important question is whether the HGIN-patients in these studies had a synchronous cancer, which was not diagnosed at the index endoscopy; the "cancer-under-diagnosis dilemma". These missed synchronous cancers will be reported as metachronous when they are discovered during follow-up. In the study by Reid *et al.* 62% of all cancers were detected within the first three surveillance endoscopies [19]. Table 25.2 shows that most studies have diagnosed a significant number of cancers during the first year of follow-up. To eliminate the "cancer-under-diagnosis dilemma" Schnell *et al.* included patients in their surveillance program only after a 1-year "hunt-for-cancer strategy" with quarterly endoscopies had not shown any cancerous lesions [5]. Most of the cancers detected in the follow-up studies are intramucosal. From a total of 80 cancers detected during follow-up in all studies listed in Table 25.2, the stage and/or cure status was reported in 52 patients. Of these, the vast majority were reported to be intramucosal, and only three had lymph node metastasis (see Table 25.2). This observation suggests that the majority of the cancers detected during follow-up for HGIN are at an early and curable stage but occasionally cancers maybe diagnosed at a more advanced stage.

Endoscopic surveillance of HGIN aims at detecting metachronous cancer at an early stage. One of the limitations of endoscopic surveillance of HGIN is the distinction between HGIN and early cancer. In the USA detection of *any* cancer will usually prompt esophagectomy, whereas in Europe HGIN and early cancers are both considered amenable to endoscopic treatment as long as they are limited to the mucosa. A detailed endoscopic work-up in an expert center, using state-of-the-art equipment, makes it unlikely that *cancers with submucosal invasion* are overlooked endoscopically. However, the endoscopic distinction between HGIN and *mucosal cancer* is more difficult. In addition, the histological differentiation of HGIN and early cancer may be difficult: Ormsby *et al.* studied the interobserver variability in the histological assessment of surgically resected specimens of patients with HGIN or early cancer [44]. They found only fair Kappa statistics (0.42) for the distinction HGIN versus intramucosal cancer and a consensus meeting

did not significantly improve this value (kappa 0.50). The difficulty in distinguishing HGIN and early cancer in biopsies is also illustrated by the results of some of the follow-up studies in patients with HGIN. Reid *et al.* reported that 39% of their patients, who had metachronous cancers detected during follow-up and subsequently underwent surgical resection, did not have cancer detected in their resection specimens [19].

Prerequisites for Endoscopic Surveillance of HGIN

The most important prerequisite for endoscopic surveillance of HGIN is to exclude the presence of a synchronous cancer. This requires that the endoscopic imaging is repeated in a specialized center by an experienced endoscopist, using state-of-the-art endoscopic imaging, and a four-quadrant 1 cm random biopsy protocol.

The focal nature of dysplasia creates the possibility of sampling error even when an intensive biopsy protocol is used [23]. In addition, the previously discussed variability between pathologists in the histological assessment of biopsy specimens adds to this problem. By obtaining a larger mucosal specimen by means of EMR these problems can be reduced. In EMR, the target lesion is lifted by injection of a fluid, usually diluted epinephrine (1 : 100 000), into the submucosal layer. Subsequently, a transparent cap is attached to the endoscope. This cap has a distal ridge that allows positioning of a special EMR-snare. The lesion is sucked into the cap creating a pseudo-polyp, which is then removed using standard electrocautery [45]. Another technique involves the use of a variceal ligating device for band ligation of the target lesion followed by removal of the resulting pseudo-polyp by standard electrosurgical polypectomy [46]. Lesions with a diameter of up to 2 cm can be removed by EMR. Studies have shown that EMR in Barrett's esophagus may change the diagnosis in up to 40% of patients [47]. Therefore, for patients with suspicious lesions, the *clinical* diagnosis HGIN should not be accepted on basis of the histological evaluation of biopsies only. In these patients EMR should be used to provide a more reliable tissue sample for the diagnosis and to exclude the presence of a synchronous cancer. The safety of EMR justifies its use as a diagnostic procedure in selected patients [46].

The endoscopic follow-up of selected patients with HGIN should preferably be carried out in a specialized center by an experienced endoscopist with a special interest in advanced endoscopic imaging techniques. As mentioned, there are many new imaging techniques that may improve the accuracy of cancer detection in selected patients with HGIN. Most of these techniques are, however, still under development, and there is no strong evidence to make a clear recommendation regarding the technique to use. High-resolution endoscopy, supplemented, if necessary, by the use of contrast staining agents such as indigo carmine or narrow band imaging (see Chapter 15) can be considered. All visible lesions, no matter how subtle, should be extensively biopsied with a low threshold to remove lesions by means of EMR for diagnostic purposes. Besides sampling visible lesions, four-quadrant biopsies every 1 cm should be obtained [19]. Based on the available literature and our own personal preference, we currently suggest high-resolution endoscopy every 4 months for the first year, and annually thereafter [5,12,19,42].

Endoscopic Treatment for HGIN

Endoscopic therapy for early esophageal neoplasia can be subdivided into two categories: EMR techniques and endoscopic ablation therapy. EMR has been shown to be a safe and effective method for complete resection of superficial lesions, with the advantage of histopathological verification [7,48]. Larger lesions, however, are less suitable for EMR since piecemeal resection is often necessary, making it impossible to be conclusive about the radicality of the resection at the lateral margins. Ablative therapy, i.e. PDT and argon plasma coagulation (APC), may allow for treatment of larger areas, but with these methods there is no specimen for histopathological evaluation and only limited depth of eradication may be achieved. In Europe and Japan, EMR is considered the mainstay of endoscopic management and ablative techniques are mainly used as an adjunct to EMR. In the USA, however, EMR is not widely used and most centers use ablation techniques for endoscopic treatment of HGIN in Barrett's

esophagus patients. The US Food and Drug Administration (FDA) has recently approved Photofrin®-PDT as an alternative to surgery for patients who have HGIN. FDA-approval was based on the results of a multicenter randomized study comparing Photofrin®-PDT with an expectant management in patients with HGIN. The study was well designed, all histology slides were read at a single center, and over 200 patients were finally randomized. PDT effectively irradiated HGIN in 77% of patients and, compared to the observation arm of the study, reduced cancer incidence from 28% to 13% [49].

PDT, however, is associated with subsquamous Barrett's mucosa and persisting genetic abnormalities that may give rise to recurrent lesions during follow-up. In addition, it is associated with esophageal stenosis in 30% of patients and cutaneous photosensitivity after administration of the photosensitizer may last up to 6 weeks [49,50].

Recent studies suggest that in the future radical endoscopic resection of the whole Barrett's segment may become the preferred treatment for selected Barrett's patients with HGIN or early cancer [51]. It allows for the complete removal of the mucosa at risk with histopathological correlation and will most likely not suffer from the drawbacks as persisting Barrett's mucosa, subsquamous Barrett's mucosa, or persisting genetic abnormalities.

Prerequisites for Endoscopic Treatment of HGIN

The prerequisites for endoscopic treatment are very similar to those of endoscopic surveillance.

The biopsies should be reviewed by an independent expert pathologist and the endoscopic imaging should be repeated in a specialized center that will also perform the treatment. A 1-cm four-quadrant biopsy protocol should be used for sampling of the Barrett's segment and to exclude advanced lesions.

The most important predictor of lymph node metastasis is the penetration depth of the tumor [52]. EMR of the most suspicious area in the Barrett's segment followed by histopathological evaluation of the EMR-specimen allows objective assessment of infiltration depth and estimation of the risk for local lymph node metastasis. Given a 25–40% change of local lymph node involvement in patients with lesions invading into the deep submucosal layers [52], endoscopic ablation should not be used in these cases. A thorough endoscopic work-up, performed in an expert center, using state-of-the-art endoscopes, a 1-cm-four-quadrant random biopsy protocol, and a low threshold to perform a diagnostic EMR, however, will make overlooking a submucosal invading cancer less likely.

Other imaging techniques can be used as well to evaluate tumor infiltration depth, local lymph node status and metastatic spread. Endoscopic ultrasonography (EUS) and computed tomography (CT) are the most widely used techniques for this purpose. EUS is superior to CT with regard to T and N staging of patients with esophageal cancer [53]. The additional value of CT scanning lies mainly in the detection of distant metastases. Since the risk for distant metastases is absent in HGIN and low (< 5%) in early cancers [52] that show no signs of deep submucosal infiltration or suspicious lymph nodes on EUS, the additional value of CT may be limited. For patients with HGIN and early cancer the reliability of EUS for T and N staging is less than for patients with advanced cancer [53]. Moreover, the additional value of EUS after an optimal endoscopic estimation of infiltration depth is limited [54]. Some experts claim that the importance of EUS lies in its high negative predictive value (> 95%) for the absence of tumor infiltration into the deeper wall layers and local lymph nodes, but one may argue that this may reflect the low pretest likelihood of these being present in patients who meet the *clinical* diagnosis of HGIN than the diagnostic accuracy of the technique. Other staging techniques such as positron emission tomography (PET) and magnetic resonance imaging (MRI) do not have a role in the work-up of patients with esophageal HGIN or early cancer.

Only surgical resection of the esophagus results in a definitive treatment of HGIN in Barrett's esophagus. After successful endoscopic treatment, recurrent lesions may develop elsewhere in the Barrett's segment during follow-up. Subsquamous cancers developing from areas of "buried Barrett's" underneath neosquamous epithelium have been described after endoscopic ablation therapy. Frequent endoscopic follow-up according to the protocol as outlined in the section on endoscopic surveillance is therefore mandatory.

Surgical Resection for HGIN

Surgical resection was for many years the treatment of choice for HGIN in Barrett's esophagus, and the 5-year survival rate after surgery in these patients is excellent (>90–95%) [4]. Of the different management strategies, surgical resection is definitely the most effective: the entire segment is removed, including not only areas of HGIN but also occult cancers that may have been missed in the endoscopic work-up as well as the local lymph nodes. Endoscopic surveillance after surgical resection is no longer necessary since the mucosa at risk has been removed. Surgical resection provides the patient with a definitive solution for their disease whereas for endoscopic surveillance and endoscopic therapy the final outcome is more uncertain. The major disadvantage of surgical resection is the invasiveness of the procedure: even in expert hands the mortality is between 3–5% and significant morbidity occurs in aproximately 40–50% of patients [6,27,32,55–57]. Furthermore, with the aging of the population, more patients are diagnosed with HGIN at an older age (with significant comorbidity), increasing the risk of surgical complications. In addition, surgical resection is associated with a permanent loss of the functional esophagus. Quality-of-life studies after esophageal resection have yielded conflicting results, but in general demonstrate a decrease in the quality-of-life scores [58].

Prerequisites for Surgical Management of HGIN

Of the aforementioned difficulties in making a clinical diagnosis of HGIN, the most important one for patients undergoing surgical resection is the issue of over-diagnosing HGIN. Follow-up studies in patients with HGIN have reported that up to 40% of patients show no further HGIN during follow-up [5]. The cause of this remains unkown. Some claim that overdiagnosis of the initial biopsies explains these findings whereas others claim that the patients probably had small foci of HGIN that were effectively removed by the biopsy that led to its diagnosis. Whatever the cause, it indicates that for some patients with HGIN a

Table 25.3 Overview of the pros and cons of the different alternatives for management of patients with high-grade intraepithelial neoplasia (HGIN) in Barrett's esophagus.

Strategy	Surgical resection	Endoscopic follow-up	Endoscopic treatment
Pros	• Complete removal of all HGIN and any occult cancer missed in the preoperative work-up • Complete removal of all Barrett's mucosa with a malignant potential • Complete removal of local lymph nodes • No need for further endoscopic surveillance	• No need for surgical treatment • Preservation of a functional esophagus • A significant number of HGIN are found not to have significant neoplasia during follow-up • The vast majority of cancers developing during follow-up are detected at an early a curable stage • Future prospective: the use of genetic markers as possible predictors for malignant progression	• No need for surgical treatment • Preservation of a functional esophagus • Success rate (eradication of HGIN) in studies >80% • Treatment is relatively safe and can be performed on outpatients' basis • In the event of failed eradication of HGIN after treatment: surgical resection is still possible without a significant delay • The vast majority of cancers developing during follow-up are detected at an early curable stage
Cons	• 3–5% mortality rate • 30–40% chance of significant morbidity • Loss of a functional esophagus: reduction in quality of life • Patients with HGIN are often old and/or have significant comorbidity	• Need for frequent endoscopic procedures • Uncertainty for the patient: 30–50% chance of developing esophageal cancer • A possible need for surgical resection in the future (at an older age, with possibly more comorbidity) • Only a limited number of follow-up series available • Available series differ in selection of patients and histological criteria used making general conclusions difficult	• Presence of residual Barrett's epithelium after treatment • Buried Barrett's under neosquamous epithelium • Need for frequent endoscopic follow-up with biopsies • A possible need for surgical resection in the future (at an older age, with possibly more comorbidity) • Only a limited number of series available

surgical resection may be an unnecessary treatment and stresses the importance of differentiating inflammatory reactive changes from "true HGIN" and thus the importance of review by an experienced pathologist.

The most important determinant for surgical outcome in patients undergoing esophagectomy for HGIN is the experience of the surgeon and the case volume of the center where the operation is performed. The difference in 30-day mortality between low-volume centers (e.g. < 5 procedures/year) and expert centers (e.g. > 25 procedures/year) may be as high as 15–20% [59,60]. This makes it imperative that surgery is performed in expert centers with a high-case volume.

Conclusions

HGIN in Barrett's esophagus is a diagnostic and a therapeutic challenge. The clinician should adhere to the five requirements for the *clinical diagnosis* of HGIN: (i) a prior histological diagnosis of HGIN; (ii) review of biopsies by an independent expert pathologist; (iii) repeated endoscopic imaging in a specialized center; (iv) using a 1-cm four-quadrant biopsy protocol for sampling; and (v) absence of endoscopic lesions suspicious for malignancy.

Adhering to such a strict definition avoids *over-diagnosis of HGIN*, which may be associated with unnecessary treatment, placing the patient at risk for complications and loss of quality of life after being stigmatized with a serious disease. On the other hand, it reduces the chances of *under-diagnosing synchronous cancers* that may require a different treatment approach. Finally, it ensures that studies describing the management of patients with HGIN can be better compared. There is considerable variation between the different continents in the frequency with which surgical resection, endoscopic surveillance, and endoscopic treatment are used for the management of HGIN in Barrett's esophagus. Each management option has its own pros and cons (Table 25.3). The choice may depend on patient characteristics (e.g. age, comorbidity, treatment preference) and local availability and experience with the different approaches. The management of these patients, however, should be performed by ex-

pert centers using a multidisciplinary approach with participation of gastroenterologists, pathologists, and surgeons.

References

1. Spechler SJ. Clinical practice. Barrett's esophagus. *N Engl J Med* 2002;**346**(11):836–42.
2. Hameeteman W, Tytgat GN, Houthoff HJ *et al*. Barrett's esophagus: development of dysplasia and adenocarcinoma. *Gastroenterology* 1989;**96**(5 Pt 1):1249–56.
3. Jankowski JA, Harrison RF, Perry I *et al*. Barrett's metaplasia. *Lancet* 2000;**356**(9247):2079–85.
4. Van Sandick JW, van Lanschot JJ, Kuiken BW *et al*. Impact of endoscopic biopsy surveillance of Barrett's oesophagus on pathological stage and clinical outcome of Barrett's carcinoma. *Gut* 1998;**43**(2):216–22.
5. Schnell TG, Sontag SJ, Chejfec G *et al*. Long-term non-surgical management of Barrett's esophagus with high-grade dysplasia. *Gastroenterology* 2001;**120**(7):1607–19.
6. Rice TW, Falk GW, Achkar E *et al*. Surgical management of high-grade dysplasia in Barrett's esophagus. *Am J Gastroenterol* 1993;**88**(11):1832–6.
7. May A, Gossner L, Pech O *et al*. Local endoscopic therapy for intraepithelial high-grade neoplasia and early adenocarcinoma in Barrett's oesophagus: acute-phase and intermediate results of a new treatment approach. *Eur J Gastroenterol Hepatol* 2002;**14**(10):1085–91.
8. Schlemper RJ, Kato Y, Stolte M. Review of histological classifications of gastrointestinal epithelial neoplasia: differences in diagnosis of early carcinomas between Japanese and Western pathologists. *J Gastroenterol* 2001;**36**(7):445–56.
9. Schlemper RJ, Hirata I, Dixon MF. The macroscopic classification of early neoplasia of the digestive tract. *Endoscopy* 2002;**34**(2):163–8.
10. Hamilton R, Aaltonen LA. *WHO Classification: Tumours of the Digestive System*. IARC press: Lyon, 2000.
11. Montgomery E, Bronner MP, Goldblum JR *et al*. Reproducibility of the diagnosis of dysplasia in Barrett esophagus: a reaffirmation. *Hum Pathol* 2001;**32**(4):368–78.
12. Buttar NS, Wang KK, Sebo TJ *et al*. Extent of high-grade dysplasia in Barrett's esophagus correlates with risk of adenocarcinoma. *Gastroenterology* 2001;**120**(7):1630–9.
13. Skacel M, Petras RE, Gramlich TL *et al*. The diagnosis of low-grade dysplasia in Barrett's esophagus and its implications for disease progression. *Am J Gastroenterol* 2000;**95**(12):3383–7.

14. Polkowski W, van Lanschot JJ, ten Kate FJ *et al*. The value of p53 and Ki67 as markers for tumour progression in the Barrett's dysplasia–carcinoma sequence. *Surg Oncol* 1995;**4**(3):163–71.

15. Hulscher JB, Haringsma J, Benraadt J *et al*. Comprehensive Cancer Centre Amsterdam Barrett Advisory Committee: first results. *Neth J Med* 2001;**58**(1):3–8.

16. Endo T, Awakawa T, Takahashi H *et al*. Classification of Barrett's epithelium by magnifying endoscopy. *Gastrointest Endosc* 2002;**55**(6):641–7.

17. Sharma P, Weston AP, Topalovski M *et al*. Magnification chromoendoscopy for the detection of intestinal metaplasia and dysplasia in Barrett's oesophagus. *Gut* 2003;**52**(1):24–7.

18. Sampliner RE. Updated guidelines for the diagnosis, surveillance, and therapy of Barrett's esophagus. *Am J Gastroenterol* 2002;**97**(8):1888–95.

19. Reid BJ, Blount PL, Feng Z *et al*. Optimizing endoscopic biopsy detection of early cancers in Barrett's high-grade dysplasia. *Am J Gastroenterol* 2000;**95**(11): 3089–96.

20. Kara MA, Bergman JJ, Tytgat GN. Follow-up for high-grade dysplasia in Barrett's esophagus. *Gastrointest Endosc Clin N Am* 2003;**13**(3):513–33.

21. Cameron AJ, Carpenter HA. Barrett's esophagus, high-grade dysplasia, and early adenocarcinoma: a pathological study. *Am J Gastroenterol* 1997;**92**(4):586–91.

22. Edwards MJ, Gable DR, Lentsch AB *et al*. The rationale for esophagectomy as the optimal therapy for Barrett's esophagus with high-grade dysplasia. *Ann Surg* 1996;**223**(5):585–9.

23. Falk GW, Rice TW, Goldblum JR *et al*. Jumbo biopsy forceps protocol still misses unsuspected cancer in Barrett's esophagus with high-grade dysplasia. *Gastrointest Endosc* 1999;**49**(2):170–6.

24. Ferguson MK, Naunheim KS. Resection for Barrett's mucosa with high-grade dysplasia: implications for prophylactic photodynamic therapy. *J Thorac Cardiovasc Surg* 1997;**114**(5):824–9.

25. Fernando HC, Luketich JD, Buenaventura PO *et al*. Outcomes of minimally invasive esophagectomy (MIE) for high-grade dysplasia of the esophagus. *Eur J Cardiothorac Surg* 2002;**22**(1):1–6.

26. Hamilton SR, Smith RR. The relationship between columnar epithelial dysplasia and invasive adenocarcinoma arising in Barrett's esophagus. *Am J Clin Pathol* 1987;**87**(3):301–12.

27. Heitmiller RF, Redmond M, Hamilton SR. Barrett's esophagus with high-grade dysplasia. An indication for prophylactic esophagectomy. *Ann Surg* 1996;**224**(1): 66–71.

28. Levine DS, Haggitt RC, Blount PL *et al*. An endoscopic biopsy protocol can differentiate high-grade dysplasia from early adenocarcinoma in Barrett's esophagus. *Gastroenterology* 1993;**105**(1):40–50.

29. McArdle JE, Lewin KJ, Randall G *et al*. Distribution of dysplasias and early invasive carcinoma in Barrett's esophagus. *Hum Pathol* 1992;**23**(5):479–82.

30. McDonald ML, Trastek VF, Allen MS *et al*. Barretts's esophagus: does an antireflux procedure reduce the need for endoscopic surveillance? *J Thorac Cardiovasc Surg* 1996;**111**(6):1135–8.

31. Nguyen NT, Schauer P, Luketich JD. Minimally invasive esophagectomy for Barrett's esophagus with high-grade dysplasia. *Surgery* 2000;**127**(3):284–90.

32. Nigro JJ, Hagen JA, DeMeester TR *et al*. Occult esophageal adenocarcinoma: extent of disease and implications for effective therapy. *Ann Surg* 1999;**230**(3): 433–8.

33. Ortiz A, Martinez de Haro LF, Parrilla P *et al*. Conservative treatment versus antireflux surgery in Barrett's oesophagus: long-term results of a prospective study. *Br J Surg* 1996;**83**(2):274–8.

34. Pera M, Cameron AJ, Trastek VF *et al*. Increasing incidence of adenocarcinoma of the esophagus and esophagogastric junction. *Gastroenterology* 1993; **104**(2):510–3.

35. Peters JH, Clark GW, Ireland AP *et al*. Outcome of adenocarcinoma arising in Barrett's esophagus in endoscopically surveyed and nonsurveyed patients. *J Thorac Cardiovasc Surg* 1994;**108**(5):813–21.

36. Reid BJ, Weinstein WM, Lewin KJ *et al*. Endoscopic biopsy can detect high-grade dysplasia or early adenocarcinoma in Barrett's esophagus without grossly recognizable neoplastic lesions. *Gastroenterology* 1988; **94**(1):81–90.

37. Schmidt HG, Riddell RH, Walther B *et al*. Dysplasia in Barrett's esophagus. *J Cancer Res Clin Oncol* 1985; **110**(2):145–52.

38. Skinner DB, Walther BC, Riddell RH *et al*. Barrett's esophagus. Comparison of benign and malignant cases. *Ann Surg* 1983;**198**(4):554–65.

39. Streitz JM, Jr, Andrews CW, Jr, Ellis FH, Jr. Endoscopic surveillance of Barrett's esophagus. Does it help? *J Thorac Cardiovasc Surg* 1993;**105**(3):383–7.

40. Zaninotto G, Parenti AR, Ruol A *et al*. Oesophageal resection for high-grade dysplasia in Barrett's oesophagus. *Br J Surg* 2000;**87**(8):1102–5.

41. Collard JM. High-grade dysplasia in Barrett's esophagus. The case for esophagectomy. *Chest Surg Clin N Am* 2002;**12**(1):77–92.

42. Weston AP, Sharma P, Topalovski M *et al*. Long-term follow-up of Barrett's high-grade dysplasia. *Am J Gastroenterol* 2000;**95**(8):1888–93.

43. Macdonald CE, Wicks AC, Playford RJ. Final results from 10 year cohort of patients undergoing surveillance for Barrett's oesophagus: observational study. *BMJ* 2000;**321**(7271):1252–5.

44. Ormsby AH, Petras RE, Henricks WH *et al*. Observer variation in the diagnosis of superficial oesophageal adenocarcinoma. *Gut* 2002;**51**(5):671–6.

45. Inoue H, Takeshita K, Hori H *et al*. Endoscopic mucosal resection with a cap-fitted panendoscope for esophagus, stomach, and colon mucosal lesions. *Gastrointest Endosc* 1993;**39**(1):58–62.

46. May A, Gossner L, Behrens A *et al*. A prospective randomized trial of two different endoscopic resection techniques for early stage cancer of the esophagus. *Gastrointest Endosc* 2003;**58**(2):167–75.

47. Nijhawan PK, Wang KK. Endoscopic mucosal resection for lesions with endoscopic features suggestive of malignancy and high-grade dysplasia within Barrett's esophagus. *Gastrointest Endosc* 2000;**52**(3):328–32.

48. Peters FP, Kara MA, Rosmolen WD *et al*. Endoscopic treatment of high-grade dysplasia and early stage cancer in Barrett's esophagus. *Gastrointest Endosc* 2005;**61**(4):506–14.

49. Overholt B, Lightdale C, Wang KK. International multicenter, partially blinded, randomized study of the efficacy of photodynamic therapy (PDT) using porfimer sodium (POR) for ablation of high-grade dysplasia (HGD) in Barrett's esophagus (BE): results of 24-month follow-up [abstract]. *Gastroenterology* 2003;**124**:A20.

50. Overholt BF, Panjehpour M, Haydek JM. Photodynamic therapy for Barrett's esophagus: follow-up in 100 patients. *Gastrointest Endosc* 1999;**49**(1):1–7.

51. Seewald S, Akaraviputh T, Seitz U *et al*. Circumferential EMR and complete removal of Barrett's epithelium: a new approach to management of Barrett's esophagus containing high-grade intraepithelial neoplasia and intramucosal carcinoma. *Gastrointest Endosc* 2003;**57**(7):854–9.

52. Buskens CJ, Westerterp M, Lagarde SM *et al*. Prediction of appropriateness of local endoscopic treatment for high-grade dysplasia and early adenocarcinoma by EUS and histopathologic features. *Gastrointest Endosc* 2004;**60**(5):703–10.

53. Bergman JJ, Fockens P. Endoscopic ultrasonography in patients with gastro-esophageal cancer. *Eur J Ultrasound* 1999;**10**(2–3):127–38.

54. May A, Gunter E, Roth F *et al*. Accuracy of staging in early oesophageal cancer using high resolution endoscopy and high resolution endosonography: a comparative, prospective, and blinded trial. *Gut* 2004;**53**(5):634–40.

55. Bonavina L, Ruol A, Ancona E, Peracchia A. Prognosis of early squamous cell carcinoma of the esophagus after surgical therapy. *Dis Esophagus* 1997;**10**:162–4.

56. Hulscher JB, Van Sandick JW, De Boer AG *et al*. Extended transthoracic resection compared with limited transhiatal resection for adenocarcinoma of the esophagus. *N Engl J Med* 2002;**347**(21):1662–9.

57. Thomas RJ, Lade S, Giles GG *et al*. Incidence trends in oesophageal and proximal gastric carcinoma in Victoria. *Aust N Z J Surg* 1996;**66**(5):271–5.

58. De Boer AG, Genovesi PI, Sprangers MA *et al*. Quality of life in long-term survivors after curative transhiatal oesophagectomy for oesophageal carcinoma. *Br J Surg* 2000;**87**(12):1716–21.

59. Birkmeyer JD, Siewers AE, Finlayson EV *et al*. Hospital volume and surgical mortality in the United States. *N Engl J Med* 2002;**346**(15):1128–37.

60. van Lanschot JJ, Hulscher JB, Buskens CJ *et al*. Hospital volume and hospital mortality for esophagectomy. *Cancer* 2001;**91**(8):1574–8.

CHAPTER 26
Esophageal and Gastroesophageal Junction Adenocarcinoma

Stuart Jon Spechler

Problems in Localizing Structures at the Gastroesophageal Junction

When a tumor straddles the gastroesophageal junction (GEJ), it can be difficult to determine whether the neoplasm arose from cells of the distal esophagus or from cells of the proximal stomach (the gastric cardia). Whereas the normal stomach is lined by a glandular, columnar epithelium that contains no squamous elements, squamous cell carcinomas that cross the GEJ are assumed to have arisen from the squamous epithelium of the distal esophagus. For glandular cancers (adenocarcinomas) that cross the junction, however, the situation is far more complex. Glandular elements that might give rise to adenocarcinomas that cross the GEJ are found in the proximal stomach, in the superficial and deep glands of the distal esophagus, in gastric-type columnar epithelium that can line a short segment of the distal esophagus, and in Barrett's esophagus (an acquired condition in which a metaplastic, intestinal-type epithelium replaces squamous mucosa that has been damaged by reflux esophagitis) [1]. Unfortunately, there is no test that establishes unequivocally the origin of adenocarcinomas at the GEJ.

One major problem that confounds investigations on the origin of tumors at the GEJ is the lack of universally accepted anatomic and histological findings that delimit the extent of the gastric cardia. The gastric cardia has been defined conceptually as the region of the stomach that adjoins the esophagus [2]. This conceptual definition is of no practical value to the endoscopist who wants to distinguish the end of the esophagus from the beginning of the stomach, however. To add to the confusion, authors have used the term "gastric cardia" to refer both to a gross anatomic region (i.e. the most proximal portion of the stomach), and to a histological finding (i.e. "cardiac epithelium"). Pathologists even dispute fundamental histological characteristics of cardiac epithelium. For example, some contend that cardiac epithelium comprises exclusively of mucus-secreting cells, and that the presence of any parietal cells in the glands precludes a histological diagnosis of cardiac epithelium [3]. Others contend that cardiac epithelium can have occasional parietal cells provided that other architectural features are typical of cardiac mucosa [4]. The terms "oxyntocardiac mucosa" or "transitional mucosa" also have been used to describe a cardiac-type epithelium that has occasional parietal cells [3].

Investigators often have assumed that the histological finding of cardiac epithelium establishes that the biopsy specimen has been obtained from the proximal stomach. However, this assumption is incorrect because cardiac mucosa clearly can line the distal esophagus [5,6]. Another widely held, but erroneous, assumption is that cardiac mucosa normally lines several centimeters of the proximal stomach. Recent studies suggest that cardiac mucosa uncommonly extends more than 2–3 mm below the junction of squamous and columnar epithelia at the end of the esophagus [7–11]. Furthermore, the junction between squamous and cardiac epithelia can be located within the esophagus a number of centimeters above the anatomic GEJ [5]. Thus, in some individuals, cardiac mucosa is found only in the esophagus and not in the stomach. Finally, some investigators contend that cardiac epithelium is not a normal mucosal structure at all, but one that is acquired as a consequence of chronic inflammation [12–15].

A study of 40 patients who had subtotal esophagectomy with esophagogastrostomy, an operation frequently complicated by severe reflux esophagitis in the esophageal remnant, supports the notion that cardiac epithelium is metaplastic [16]. Endoscopic examinations performed at a median of 36 months postoperatively showed that 19 of the 40 patients had developed columnar metaplasia in the esophageal remnant (10 cardiac epithelium, nine intestinal metaplasia). Seven patients who had serial endoscopic examinations progressed from cardiac epithelium on the initial postoperative endoscopy to specialized intestinal metaplasia (typical of Barrett's esophagus) on subsequent studies. The median time to the development of cardiac epithelium was 14 months, whereas specialized intestinal metaplasia was found at a median of 27 months postoperatively. These findings suggest that cardiac epithelium is not only metaplastic, but maybe the precursor of intestinal metaplasia in the esophagus. It is not clear whether cardiac epithelium can become malignant directly without an intervening stage of intestinal metaplasia.

Problems in Defining Cancer of the Gastric Cardia

The above-described difficulties in identifying the GEJ and in delimiting the gastric cardia create major problems for investigators designing studies on tumors of this region, and for clinicians interpreting the results of published reports. When reading these reports it is important to determine what the authors mean specifically when they use the term "cancer of the gastric cardia"? Does the term refer merely to the anatomic location of the tumor, or does it imply that the cancer arose from cardiac epithelium? Authors frequently are not clear on this issue, perhaps because they have mistakenly assumed that tumors of the proximal stomach must have arisen from cardiac epithelium. Recent studies have shown that the proximal stomach normally is lined predominantly, if not exclusively, by oxyntic (acid-producing) epithelium [7,12–15]. Therefore, even a tumor that is unquestionably "cardiac" in anatomic location may not have arisen from cardiac epithelium. Conversely, a tumor that clearly is located in the distal esophagus conceivably could have arisen from esophageal cardiac epithelium.

Table 26.1 lists some of the published criteria that have been used to categorize tumors in the region of the GEJ as cancers of the gastric cardia [17–23]. In these classification systems, the anatomic location of the epicenter or predominant mass of the tumor is used to determine whether the neoplasm is esophageal or gastric in origin. These criteria are arbitrary, and it is not clear that the predominant location of the tumor is a useful predictor of the cell of origin. Conceivably, a cancer of the distal esophagus might exhibit a predominantly distal pattern of growth (into the stomach), whereas a tumor of gastric origin might grow proximally to involve the esophagus predominantly. The use of these arbitrary classification systems virtually guarantees that the patient population in studies on cancers of the gastric cardia will be heterogeneous, including some patients with gastric tumors and others with tumors of esophageal origin. Siewert *et al.* has suggested that GEJ tumors should be classified as type I if the tumor epicenter is located above the proximal extent of the

Table 26.1 Published criteria that have been used to classify a tumor as "cardiac."

1 Epicenter located within 1 cm proximal and 2 cm distal to the esophagogastric junction [17]
2 Epicenter located at the gastroesophageal junction [18]
3 Within or immediately below the gastroesophageal junction [19]
4 Epicenter located within 2 cm of the cardioesophageal junction [20]
5 Originating from cardial glands 3 cm distal to the gastroesophageal junction [21]
6 A carcinoma of the fundus which has reached the cardia or has crossed over to the distal esophagus [22]
7 Involves the proximal one-third of the stomach [23]

gastric folds, type II if the epicenter is at the top of the folds, and type III if the epicenter is below the proximal extent of the folds [24]. Although this classification system does not obviate the problems discussed above, it may have implications regarding surgical therapy.

Intestinal Metaplasia as a Risk Factor for Cancer of the Esophagogastric Junction

Intestinal metaplasia is judged to be the precursor of adenocarcinoma both in the esophagus and in the stomach [1,25]. However, there appear to be substantial differences in the pathogenesis, morphological and histochemical characteristics, and clinical importance of intestinal metaplasia in the two organs (Table 26.2). Gastroesophageal reflux disease (GERD) is a strong risk factor for adenocarcinoma of the esophagus [26], presumably because GERD causes chronic reflux esophagitis that leads to intestinal metaplasia (Barrett's esophagus). In the body and antrum of the stomach, *Helicobacter pylori* infection causes chronic gastritis that leads to intestinal metaplasia [27–29]. In contrast to the stomach, infection with *H. pylori* does not appear to play a direct role in the pathogenesis of esophageal inflammation and metaplasia [30–37]. Indeed, a number of reports suggest that gastric infection with *H. pylori* actually may protect the esophagus from cancer by preventing the development of reflux esophagitis and Barrett's esophagus [38–43]. Intestinal metaplasia in the stomach often is of the "complete" (type I) variety that strongly resembles the epithelium of the normal small intestine, whereas intestinal metaplasia in Barrett's esophagus usually is incomplete (type

II or III), exhibiting gastric and colonic features [44–50]. In biopsy specimens taken from the squamocolumnar junction (SCJ) of patients with Barrett's esophagus, investigators have found a peculiar hybrid cell that has both microvilli (a feature of columnar cells) and intercellular ridges (a feature of squamous cells) on its surface [51]. Some studies also show that the cytokeratin staining pattern of intestinal metaplasia in the esophagus differs from that of intestinal metaplasia in the stomach [52–56]. Finally, the risk of dysplasia and cancer for patients with intestinal metaplasia in the esophagus appears to be substantially higher than for patients with intestinal metaplasia in the stomach [1,57].

The observations noted above suggest that intestinal metaplasia in the esophagus differs substantially from that in the body and antrum of the stomach. It is not clear how cardiac epithelium fits into this scheme. Intestinal metaplasia arising from gastric cardiac epithelium conceivably might have unique epidemiologic and clinical characteristics, but few data are available to address this issue. Cancers of the gastric cardia are said to resemble esophageal adenocarcinomas in terms of their associations with GERD and *H. pylori* [58–60]. It is not clear whether these tumors share epidemiologic features because many so-called cardiac tumors are in fact esophageal in origin, or because gastric cardiac epithelium shares the same cancer risk factors as Barrett's esophagus.

Criteria for Identifying Cancers of the Esophagogastric Junction

Figure 26.1 shows endoscopically recognizable landmarks that can be used to identify structures at the GEJ. The SCJ (or Z line) is the visible line formed by

	IM stomach	IM esophagus
Helicobacter pylori association	Positive	Negative
GERD association	No	Yes
Common type of IM	Complete	Incomplete
Barrett's cytokeratin pattern	Uncommon	Common
Cancer risk	Lower	Higher

Table 26.2 Features of intestinal metaplasia in the stomach and esophagus.

GERD, gastroesophageal reflux disease; IM, intestinal metaplasia.

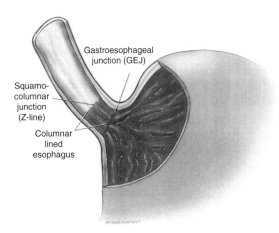

Fig. 26.1 Landmarks at the gastroesophageal junction (GEJ) region. The squamocolumnar junction (SCJ or Z line) is the visible line formed by the juxtaposition of squamous and columnar epithelia. The GEJ is the imaginary line at which the esophagus ends and the stomach begins. The GEJ corresponds to the most proximal extent of the gastric folds, and marks the proximal extent of the gastric cardia. When the SCJ is located proximal to the GEJ, there is a columnar-lined segment of esophagus. Adapted from Spechler [1].

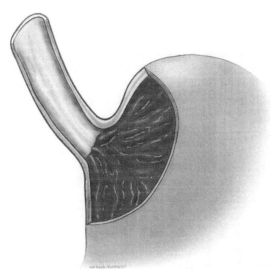

Fig. 26.2 The squamocolumnar junction (SCJ) and gastroesophageal junction (GEJ) coincide. In this situation, the entire esophagus is lined by squamous epithelium. Adapted from Spechler [1].

the juxtaposition of pale, glossy squamous epithelium and red, velvet-like columnar mucosa. The GEJ is the imaginary line at which the esophagus ends and the stomach begins anatomically. Endoscopists have defined the GEJ, somewhat arbitrarily, as the level of the most proximal extent of the gastric folds [61]. In normal individuals, the proximal extent of the gastric folds generally corresponds to the point at which the tubular esophagus flares to become the sack-shaped stomach in the region of the lower esophageal sphincter. In patients with hiatal hernias whose lower esophageal sphincters are weak and in whom there may be no clear-cut flare at the esophagogastric junction, the proximal margin of the gastric folds is determined when the distal esophagus is minimally inflated with air because overinflation obscures this landmark [62]. When the SCJ is located proximal to the GEJ, there is a columnar-lined segment of esophagus. When the SCJ and GEJ coincide (Fig. 26.2), the entire esophagus is lined by squamous epithelium. The gastric cardia, by definition, starts at the GEJ, but there are no gross anatomic structures that mark the distal extent of the cardia.

Investigators should be encouraged to use the landmarks described above whenever possible for localizing tumors in the region of the GEJ. Tumors located entirely above the junction can be considered esophageal, whereas tumors entirely below the GEJ can be considered gastric in origin. When describing these tumors, the use of the ambiguous and often misleading term "gastric cardia" should be discouraged. Adenocarcinomas that cross the junction can be called adenocarcinomas of the GEJ, regardless of where the bulk of the tumor lies. Presently, there is no way to ascertain the origin of adenocarcinomas of the GEJ, although the finding of intestinal metaplasia with dysplastic changes in either the esophagus or stomach surrounding the tumor strongly suggests an esophageal or gastric origin, respectively.

Clinical Features, Diagnosis, and Staging

Adenocarcinomas of the esophagus and GEJ are tumors that affect older White men predominantly [58,59]. Common presenting symptoms for patients with these cancers include dysphagia, weight loss, and abdominal pain. Gastroesophageal metaplasia and dysplasia, and early GEJ cancers generally cause no symptoms. Consequently, the presence of symptoms usually indicates that the patient has advanced, incurable disease. Uncommonly, cancers of the esophagus and GEJ are discovered in an early, curable stage during endoscopic surveillance for patients known to have Barrett's esophagus.

The diagnosis of cancer of the esophagus and the GEJ usually is established by endoscopic examination with biopsy. Barium swallow usually has a limited role as a diagnostic test for these tumors [63,64], but a barium esophagram may be very helpful in the analysis of malignant stenoses that are too narrow to be traversed by the endoscope. Computed tomography (CT) is used to assess local invasion and, especially, to detect distant thoracic and abdominal metastases. Similar information can be obtained with magnetic resonance imaging (MRI), but CT usually is recommended because it is more readily available, more familiar to clinicians, and less expensive than MRI [65]. Endoscopic ultrasonography (EUS) appears to be the most accurate modality for local tumor staging, especially when high frequency (20 or 30 MHz) miniprobe transducers are used [66,67]. EUS also can be useful in assessing the proximal extent of submucosal tumor invasion in the esophagus. A number of reports suggest that EUS accurately identifies the depth of tumor invasion and the presence of regional lymph node involvement in approximately 77% and 78% of cases, respectively [67,68]. However, the studies that describe such excellent results often comprise predominantly patients with advanced tumors. Recent reports suggest that the accuracy of endosonography may be substantially less for determining whether small tumors are limited to the mucosa [69,70]. The role of positron emission tomography (PET) for the staging of adenocarcinoma of the GEJ remains controversial, but the procedure appears to add little to the staging of locoregional disease [71].

Few studies on cancer staging and therapy have focused exclusively on cancers of the GEJ [72]. Rather, investigators generally have pooled data on patients with junctional tumors together with data on patients who have cancer of the esophagus. Furthermore, relatively few studies on cancer of the esophagus have focused specifically on the treatment of adenocarcinomas. Many investigations on esophageal cancer have included patients with squamous cell carcinoma in addition to those with adenocarcinoma. Consequently, the management of adenocarcinomas of the esophagus and GEJ has been based on principles established largely for patients with squamous cell carcinoma of the esophagus. This approach may be inappropriate and, consequently, it is difficult to draw firm conclusions on the optimal management strategy for patients with adenocarcinomas of the esophagus and GEJ [73].

Survival for patients with adenocarcinomas of the esophagus and GEJ clearly is related to the stage of the disease at the time of presentation [74]. A number of different systems have been proposed for the staging of these cancers, and all of the systems have certain deficiencies. Perhaps the most popular system is a modifications of the TNM staging classification proposed by the American Joint Committee on Cancer (AJCC) [60] (Table 26.3). Preoperative use of this system generally requires esophageal endosonography. Endosonographic study of the wall of the esophagus commonly reveals five distinct layers [75]. There are three hyperechoic layers that are separated by two layers that are hypoechoic. The inner and external hyperechoic layers correspond to the interfaces of the esophageal wall with the gut lumen and surrounding tissues, respectively. The intermediate hyperechoic layer reflects the submucosa. The inner and outer hypoechoic layers represent part of

Table 26.3 TNM staging.

Primary tumor (T)	
T1	Invades lamina propria or submucosa
T2	Invades muscularis propria
T3	Invades adventitia (esophagus) or serosa (stomach)
T4	Invades adjacent structures
Regional lymph nodes (N)	
N0	No lymph node metastases
N1	Lymph node metastases
Distant metastases	
M0	No distant metastases
M1	Distant metastases

the muscularis mucosae and the muscularis propria, respectively. Superficial (T1) tumors do not invade the outer hypoechoic layer (the muscularis propria), whereas advanced (T3) tumors, interrupt the external hyperechoic layer (the adventitia or serosa). Even though tumors of the GEJ often are included in series of patients with esophageal cancer, the AJCC has considered junctional cancers to be tumors of the stomach (the gastric cardia). There are differences in the criteria for stage grouping esophageal and gastric malignancies, and the pathologic staging recommended by the AJCC for lymph node involvement by gastric cancers is not easily adapted for use by endosonographers. Another consideration in staging these tumors is the fact that involvement of the celiac lymph nodes is usually deemed regional disease for gastric cancers (sometimes designated as N2), whereas celiac node involvement is considered distant metastatic disease (M1) for cancers of the thoracic esophagus.

Treatment

Series of patients treated for adenocarcinoma of the esophagus and GEJ often have included many patients with advanced disease whose median survival can be measured in months [76–78]. For patients with early stage disease, however, long-term survival rates with treatment may exceed 80% [79]. Localized esophageal cancers usually are removed surgically using either a transthoracic approach (which combines laparotomy and right thoracotomy to effect wide excision of the tumor, peritumoral tissue and mediastinal lymph nodes) or a transhiatal approach (which involves laparotomy with blunt dissection of the thoracic esophagus without formal lymphadenectomy). In the transthoracic approach the esophagogastric anastomosis can be placed either in the upper chest or in the neck, whereas the anastomosis is placed in the neck with the transhiatal approach. It is not clear whether the potential benefit of the transthoracic approach in eradicating local disease warrants its higher morbidity and cost compared to the transhiatal route. One recent study randomized 220 patients with adenocarcinoma of the esophagus or cardia to either transhiatal or transthoracic esophagectomy [80]. Perioperative morbidity

was higher in the transthoracic esophagectomy group, but there were no significant differences between the groups in in-hospital mortality and long-term survival rates. However, there appeared to be a trend toward a survival benefit in the transthoracic group at 5 years.

For patients whose tumors recur after surgery, the recurrence pattern is local–regional in less than one-third of cases, whereas the large majority of recurrences are in the form of distant metastases. These observations suggest that curative treatment ideally should have some component of systemic therapy aimed at eradicating metastases. Survival rates are especially poor for patients with advanced disease who are treated with surgery, radiation, or chemotherapy alone as the sole therapeutic modality [76–78]. Consequently, a number of studies have explored the use of combined modality therapies for adenocarcinomas of the esophagus and esophagogastric junction.

Preoperative radiotherapy appears to provide no survival benefit over surgery alone [81]. Data on the role of preoperative chemotherapy (usually a combination of cisplatin and 5-fluorouracil) are contradictory. A large US study comparing neoadjuvant chemotherapy followed by surgery to immediate surgery without chemotherapy for patients with localized cancer of the esophagus (many of whom had adenocarcinomas) showed no significant differences between the groups in median survival (14.9 months for the neoadjuvant group, 16.1 months for the surgery alone group) [82]. In contrast, a large UK study found a small survival advantage at 2 years for the patients who received preoperative chemotherapy (43% survival) compared to those who received surgery alone (34% survival) [83]. These findings do not support the routine use of neoadjuvant chemotherapy for patients with adenocarcinoma of the GEJ.

For reasons that are not entirely clear, the combination of chemotherapy and radiotherapy (chemoradiotherapy) prior to surgery has become popular as a treatment for localized esophageal cancer. At least eight randomized trials have compared neoadjuvant chemoradiotherapy with surgery alone for esophageal cancer [84]. Only one of those eight studies demonstrated a clear survival advantage for

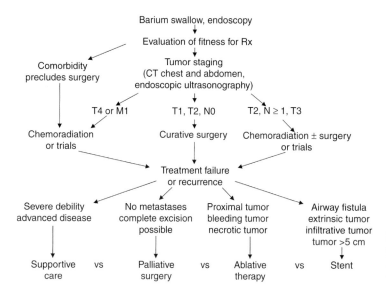

Fig. 26.3 Management approach for patients with adenocarcinoma of the esophagus and esophagogastric junction. CT, computed tomography.

neoadjuvant chemoradiotherapy [85], and that study suffered from a number of deficiencies that limit its utility [84]. Relatively few data are available on chemoradiation without surgery as primary therapy for adenocarcinoma of the GEJ. Some investigators have compared chemoradiation to radiation therapy alone, primarily in patients with squamous cell carcinoma of the esophagus [86]. Although available data suggest a survival advantage for chemoradiation over radiation therapy alone, it is not clear that these results can be extrapolated to patients with adenocarcinoma of the esophagus and GEJ. A number of systematic reviews have been conducted recently on the treatment of esophageal cancer, but none of these provide definitive results because the trials are heterogeneous and the sample sizes are small even when data are pooled [87]. Trials are underway evaluating the role of promising newer chemotherapy agents such as paclitaxel and irinotecan. Experimental ablative treatment modalities such as photodynamic therapy and endoscopic mucosal resection for localized adenocarcinoma of the esophagus are discussed elsewhere in this book.

Management Recommendations

Optimal management for patients with adenocarcinoma of the esophagus and GEJ remains disputed.

Whenever possible, therefore, the use of research protocols for patient management is recommended. If such protocols are not available, one suggested management approach is summarized in Fig. 26.3. This approach is a modification of the management guidelines prepared for the 1994 AGA Clinical Practice Section symposium on esophageal cancer conducted by Drs DeMeester, Kimmey, Kozarek, Levin, Spechler, and Tytgat. After the diagnosis has been established by barium swallow and endoscopy, the next step involves a decision regarding the patient's fitness to undergo surgery. If comorbidity precludes surgery, then primary therapy might include chemoradiation or, preferably, the patient can be enrolled in a clinical trial. If the patient is reasonably fit, then the next step is tumor staging with CT scan and, if available, EUS. Surgery generally is not recommended for patients with T4 tumors that invade adjacent structures, or for patients with metastases (M1). Primary therapy for these patients might include chemoradiation or clinical trials. For tumors that do not invade beyond the muscularis propria (T1,T2), and do not involve local lymph nodes (N0), surgery appears to offer the best hope for cure. For lesions that are more advanced due to lymph node involvement (N_1) or invasion to the adventitia (T3), the choices for primary therapy include chemoradiation with or without surgery or, preferably, enrollment in an established clinical trial. If these primary treatments fail, or if the tumor recurs, there are a number of treatment options. For patients who are severely debilitated and who have advanced disease, the most humane option may be only supportive care with careful attention to pain control. If there are no apparent metastases, and complete excision of the tumor is possible, then surgery can provide excellent palliation. Other options include ablative therapies (e.g. photodynamic therapy, Nd : YAG laser) or stents. The placement of a stent across the GEJ often results in severe gastroesophageal reflux, although this problem sometimes can be controlled adequately with proton pump inhibitors. Stents also may not provide good palliation for patients who have tumors that are necrotic or bleeding, and ablative therapy may be preferable in these circumstances. Although esophago-bronchial fistulas are uncommon for tumors of the GEJ, such fistulas are best managed with a stent. Also, stents may be preferable to ablative therapy for infiltrative (submucosal) tumors that are causing dysphagia.

References

1. Spechler SJ. The role of gastric carditis in metaplasia and neoplasia at the gastroesophageal junction. *Gastroenterology* 1999;**117**:218–8.
2. Redel CA, Zwiener RJ. Anatomy and anomalies of the stomach and duodenum. In: Feldman F, Scharschmidt BF, Sleisenger MH, eds. *Sleisenger and Fordtran's Gastrointestinal and Liver Disease*, 6th edn. Philadelphia: W. B. Saunders Co., 1998:557–71.
3. Chandrasoma P. Pathophysiology of Barrett's esophagus. *Semin Thorac Cardiovasc Surg* 1997;**9**:270–8.
4. Goldblum JR, Vicari JJ, Falk GW *et al.* Inflammation and intestinal metaplasia of the gastric cardia: the role of gastroesophageal reflux and *H. pylori* infection. *Gastroenterology* 1998;**114**:633–9.
5. Paull A, Trier JS, Dalton MD *et al.* The histologic spectrum of Barrett's esophagus. *N Engl J Med* 1976;**295**:476–80.
6. Hayward J. The lower end of the oesophagus. *Thorax* 1961;**16**:36–41.
7. Kilgore SP, Ormsby AH, Gramlich TL *et al.* The gastric cardia: fact or fiction? *Am J Gastroenterol* 2000;**95**:921–4.
8. Sarbia M, Donner A, Gabbert HE. Histopathology of the gastroesophageal junction. A study on 36 operation specimens. *Am J Surg Pathol* 2002;**26**:1207–12.
9. Chandrasoma PT, Der R, Ma Y, Dalton P, Taira M. Histology of the gastroesophageal junction. An autopsy study. *Am J Surg Pathol* 2000;**24**:402–9.
10. Zhou H, Greco A, Daum F, Kahn E. Origin of cardiac mucosa: ontogenic consideration. *Pediatr Dev Pathol* 2001;**4**:358–63.
11. Park YS, Park HJ, Kang GH, Kim CJ, Chi JG. Histology of the gastroesophageal junction in fetal and pediatric autopsy. *Arch Pathol Lab Med* 2003;**127**:451–5.
12. Chandrasoma PT, Der R, Ma Y, Dalton P, Taira M. Histology of the gastroesophageal junction: an autopsy study. *Am J Surg Pathol* 2000;**24**:402–9.
13. Öberg S, Peters JH, DeMeester TR *et al.* Inflammation and specialized intestinal metaplasia of cardiac mucosa is a manifestation of gastroesophageal reflux disease. *Ann Surg* 1997;**226**;522–32.
14. Chandrasoma P. Pathophysiology of Barrett's esophagus. *Semin Thorac Cardiovasc Surg* 1997;**9**:270–8.
15. Chandrasoma PT, Lokuhetty DM, DeMeester TR *et al.* Definition of histopathologic changes in gastroesophageal reflux disease. *Am J Surg Pathol* 2000;**24**:344–51.
16. Dresner SM, Griffin SM, Wayman J *et al.* Human model of duodenogastro-oesophageal reflux in the development of Barrett's metaplasia. *Br J Surg* 2003;**90**:1120–8.
17. Misumi A, Murakami A, Harada K, Baba K, Akagi M. Definition of carcinoma of the gastric cardia. *Langenbecks Arch Chir* 1989;**374**:221–6.
18. Clark GWB, Smyrk TC, Burdiles P *et al.* Is Barrett's metaplasia the source of adenocarcinomas of the cardia? *Arch Surg* 1994;**129**:609–14.
19. Kalish RJ, Clancy PE, Orringer MB, Appelman HD. Clinical, epidemiologic, and morphologic comparison between adenocarcinomas arising in Barrett's esophageal mucosa and in the gastric cardia. *Gastroenterology* 1984;**86**:461–7.
20. Mori M, Kitagawa S, Iida M *et al.* Early carcinoma of the gastric cardia. A clinicopathologic study of 21 cases. *Cancer* 1987;**59**:1758–66.
21. Guanrei Y, Sunglian Q. Incidence rate of adenocarcinoma of the gastric cardia, and endoscopic classifications of early cardial carcinoma in Henan Province, the People's Republic of China. *Endoscopy* 1987;**19**:7–10.
22. Husemann B. Cardia carcinoma considered as a distinct clinical entity. *Br J Surg* 1989;**76**:136–9.
23. Heidl G, Langhans P, Krieg V *et al.* Comparative studies of cardia carcinoma and infracardial gastric carcinoma. *J Cancer Res Clin Oncol* 1993;**120**:91–4.

24. Siewert RJ, Feith M, Stein HJ. Biologic and clinical variations of adenocarcinoma at the esophago-gastric junction: relevance of a topographic-anatomic subclassification. *J Surg Oncol* 2005;**90**:139–46.

25. Ruol A, Parenti A, Zaninotto G *et al*. Intestinal metaplasia is the probable common precursor of adenocarcinoma in Barrett esophagus and adenocarcinoma of the gastric cardia. *Cancer* 2000;**88**:2520–8.

26. Lagergren J, Bergström R, Lindgren A, Nyrén O. Symptomatic gastroesophageal reflux as a risk factor for esophageal adenocarcinoma. *N Engl J Med* 1999;**340**: 825–31.

27. Stemmermann GN. Intestinal metaplasia of the stomach. A status report. *Cancer* 1994;**74**:556–64.

28. Asaka M, Takeda H, Sugiyama T, Kato M. What role does *Helicobacter pylori* play in gastric cancer. *Gastroenterology* 1997;**113**:556–60.

29. Correa P. *Helicobacter pylori* and gastric carcinogenesis. *Am J Surg Pathol* 1995;**19**(suppl 1):S37–43.

30. O'Connor HJ, Cunnane K. *Helicobacter pylori* and gastro-oesophageal reflux disease—a prospective study. *Ir J Med Sci* 1994;**163**:369–73.

31. Liston R, Pitt MA, Banerjee AK. Reflux oesophagitis and *Helicobacter pylori* infection in elderly patients. *Postgrad Med J* 1996;**72**:221–3.

32. Rosioru C, Glassman MS, Halata MS, Schwarz SM. Esophagitis and *Helicobacter pylori* in children: incidence and therapeutic implications. *Am J Gastroenterol* 1993;**88**:510–3.

33. Talley NJ, Cameron AJ, Shorter RG, Zinsmeister AR, Phillips SF. *Campylobacter pylori* and Barrett's esophagus. *Mayo Clin Proc* 1988;**63**:1176–80.

34. Ursua I, Ramos R, Val-Bernal JF. *Helicobacter pylori* in Barrett's esophagus. *Histol Histopathol* 1991;**6**:403–8.

35. Loffeld RJLF, Ten Tije BJ, Arends JW. Prevalence and significance of *Helicobacter pylori* in patients with Barrett's esophagus. *Am J Gastroenterol* 1992;**87**:1598–1600.

36. Abbas Z, Hussainy AS, Ibrahim F *et al*. Barrett's oesophagus and *Helicobacter pylori*. *J Gastroenterol Hepatol* 1995;**10**:331–3.

37. Ricaurte O, Fléjou JF, Vissuzaine C *et al*. *Helicobacter pylori* infection in patients with Barrett's oesophagus: a prospective immunohistochemical study. *J Clin Pathol* 1996;**49**:176–7.

38. Werdmuller BFM, Loffeld RJLF. *Helicobacter pylori* infection has no role in the pathogenesis of reflux esophagitis. *Dig Dis Sci* 1997;**42**:103–5.

39. Labenz J, Blum AL, Bayerdörffer E *et al*. Curing *Helicobacter pylori* infection in patients with duodenal ulcer may provoke reflux esophagitis. *Gastroenterology* 1997; **112**:1442–7.

40. Weston AP, Badr AS, Topalovski M, Cherian R, Dixon A. Prospective evaluation of the association of gastric *H. pylori* infection with Barrett's dysplasia and Barrett's adenocarcinoma. *Gastroenterology* 1998;**114**:A703.

41. Chow WH, Blaser MJ, Blot WJ *et al*. An inverse relation between *cag*A+ strains of *Helicobacter pylori* infection and risk of esophageal and gastric cardia adenocarcinoma. *Cancer Res* 1998;**58**:588–90.

42. Vicari JJ, Peek RM, Falk GW *et al*. The seroprevalence of *cag*A-positive *Helicobacter pylori* strains in the spectrum of gastroesophageal reflux disease. *Gastroenterology* 1998;**115**:50–7.

43. Graham DY, Yamaoka Y. *H. pylori* and *cag*A: relationships with gastric cancer, duodenal ulcer, and reflux esophagitis and its complications. *Helicobacter* 1998;**3**:145–50.

44. Filipe MI, Potet F, Bogomoletz WV *et al*. Incomplete sulphomucin-secreting intestinal metaplasia for gastric cancer. Preliminary data from a prospective study from three centers. *Gut* 1985;**26**:1319–26.

45. Craanen ME, Blok P, Dekker W, Ferwerda J, Tytgat GNJ. Subtypes of intestinal metaplasia and *Helicobacter pylori*. *Gut* 1992;**33**:597–600.

46. Filipe MI, Munoz N, Matko I *et al*. Intestinal metaplasia types and the risk of gastric cancer: a cohort study in Slovenia. *Int J Cancer* 1994;**57**:324–9.

47. Tosi P, Filipe MI, Luzi P *et al*. Gastric intestinal metaplasia type III cases are classified as low-grade dysplasia on the basis of morphometry. *J Pathol* 1993;**169**:73–8.

48. Zwas F, Shields HM, Doos WG *et al*. Scanning electron microscopy of Barrett's epithelium and its correlation with light microscopy and mucin stains. *Gastroenterology* 1986;**90**:1932–41.

49. Jass JR. Mucin histochemistry of the columnar epithelium of the oesophagus: a retrospective study. *J Clin Pathol* 1981;**34**:866–70.

50. Trier JS. Morphology of the columnar cell-lined (Barrett's) esophagus. In: Spechler SJ, Goyal RK, eds. *Barrett's Esophagus: Pathophysiology, Diagnosis, and Management*. New York: Elsevier Science, 1985:19–28.

51. Shields HM, Zwas, F, Antonioli DA *et al*. Detection by scanning electron microscopy of a distinctive esophageal surface cell at the junction of squamous and Barrett's epithelium. *Dig Dis Sci* 1993;**38**:97–108.

52. Ormsby AH, Goldblum JR, Rice TW *et al*. Cytokeratin subsets can reliably distinguish Barrett's esophagus from intestinal metaplasia of the stomach. *Hum Pathol* 1999;**30**:288–94.

53. Salo JA, Kivilaakso EO, Kiviluoto TA, Virtanen IO. Cytokeratin profile suggests metaplastic epithelial transformation in Barrett's oesophagus. *Ann Med* 1996;**28**: 305–9.

54. Boch JA, Shields HM, Antonioli DA *et al*. Distribution of cytokeratin markers in Barrett's specialized columnar epithelium. *Gastroenterology* 1997;**112**:760–5.

55. Morales CP, Spechler SJ. Intestinal metaplasia at the gastroesophageal junction: Barrett's, bacteria, and biomarkers. *Am J Gastroenterol* 2003;**98**:759–62.

56. Glickman JN, Ormsby AH, Gramlich TL, Goldblum JR, Odze RD. Interinstitutional variability and effect of tissue fixative on the interpretation of a Barrett cytokeratin 7/20 immunoreactivity pattern in Barrett esophagus. *Hum Pathol* 2005;**36**:58–65.

57. Sharma P, Weston AP, Morales T *et al*. Relative risk of dysplasia for patients with intestinal metaplasia in the distal oesophagus and in the gastric cardia. *Gut* 2000;**46**:9–13.

58. MacDonald WC, MacDonald JB. Adenocarcinoma of the esophagus and/or gastric cardia. *Cancer* 1987;**60**:1094–8.

59. Zhang ZF, Kurtz RC, Sun M *et al*. Adenocarcinomas of the esophagus and gastric cardia: medical conditions, tobacco, alcohol, and socioeconomic factors. *Cancer Epidemiol Biomarkers Prev* 1996;**5**:761–8.

60. Parsonnet J, Friedman GD, Vandersteen DP *et al*. *Helicobacter pylori* infection and the risk of gastric carcinoma. *N Engl J Med* 1991;**325**:1127–31.

61. McClave SA, Boyce HW, Jr, Gottfried MR. Early diagnosis of columnar-lined esophagus: a new endoscopic criterion. *Gastrointest Endosc* 1987;**33**:413–6.

62. Sharma P, Morales TG, Sampliner RE. Short segment Barrett's esophagus—the need for standardization of the definition and of endoscopic criteria. *Am J Gastroenterol* 1998;**93**:1033–6.

63. Levine MS, Chu P, Furth EE *et al*. Carcinoma of the esophagus and esophagogastric junction:sensitivity of radiographic diagnosis. *Am J Roentgenol* 1997;**168**:1423–6.

64. Maruyama M, Baba Y. Gastric carcinoma. *Radiol Clin North Am* 1994;**32**:1233–52.

65. Dave UR, Williams AD, Wilson JA *et al*. Esophageal cancer staging with endoscopic MR imaging: pilot study. *Radiology* 2004;**230**:281–6.

66. Harris KM, Kelly S, Berry E *et al*. Systematic review of endoscopic ultrasound in gastro-oesophageal cancer. *Health Technol Assess* 1998;**2**:1–134.

67. Lowe AS, Kay CL. Noninvasive competition for endoscopic ultrasound. *Gastrointest Endosc Clin N Am* 2005;**15**:209–24.

68. Murata Y, Oguma H, Kitamura Y *et al*. The role of endoscopic ultrasonography for gastric cancer in the cardiac area [Japanese]. *Nippon Geka, Gakkai Zasshi* 1998;**9**:564–8.

69. Zuccaro G, Jr, Rice TW, Vargo JJ *et al*. Endoscopic ultrasound errors in esophageal cancer. *Am J Gastroenterol* 2005;**100**:601–6.

70. May A, Gunter E, Roth F *et al*. Accuracy of staging in early oesophageal cancer using high resolution endoscopy and high resolution endosonography: a comparative, prospective, and blinded trial. *Gut* 2004;**53**:634–40.

71. Sihvo EIT, Rasanen JV, Knuuti MJ *et al*. Adenocarcinoma of the esophagus and the esophagogastric junction: positron emission tomography improves staging and prediction of survival in distant but not in locoregional disease. *J Gastrointest Surg* 2004;**8**:988–96.

72. Spechler SJ. Adenocarcinoma of the gastroesophageal junction. *Clinical Perspectives in Gastroenterology* 1999;**2**:93–9.

73. Mariette C, Finzi L, Piessen G, Van Seuningen I, Triboulet JP. Esophageal carcinoma: prognostic differences between squamous cell carcinoma and adenocarcinoma. *World J Surg* 2005;**29**:39–45.

74. Hiele M, De Leyn P, Schurmans P *et al*. Relation between endoscopic ultrasound findings and outcome of patients with tumors of the esophagus or esophagogastric junction. *Gastrointest Endosc* 1997;**45**:381–6.

75. American Joint Committee on Cancer. *Cancer Staging Manual*, 6th edn. 2002.

76. Kelsen D. Multimodality therapy for adenocarcinoma of the esophagus. *Gastroenterol Clin North Am* 1997;**26**:635–45.

77. Kelsen DP. Multimodality therapy of esophageal cancer: an update. *Cancer J Sci Am* 2000;**6**(suppl 2):S177–81.

78. Anderson SE, Minsky BD, Bains M, Kelsen DP, Ilson DH. Combined modality therapy in esophageal cancer: the Memorial experience. *Semin Surg Oncol* 2003;**21**:228–32.

79. Van Sandick JW, van Lanschot JJB, ten Kate JFW *et al*. Pathology of early invasive adenocarcinoma of the esophagus or esophagogastric junction. *Cancer* 2000;**88**:2429–37.

80. Hulscher JBF, van Sandick JW, de Boer AGEM *et al*. Extended transthoracic resection compared with limited transhiatal resection for adenocarcinoma of the esophagus. *N Engl J Med* 2002;**347**:1662–9.

81. Arnott SJ, Duncan W, Gignoux M *et al*. Oeosphageal Cancer Collaborative Group. Preoperative radiotherapy for esophageal carcinoma. *Cochrane Database Syst Rev* 2000;**4**:CD001799.

82. Kelsen DP, Ginsberg R, Pajak TF *et al*. Chemotherapy followed by surgery compared with surgery alone for localized esophageal cancer. *N Engl J Med* 1998;31;**339**:1979–84.

83. Medical Research Council Oesophageal Cancer Working Party. Surgical resection with or without preoperative chemotherapy in oesophageal cancer: a randomised controlled trial. *Lancet* 2002;**359**:1727–33.

84. Enzinger PC, Mayer RJ. Esophageal cancer. *N Engl J Med* 2002;**349**:2241–52.

85. Walsh TN, Noonan N, Hollywood D *et al.* A comparison of multimodal therapy and surgery for esophageal adenocarcinoma. *N Engl J Med* 1996;**335**:462–7.

86. Herskovic A, Martz K, Al-Sarraf M *et al.* Combined chemotherapy and radiotherapy compared with radiotherapy alone in patients with cancer of the esophagus. *N Engl J Med* 1992;**326**:1593–8.

87. Munro AJ. Oesophageal cancer: a view over overviews. *Lancet* 2004;**364**:566–8.

CHAPTER 27

The Options for Palliation of Esophageal Adenocarcinoma

Shyam Varadarajulu and C. Mel Wilcox

Introduction

Esophageal cancer accounts for approximately 7% of all gastrointestinal malignancies and worldwide is the sixth leading cause of cancer death [1]. Despite advances in its diagnosis and treatment, up to 50% of patients have incurable disease at presentation, therefore necessitating palliative measures [2–4]. The goal of palliative therapy in patients with unresectable esophageal carcinoma is to ameliorate symptoms and treat complications thereby improving their quality of life. A variety of therapies have been employed to palliate dysphagia in patients with esophageal carcinoma including esophageal dilation, radiation therapy, neodinium yttrium argon (YAG) laser, thermal electrocoagulation, photodynamic therapy (PDT), and sclerotherapy of the tumor [5]. Esophageal prostheses (stents) have also been used for several decades as a method for palliation of malignant dysphagia [6]. The use of plastic stents has never become widely popularized because of substantial morbidity related to stent insertion and migration [7]. Because of improved design, materials, and deployment systems, self-expandable metal stents (SEMS) have become an attractive alternative to palliate esophageal carcinoma. The aim of this chapter is to review the multiple modalities available for palliation of esophageal cancer focusing on adenocarcinoma (Table 27.1).

Surgical Therapy

For the patient presenting with esophageal carcinoma, tumor resection should be initially considered when the surgical risk is acceptable and metastatic disease is not identified. Not only will surgery provide the potential for cure, but reliable palliation of esophageal complaints can also be achieved. Nevertheless, it is well recognized that esophageal adenocarcinoma may relapse at the surgical anastomosis, likely because of the high frequency of locally advanced disease [8]. In addition, despite negative preoperative staging, metastatic disease may be found at the time of exploration in up to 95% of patients [9]. In a recent prospective study, Walsh *et al.* found that of 55 patients with esophageal carcinoma undergoing resection, 45 (82%) had positive lymph nodes or identifiable metastasis at the time of exploration despite negative preoperative imaging with CT [10]. However, with the increasing use of endoscopic ultrasonography and positron emission tomography (PET) scans for staging, the number of patients undergoing resection with occult metastatic disease is reduced [11,12] and the prognosis following resection has improved [13]. Although esophageal resection can usually be performed successfully even when disease is locally advanced, the high frequency of metastatic disease at diagnosis suggests that multimodality therapy will be necessary to more adequately treat the tumor burden. Another major concern regarding surgery is morbidity and potential mortality. Over the last several decades, however, both morbidity and mortality have substantially decreased [13] with some series reporting very low mortality [14]. In addition, recent evidence has shown that surgical therapy in high-volume centers reduces perioperative mortality [8]. Nevertheless, postoperative morbidity is difficult to qualitate and has received little attention.

Table 27.1 Palliative therapies for esophageal adenocarcinoma.

Method
Endoscopic
a. Dilation
Savary–Gillard (over a guidewire)
Olive (Eder–Puestow)
Lead-filled rubber bougie (Maloney)
Balloon
b. Laser
Nd : YAG laser
Photodynamic electrocoagulation
c. Sclerotherapy
Thermal: Bicap, electrocoagulation
Chemical (absolute alcohol, sodium morrhuate, ethynil alcohol)
d. Radiation therapy
External
Intracavitary

Bicap, bipolar electrocoagulation.

Although surgical therapy alone will usually ameliorate dysphagia, routine surgical exploration must be tempered by the poor long-term prognosis. In studies reporting follow-up after curative resection of esophageal adenocarcinoma, the median survival is 10 months with a 5-year survival of 15% for those with stage III disease [15]. More recently median survival following surgery of 17 or more months has been reported [2,13]. It should be remembered that although surgical therapy has been the cornerstone of therapy for esophageal adenocarcinoma for years, there are scant data documenting a survival advantage of surgery as compared to radiation and/or combined modality therapy of radiation and chemotherapy for patients with locally advanced disease.

Radiation Therapy and Chemotherapy

Given the pathologic findings of locally advanced disease and metastatic disease in many patients un-dergoing surgical exploration for adenocarcinoma, multimodality therapy that combines radiation therapy and chemotherapy, either preoperatively and/or postoperatively, has been extensively evaluated. Theoretically, radiation therapy may "prime" tumor cells, which then makes subsequent chemotherapy more successful. This multimodality approach has been effective in the treatment of other tumors [16].

When evaluating studies of both surgery as well as radiation combined with chemotherapy for esophageal cancer, it is critical that the specific histologic subtype of the tumor is noted. A number of studies suggest that the response to both radiation and chemotherapy is better with squamous cell carcinoma of the esophagus than adenocarcinoma [10,17]. Thus, the results of trials reporting a significant response from aggressive therapy for "esophageal cancer" that consists primarily of squamous cell cancer cannot be extrapolated to adenocarcinoma. Furthermore, as endoscopic ultrasound (EUS) has emerged as the superior staging modality for esophageal carcinoma, the results of trials that use EUS for staging, thereby determining those most likely to have local disease, is not comparable to prior studies. Finally, it is important that studies evaluating palliative therapies clearly define the relief of dysphagia as well as quality of life. These are missing from many trials and can better help determine the best therapies to achieve palliation.

A number of studies have evaluated the role of preoperative chemotherapy and radiation for localized esophageal adenocarcinoma [17]. These observations suggest that high-dose radiation therapy combined with chemotherapy may reduce local disease and improve the chance for resectability; an impact on survival has not been uniformly shown [17,18]. A variety of different radiation and chemotherapy regimens have been used making comparisons between studies difficult. Although some studies have suggested improvements as compared to historical controls, other trials report no differences as well as significant toxicity [19].

In a study of esophageal adenocarcinoma, Walsh *et al.* randomized 58 patients to multimodality therapy and 52 to surgery [10]. Two courses of 5-FU and mitomycin C with 4000 cGy were given preoperatively. Of the patients undergoing multimodality therapy, 42% had positive nodes or metastatic disease at the time of surgery as compared to 82% undergoing surgery alone. Only 13 patients (25%) undergoing surgery after radiation and chemotherapy had a complete histological response. The median survival for patients receiving multimodality therapy was 16 months as compared to 11 months for those receiving surgery alone. These favorable results suggested a benefit from preoperative therapy in patients considered surgical candidates. Treatment related morbidity in this study was low, and the in-hospital mortality rate was 6%.

In contrast, Kelsen *et al.* compared preoperative chemotherapy to surgery alone in a large cohort of patients with esophageal cancer [20]. This trial included patients with both squamous cell carcinoma and adenocarcinoma. In contrast to the findings of Welsh *et al.*, no difference in overall survival was observed between the two groups, and subgroup analysis based on histologic type also revealed no differences. Urba *et al.* randomized 100 patients to either surgery or preoperative chemoradiotherapy followed by esophagectomy [21]. Median survival was no different between the groups (17.6 vs. 16.9 months).

It is well recognized that patients who are poor surgical candidates are those most likely to have a poor response from aggressive therapy. Several trials suggest some benefit from radiation and chemotherapy in patients with inoperable locally advanced disease [22–25]. Harvey *et al.* treated 106 patients with palliation chemoradiotherapy and showed a significant improvement in dysphagia [22]. Fifty-one percent maintained improved swallowing at last follow-up. Treatment was well tolerated with a treatment-related mortality of 6%.

In another study, Keller *et al.* evaluated preoperative radiation with 5-FU and mitomycin [24]. Overall, 18 patients (39%) achieved a complete clinical response; however, 20% developed progressive disease during chemoradiotherapy, and 20% of patients did not undergo surgery for a variety of reasons which emphasizes the importance of palliation. Postoperative complications were significant (41%).

Overall, the radiation and chemotherapy regimen was well tolerated. No survival advantage was noted with this regimen.

Thus, in summary, the data evaluating the role of multimodality therapy for the treatment of esophageal adenocarcinoma is mixed. Small randomized trials suggest efficacy while large studies fail to document improvement. Nevertheless, the available data does suggest some potential benefit of radiation and chemotherapy for patients in whom surgical therapy cannot be undertaken because of comorbidity or metastatic disease. Further study trials focusing on adenocarcinoma with attention to symptom improvement and quality of life are needed.

Tissue Ablation

Various methods of tissue ablation have been employed to palliate dysphagia in patients with esophageal adenocarcinoma [26]. Thermal ablation of tumor tissue (bipolar electrocoagulation [Bicap] or diathermy can be applied via the electrocantery probe device [27]. This method is less expensive than laser, but its success rate has not been high. Although this technique enjoyed a modest popularity in the early 1980s, its popularity has decreased with the availability of other modalities. It is most effective in managing circumferential tumors; however, most esophageal cancers are asymmetric and tortuous. The major complications of this therapy are perforation (occurring in 20% of patients) and fistula formation [26]. Argon plasma coagulation (APC) is another method for ablating esophageal cancer. In a study comparing outcomes in those who underwent thermal ablation using APC versus esophageal metal stenting, the median survival was longer for patients who underwent APC [27]. However, the median length of hospital stay and cost were significantly higher for those palliated with APC [27]. The superficial nature of the thermal energy as well as the inability to control the orientation of the tumor probes have led to limited use of thermal ablative modalities. These techniques are often used today as "salvage" methods to treat the tissue hyperplasia and tumor ingrowth/outgrowth at the margins of previously placed stents and for local control of bleeding from these tumors that tend to be vascular.

Ablation of tumors can also be achieved with the injection of chemicals or sclerosing agents, resulting in tumor necrosis and partial restoration of esophageal luminal patency. Tumors have been injected with cytotoxic agents, absolute alcohol, polidocanol, and sodium morrhuate. Despite the ease of performing this technique, injection sclerotherapy has not gained popularity for the palliative therapy of esophageal adenocarcinoma because the response is partial and only temporary. To overcome these shortcomings, mitomycin absorbed into activated carbon particles, for prolonging the effect of local therapy, was injected into the tumor site in a pilot study of 10 patients [28]. Preliminary results revealed an increase in median survival time, improved dysphagia and Karnofsky scores.

Esophageal Dilation

Dilation is an effective method for providing temporary relief of dysphagia. Most clinicians prefer to use over-a-wire bougie dilators (e.g. Savary–Gillard) due to its lower incidence of esophageal perforation. Other dilation devices include hydrostatic balloon devices, mercury filled rubber bougies (Maloney, Hurst) and metal olives (Eder–Puestow) [29–31]. These methods are generally simple to use and inexpensive. The major drawback of peroral dilation in the setting of advanced esophageal adenocarcinoma is its short-term relief of dysphagia, the need for frequent dilation sessions and associated complications (perforation). Perforation in the setting of malignancy may occur more frequently than with dilation of other strictures, perhaps due to lack of tissue compliance and decreased tissue tensile strength resulting from tumor infiltration of the esophageal wall [30]. Techniques for performing peroral dilation in patients with malignant strictures differ very little from techniques used for patients with benign strictures [30]. Balloon dilators have several theoretical advantages over bougie dilators, the most important being that applied force is directed only radially. Graham and Smith evaluated balloon dilation in 12 consecutive patients with malignant strictures and were able to dilate every patient to a desired esophageal di-

ameter of 15 mm without any complications [31]. The ideal size to which a stricture needs to be dilated remains unclear. With increasing use of EUS for staging esophageal cancer, a minimum of 14 mm has been shown to be a prerequisite for safe and satisfactory staging [32].

Photodynamic Therapy

PDT is based on the principle that a photosensitizing agent administered intravenously, usually a porphyrin derivative, accumulates selectively in malignant or dysplastic tissue (e.g. esophageal adenocarcinoma). Porphyrin is then activated by light administered through the endoscope, and a subsequent chemical reaction selectively destroys tumor cells. Contraindications to PDT include pregnancy, porphyrias, and known tracheoesophageal fistula or porphyrin hypersensitivity. Fertile females should be practicing birth control.

The use of PDT for unresectable cancer of the gastroesophageal junction (GEJ) has gained in popularity due to its success in improving dysphagia, quality of life and nutritional status, with benefits lasting from 1–3 months [33–35]. In an early experience using PDT, McCaughan *et al.* treated 19 patients with unresectable adenocarcinoma of the esophagus [33]. The average improvement in esophageal diameter was from 6 to 9 mm, an improvement in food intake from liquid to soft diet was noted in most patients, and the average survival was 7.7 months. In another open study, Patrice *et al.* showed favorable results with PDT for palliation of esophageal adenocarcinoma [36]. Ten of 14 patients had a partial or complete response to PDT. Five patients were free of tumor at an average follow-up of 15.5 months. In the largest series [37] reported to date of 215 esophageal cancer patients, PDT offered effective palliation for patients with obstructing cancer in 85% of treatment courses. The ideal patients for PDT palliation were those with obstructing endoluminal cancer. Patients living more than 2 months required re-intervention to maintain palliation of malignant dysphagia. However, PDT has usually been one component of a multimodality approach.

The most common side effects from PDT in these studies were the development of esophageal strictures, pleural effusions, fever, esophageal perforation, and sunburn. Studies evaluating the efficacy of steroids in preventing post-PDT strictures have been mostly disappointing [38]. Due to the theoretical advantage of selective tumor destruction, PDT appears more efficacious than YAG laser for tumors of the upper and lower esophagus, long tumors, and patients who have received previous palliative therapies [39]. Two multicenter trials comparing YAG laser therapy to PDT showed small differences in clinical efficacy favoring PDT over laser therapy for palliation of esophageal adenocarcinoma [40,41]. In the first study, 22 patients were randomized to PDT and 20 to YAG laser [40]. Both PDT and laser therapy relieved dysphagia, but PDT resulted in an improved Karnofsky performance status at 1 month and a longer duration of response. Another important difference was that patients assigned to laser required more therapy sessions than those patients assigned to PDT. The duration of response was also longer with PDT (84 vs. 53 days). Survival was similar amongst both groups of patients. In the largest multicenter randomized study comparing PDT to YAG laser, Lightdale *et al.* randomized 110 patients to receive PDT and 108 to YAG laser [41]. Improvement in dysphagia was equivalent between the two treatment groups. Objective tumor response was also equivalent at 1 week, but at 1 month tumor response was 32% after PDT and 20% after YAG. Nine complete tumor responses occurred after PDT and two after YAG. Trends for improved responses for PDT were seen in tumors located in the upper and lower third of the esophagus, in long tumors, and in patients who had prior therapy. More mild to moderate complications followed PDT but severe complications (e.g. perforation) were more common in YAG treated patients (1% vs. 7%).

Laser

Endoscopic laser therapy of esophageal cancer was first described in 1982 [39]. Laser light is monochromatic and collimated; therefore, it can be directly aimed at the tumor target and has predictable interaction with tissue. YAG is a gem quality solid crystal, which has a wavelength of 1.06 μm. It penetrates the normal gastrointestinal mucosa to a depth of

1–2 mm [26,42]. Laser therapy was the predominant form of palliative endoscopic therapy for esophageal carcinoma in the 1980s, but since then PDT and self-expanding esophageal stents have become more popular. Although laser therapy is useful for exophytic and polypoid lesion, it can be applied to almost any type of tumor leading to esophageal obstruction. Submucosal or extrinsic lesions and malignancies approximating the cricopharyngeus or those in severely angulated lumens are generally not amenable to this type of treatment. Luminal patency is achieved in almost every patient with relief of dysphagia achieved in 75–90%; however, relief is not long lasting, with only 30% of patients symptom-free at 3 months, thus requiring repeated sessions [26,42].

YAG laser is usually applied in several sessions. On day 1, the patient should undergo a detailed endoscopic exam of the esophagus and stomach, preferably using a small diameter endoscope. If the endoscope cannot be passed through the stricture, dilation over a wire should be attempted. The application of laser is performed starting at the most distal end of the tumor and slowly proceeding proximally. Treatment of the normal esophageal mucosa should be always avoided. The endpoint of laser therapy is to vaporize the tumor. Upon application of the laser light, the endoscopist will first observe a whitening of the tumor tissue (coagulation), and upon further application the endoscopist will observe black charring, formation of divots and evaporation of tissue (vaporization). A second session is usually scheduled on day 3. At this point an endoscopy is performed to evaluate the efficacy of the previous application. The endpoint of laser therapy is to achieve a luminal diameter that will prevent ongoing dysphagia; this diameter is usually the one that allows passage of a 9 mm endoscope [26].

A major disadvantage is the availability of laser equipment and the expense of therapy. The most serious complication is perforation, which occurs in 2–7% of cases [41,42]. Minor complications are infrequent and include transient bacteremia, fever, pain, and abdominal distention from air insufflated during the procedure [26].

Esophageal Stents

Placement of esophageal prostheses is a well-established, reliable, inexpensive, and durable method for palliation of malignant dysphagia [43] (Table 27.2). Two main types of esophageal stents are available: rigid (plastic) and expandable (metallic). Plastic stents have lost popularity because of their high complication rate [44] and the commercial availability of the newer, easier-to-insert SEMS [45].

To date, three prospective randomized controlled trials have compared metallic and plastic stents [7,45,46]. Knyrim *et al.* randomized 42 patients with malignant esophageal obstruction to either plastic Wilson–Cook esophageal stents with an internal diameter of 12 mm or Wallstents with an internal diameter of 16 mm [46]. In both treatment groups there was similar improvement in dysphagia scores as well as 30-day mortality rates, but complications were significantly less frequent in the metal stent group. It is important to note that in this study [46], all patients receiving a plastic stent underwent general anesthesia and also required esophageal dilation to 20 mm before stent insertion (in contrast to 10 mm for the metallic stents). These factors may not have allowed for a fair comparison of both devices.

DePalma *et al.* recently published a prospective controlled study comparing plastic versus Ultraflex esophageal prosthesis (Microvasive, Nattick, MA) [45]. Thirty-nine patients with esophageal cancer were prospectively randomized to either plastic stent (20 patients) or metallic stent (19 patients). Techni-

cal success was similar in both groups. Dysphagia scores improved significantly and were similar in both groups. Nevertheless, complications and mortality related to deployment were significantly less frequent with metal stents than with plastic prosthesis (complications 0% vs. 21%, mortality 0% vs. 15.8%). Late complications (food obstruction, tumor ingrowth, and migration) were not significantly different between the groups. The higher short-term complication rate and mortality were associated with the technique of stent insertion, which required greater esophageal dilation prior to plastic stent insertion.

The third randomized trial [7] was specifically designed to evaluate the usefulness of stents for GEJ tumors (i.e. adenocarcinoma). Siersema *et al.* compared the effectiveness of SEMS compared to plastic stents [7]. Although technical success and improvement of dysphagia scores were similar in both groups, major complications were more frequent with plastic prostheses (47%) than with metal stents (16%). Also, the hospital stay was longer in patients who underwent placement of a plastic prosthesis.

There exist a large variety of self-expanding metal stents, each with its own characteristics (Table 27.3). It is difficult to compare different metal stents because every stent has its own physical characteristics [47]. On the other hand, the patient's underlying pathology (e.g. malignant stricture at GEJ, tracheoesophageal fistula, etc.) will dictate the type or types of stent that will be required. Several uncovered and most covered stents are useful to palliate malignant tracheoesophageal fistulas secondary to esophageal cancer [48].

To summarize a decade of literature on SEMS, successful deployment is reported in 85–100% of series, although up to 22% require a second prosthesis at the time of initial stenting [49–51]. Covered stents are associated with prolonged patency when compared with uncovered ones [52]. Stents with flange diameters of 25 mm or larger are associated with lesser degrees of prosthetic migration [53]. An improvement in quality of life as well as cost-effectiveness has been shown from the use of SEMS [54].

Before stent insertion, an appropriate esophageal luminal diameter will be required to introduce the

Table 27.2 Indications for placement of esophageal prosthesis.

Esophageal cancer with stricture
Benign stricture
Tracheoesophageal fistula
  a. Malignant
  b. Benign
Malignant compression of gastroesophageal junction
  a. Bronchial carcinoma
  b. Metastatic tumors
  c. Lymphadenopathy

Table 27.3 US Food and Drug Administration (FDA) approved self-expandable metal stents (SEMS).

Stent type	Flanges	Length (cm)	Coating (cm)	Delivery catheter size (Fr)	Minimum lumen diameter (mm)	Maximum flange diameter (mm)
Ultraflex (Microvasive)	Proximal	10, 15	None	15	18	23
Ultraflex (Microvasive)	Proximal	10, 15	Yes 7, 12	15	18	23
Wallstent Esophageal (Schneider)	Proximal distal	8, 10, 13	Permalume 4, 6, 9	38	18	20–28
Wallstent Esophageal II (Schneider)	Proximal distal	10, 15	Permalume 8, 13	18	19	20–28
Wallstent Enteral (Schneider)	None	6, 9	None	10	18, 20, 22	18, 20, 22
Z-stent (Wilson–Cook)	Proximal distal	6, 8, 10, 12, 14	Polyurethane 6, 8, 10, 12, 14	31	18	21–15
Esophacoil (Instent) (Bard)	Proximal distal	10, 15	Coil	32	16–18	21–24

delivery catheter. If the esophagus cannot be dilated to the minimum diameter, damage to the esophagus may occur. Conversely, overdilation may increase the chance of stent migration. Relative contraindications include: uncooperative patients, tracheobronchial compression (especially with cuffed stents), significant coagulopathy, recent myocardial infarction, and presence of a fixed cervical spine or cervical arthritis [47]. If the esophageal tumor has significant necrosis, the chances of perforation and stent migration increase. Some stents (e.g. Gianturco) cannot be placed in areas of acute angled stenosis because the prosthesis may kink leading to obstruction. The concomitant presence of gastric outlet obstruction will negate the efficacy of any esophageal stent. If a patient is deemed a surgical candidate, no attempt should be made to place a prosthesis.

Types of Stents

Wallstents are prosthesis woven in the form of a tubular mesh made from surgical-grade stainless steel alloy filaments. These stents are pliable, self-expanding, and flexible in the longitudinal axis. The stent is maintained in its compressed from by an invaginated rolling membrane with an 18 Fr diameter, and it can be loaded on a 0.035″ guidewire [55,56]. Numerous studies have evaluated the use of uncovered Wallstents [55–59]. Neuhaus *et al.* prospectively evaluated 10 patients with malignant dysphagia using Wallstents after dilation of the stricture [56]. All patients had immediate improvement of dysphagia. One perforation was reported whereas stent occlusion secondary to food impaction or tumor ingrowth occurred in 40%.

The Z-stent is also a self-expanding tubular prosthesis. The basic structure consists of variable number of interconnected cages of 2 cm length. Each cage is composed of Z-shaped stainless steel wire. It can be compressed and placed inside a delivery catheter. The stent is available in several lengths (6, 8, 10, and

12 cm) with an 18 mm diameter [59]. There are several modifications that evolved from the original uncovered prototype. Its silicone covering decreases the exposure of the metal to surrounding neoplastic tissue and hence decreases tumor ingrowth. Due to its silicone membrane, the Z-stent is also useful to palliate esophagotracheal fistulas [60]. In order to avoid dislodgement or migration (due to the silicone coating), special anchoring hooks ("barbs") have been placed on the external surface (European model). This stent with anchoring hooks recently became available in the USA. For the same reason, new versions of the stent have flared distal and proximal ends (25 mm) for greater anchoring to the esophagus (Wilson–Cook, USA). A potential advantage of having a barbless Z-stent is that it is easier to extract it if the stent migrates into the stomach. The radial force exerted by the Z-stent is considerable, making it suitable for tight strictures.

Kozarek *et al.* have reported the largest prospective USA experience with this stent [53]. Fifty-four patients with refractory dysphagia or malignant esophagoairway fistulas had 73 Z-stents successfully inserted. Incomplete stent expansion was noted in 17% of patients. The short-term complication rate was 11% (severe pain, bleeding from necrotic tumor, hiatal hernia, intussusception). No perforations occurred. Adequate tracheoesophageal fistula closure was noted in 73% of patients. Stent migration occurred in 27% of patients. Three patients had stent-induced esophageal erosion resulting in bleeding (exsanguination) or fistula formation. A major issue to be addressed with this stent is its tendency for distal migration, noted primarily in neoplasms that bridged the esophagogastric junction; this complication has been reported to occur in 25% of patients at a mean of 1 month after placement.

The Ultraflex stent, which is knitted from a single wire of elastic alloy of nickel–titanium (nitinol), is embedded in gelatin that keeps it in a compressed state [61]. When deployed, the gelatin dissolves slowly and the stent expands, but deployment may take as long as 9 min. Injecting warm water through the biopsy channel accelerates the process, but carries the risk of aspiration. The expanded stent varies in length (7, 10, or 15 cm). Incomplete expansion is a significant problem due to its low radial expansile force. Thus, balloon dilation of the stent may be needed to achieve full expansion. The Ultraflex stent is mounted on a stabilizer with an outer diameter of 8 mm. Within the stabilizer, the stent is localized by four radiopaque markers. The two outer markers indicate the length of the stent in the compressed state; the two inner markers indicate the position of the ends of the stent after expansion (i.e. when it is shortened). The Ultraflex is the most extensively studied SEMS [44,61,62]. May *et al.* treated 30 patients with incurable tumors of the esophagus, and most tumors (84%) were located at the level of the esophagogastric junction [62]. Stent placement was successful in all patients. One week after placement, 83% of patient reported an improvement in dysphagia. No severe early complications occurred. Minor complications were reported in 70% of patients; these included insufficient stent expansion, retrosternal pain, and pyrosis. Twelve patients required further dilations to expand the prosthesis. In nine patients, recurrent dysphagia was noted at 9 weeks, six of them had endoscopically proven tumor ingrowth.

The Esophacoil stent consists of a single coiled flat wire made of nickel–titanium alloy [63,64]. This stent is unique in that it is a simple coil with a tight loop. It has a high radial force and almost no dilation is necessary prior to implantation. The ends of the stent are wide to prevent migration. The soft spherical wire ends avoid epithelial injury. The stent's flexibility allows adaptation to the wall of the tumor, diminishing significantly retrosternal pain and foreign body sensation. The very close loops of the spring prevent tumor ingrowth and impart appropriate wall permeability. For this reason this stent can also be used to palliate esophagorespiratory fistula. During deployment a piece of esophageal wall may become entrapped between the coil with partial or complete obstruction of the lumen. Wengrower *et al.* has published the largest experience with this stent [64]. During a 4-year period they placed 84 stents in 81 patients. In a long-term follow-up, Esophacoil was effective in the palliative treatment of dysphagia caused by malignant strictures. In their experience, the complications were low, but other authors have not had similar good results with this stent [65].

Complications of SEMS

Complications of stent placement can occur immediately in the postprocedure period, early and late after stent deployment (Table 27.4). Perforation is one of the most feared complications, and has been reported with almost every type stent. The risk of perforation appears greatest in patients who have received chemotherapy and/or radiation therapy, those with long strictures, inadequately dilated strictures, and with poor technique. Migration (proximal or distal) has been reported in 1–20% of cases [66]. Food impaction can result if the inner lumen of the stent does not reach proper diameter [47]. Most often, food impaction occurs because of a patient's carelessness in food selection, either from lack of knowledge or noncompliance with instructions. Stent occlusion can also occur either from tumor overgrowth (tumor extending proximally and distally to stent margins) or from tumor ingrowth [67,68]. Bleeding secondary to stent placement is uncommon (2%) [66], and is most commonly due to injury to the esophageal wall or mucosa. Late bleeding can result from mucosal necrosis or erosion into major vessels. Retrosternal pain may occur following uncomplicated esophageal stent placement due to impaction of the prosthesis against the esophageal wall. Its occurrence is unpredictable. Reflux esophagitis occurs mainly for stents placed across the GEJ. The most common causes of stent-related death are perforation, bleeding, and airway occlusion [47,65–67,69]. In patients with advanced esophageal cancer complicated by airway compression (as may be seen with tracheoesophageal fistula), it is either impossible or very difficult to extract the stent immediately from the esophagus once airway obstruction occurs. To avoid this serious complication, the potential for airway compression by an esophageal stent can be assessed by passing a bougie of a similar size into the esophagus while monitoring the airways by bronchoscopy. If significant airway compromise occurs, consideration should be given to endobronchial stent placement prior to esophageal stenting [70,71].

Table 27.4 Complications of esophageal stents.

Early (< 30 days)	Late (> 30 days)
Pain	Tumor ingrowth
Food impaction	Bleeding
Tumor ingrowth	Food impaction
Bleeding	Pain
Fistula	Fistula
Stridor	Esophageal reflux
Esophageal ulceration	Migration
Esophageal erosion	Foreign body sensation
Esophageal reflux	
Migration	
Foreign body sensation	
Perforation	
Airway compromise	

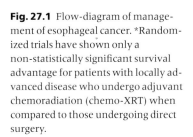
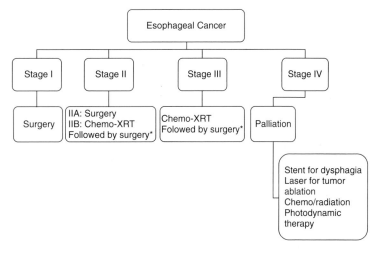

Fig. 27.1 Flow-diagram of management of esophageal cancer. *Randomized trials have shown only a non-statistically significant survival advantage for patients with locally advanced disease who undergo adjuvant chemoradiation (chemo-XRT) when compared to those undergoing direct surgery.

Conclusions

Esophageal adenocarcinoma remains a deadly disease with most patients being incurable at the time of initial presentation. A variety of measures are available which offer excellent palliation and the management strategy must be individualized depending on the stage of disease (Fig. 27.1). Surgical resection should be considered in the fit patient without evidence of metastatic disease. In contrast, for those with poor performance status and/or metastatic disease, endoscopic measures may be most appropriate, and a wide variety of endoscopic prostheses are available which can be placed with minimal morbidity and offer improvement in dysphagia. Chemoradiation should be coupled with surgical therapy, but may be used as primary palliation for patients with incurable disease, reasonable short-term life expectancy, and adequate performance status.

References

1. Jemal A, Tiwari RC, Murray T *et al*. Cancer statistics, 2004. *CA Cancer J Clin* 2004;**54**:8–29.
2. Sihvo EI, Luostarinen ME, Salo JA. Fate of patients with adenocarcinoma of the esophagus and the esophagogastric junction: a population-based analysis. *Am J Gastroenterol* 2004;**99**:419–24.
3. Mayoral W, Fleischer DE. Laser therapy for malignant esophageal strictures. *Tech Gastrointest Endosc* 1999;**1**:82–5.
4. Polee MB, Hop WC, Kok TC *et al*. Prognostic factors for survival in patients with advanced oesophageal cancer treated with cisplatin-based combination chemotherapy. *Br J Cancer* 2003;**89**:2045–50.
5. Likier H, Levine J, Lightdale C. Photodynamic therapy for completely obstructing esophageal carcinoma. *Gastrointest Endosc* 1991;**37**:175–8.
6. Schaer J, Katon RM, Ivancev K *et al*. Treatment of malignant esophageal obstruction with silicone-coated metallic self-expanding stents. *Gastrointest Endosc* 1992;**38**:7–11.
7. Siersema PD, Hop WCP, Dees J, Tilanus H, van Blankenstein M. Coated self-expanding metal stents versus latex prostheses for esophagogastric cancer with special reference to prior radiation and chemotherapy: a controlled, prospective study. *Gastrointest Endosc* 1998;**47**:113–20.
8. Hartel M, Wente MN, Büchler MW, Friess H. Surgical treatment of oesophageal cancer. *Dig Dis* 2004;**22**:213–20.
9. Lund O, Hasenkam JM, Agaard MT, Kimose HH. Time-related changes in characteristics of prognostic significance in carcinoms of the oesophagus and cardia. *Br J Surg* 1989;**76**:1301–7.
10. Walsh TN, Noonan N, Hollywood D *et al*. A comparison of multimodal therapy and surgery for esophageal adenocarcinoma. *N Engl J Med* 1996;**335**:462–7.
11. Sihvo EIT, Rasanen JV, Knuuti J *et al*. Adenocarcinoma of the esophagus and the esophagogastric junction: positron emission tomography improves staging and prediction of survival in distant but not in locoregional disease. *J Gastrointest Surg* 2004;**8**:988–96.
12. Rasanen JV, Sihvo EI, Knuuti MJ *et al*. Prospective analysis of accuracy of positron emission tomography and endoscopic ultrasonography in staging of adenocarcinoma of the esophagus and the esophagogastric junction. *Ann Surg Oncol* 2003;**10**:954–60.
13. Stein JH, Siewert J-R. Improved prognosis of resected esophageal cancer. *World J Surg* 2004;**18**:520–5.
14. Stewart JR, Hoff SJ, Johnson DH *et al*. Improved survival with neoadjuvant therapy and resection for adenocarcinoma of the esophagus. *Ann Surg* 1993;**218**:571–8.
15. Simon YK, Fok M, Cheng SWK, Wong J. A comparison of outcome after resection for squamous cell carcinomas and adenocarcinomas of the esophagus and cardia. *Surg Gynecol Obstet* 1992;**175**:107–12.
16. Poplin EA, Parvinderjit SK, Kraut MJ *et al*. Chemoradiotherapy of esophageal carcinoma. *Cancer* 1994;**74**:1217–24.
17. Enzinger PC, Mayer RJ. Esophageal cancer. *N Engl J Med* 2003;**349**:2241–52.
18. Zacherl J, Sendler A, Stein JH *et al*. Current status of neoadjuvant therapy for adenocarcinoma of the distal esophagus. *World J Surg* 2003;**9**:1067–74.
19. Imdahl A, Schoffel U, Ruf G. Impact of neoadjuvant therapy of perioperative morbidity in patients with esophageal cancer. *Am J Surg* 2004;**187**:64–8.
20. Kelsen DP, Ginsberg R, Pajak TF *et al*. Chemotherapy followed by surgery compared with surgery alone for localized esophageal cancer. *N Engl J Med* 1998;**339**:1979–84.
21. Urba SG, Orringer MB, Turrisi A *et al*. Randomized trial of preoperative chemoradiation versus surgery alone in patients with locoregional esophageawl carcinoma. *J Clin Oncol* 2001;**19**:305–13.
22. Harvey JA, Bessell JR, Beller E *et al*. Chemoradiation

therapy is effective for the palliative treatment of malignant dysphagia. *Dis Esophagus* 2004;**17**:260–5.

23. Liao Z, Zhang Z, Jin J *et al.* Esophagectomy after concurrent chemoradiotherapy improves locoregional control in clinical stage II or III esophageal cancer patients. *Int J Radiation Oncol Biol Phys* 2004;**5**:1484–93.

24. Keller SM, Ryan LM, Coia LR *et al.* High dose chemoradiotherapy followed by esophagectomy for adenocarcinoma of the esophagus and gastroesophageal junction. *Cancer* 1998;**83**:1908–16.

25. Hejna M, Kornek GV, Schratter-Sehn AU *et al.* Effective radiochemotherapy with cisplatin and etoposide for the management of patients with locally inoperable and metastatic esophageal carcinoma. *Cancer* 1996;**78**:1646–50.

26. Dallal HJ, Smith GD, Grieve DC *et al.* A randomized trial of thermal ablative therapy versus expandable metal stents in the palliative treatment of patients with esophageal carcinoma. *Gastrointest Endosc* 2001;**54**(5):549–57.

27. Johnston J, Quint R, Petruzzi C. The development and testing of a large Bicap probe for treatment of obstructing esophageal and rectal malignancy. *Gastrointest Endosc* 1985;**31**:156–63.

28. Ortner MA, Taha AA, Schreiber S *et al.* Endoscopic injection of mitomycin adsorbed on carbon particles for advanced esophageal cancer: a pilot study. *Endoscopy* 2004;**36**(5):421–5.

29. Kadakia SC, Cohan CF, Starnes EC. Esophageal dilation with polyvynil bougies usng a guidewire with markings without the aid of fluoroscopy. *Gastrointest Endosc* 1991;**37**:183–7.

30. McClave SA, Wright RA, Brady PG. Prospective randomized study of Maloney esophageal dilation: blinded versus fluoroscopic guidance. *Gastrointest Endosc* 1990;**36**:272–5.

31. Graham DY, Smith JL. Balloon dilation of benign and malignant esophageal strictures. *Gastrointest Endosc* 1985;**31**:171–4.

32. Wallace MB, Hawes RH, Sahai AV, Van Velse A, Hoffman BJ. Dilation of malignant esophageal stenosis to allow EUS guided fine-needle aspiration: safety and effect on patient management. *Gastrointest Endosc* 2000;**51**(3):309–13.

33. McCaughan JS, Nims TA, Guy JT *et al.* Photodynamic therapy for esophageal tumors. *Arch Surg* 1989;**124**:74–80.

34. Calzavara F, Tomio L, Corti P *et al.* Oesophageal cancer treated b photodynamic therapy alone or followed by radiation therapy. *J Photochem Photobiol* 1990;**6**:167–94.

35. McCaughn JB, William TE, Bethel BH. Palliation of esophageal malignancy with photodynamic therapy. *Ann Thorac Surg* 1985;**40**:113–22.

36. Patrice T, Foultier MT, Yactayo S *et al.* Endoscopic photodynamic therapy with hematoporphyrin derivative for primary treatment of gastrointestinal neoplasms in inoperable patients. *Dig Dis Sci* 1990;**35**:545–52.

37. Litle VR, Luketich JD, Christie NA *et al.* Photodynamic therapy as palliation for esophageal cancer: experience in 215 patients. *Ann Thorac Surg* 2003;**76**(5):1687–92.

38. Panjehpour M, Overholt BF, Haydek JM, Lee SG. Results of photodynamic therapy for ablation of dysplasia and early cancer in Barrett's esophagus and effect of oral steroids on stricture formation. *Am J Gastroenterol* 2000;**95**(9):2177–84.

39. Fleischer D, Kessler F, Haye O. Endoscopic Nd : YAG lser therapy for carcinoma of the esophagus. A new palliative approach. *Am J Surg* 1982;**143**:280–3.

40. Heier SK, Rothman KA, Heier LM, Rosenthal WS. Photodynamic therapy for obstructing esophageal cancer: light dosimetry and randomized comparison with Nd : YAG laser therapy. *Gastroenterology* 1995;**109**:63–75.

41. Lightdale CJ, Heier SJ, Marcon NE *et al.* Photodynamic therapy with porfimer sodium versus thermal ablation therapy with Nd : YAG laser for palliation of esophageal cancer: a multicenter randomized trial. *Gastrointest Endosc* 1995;**42**:507–12.

42. Nath G, Gorish W, Kiefhaber P. First laser endoscopy via fiberoptic transmission system. *Endoscopy* 1973;**5**:208–12.

43. Wu WC, Katon RM, Saxon RR *et al.* Silicone-covered self-expanding metallic stents for the palliation of malignant esophageal obstruction and esophagorespiratory fistulas: experience in 32 patients and a review of the literature. *Gastrointest Endosc* 1994;**40**:22–33.

44. Vermeijden JR, Bartelsman JFWM, Fockens P, Meijer RC, Tytgat GNJ. Self-expanding metal stents for palliation of esophagocardial malignancies. *Gastrointest Endosc* 1995;**41**:58–63.

45. DePalma GD, Galloro G, Sivero L *et al.* Self-expandable metal stents for palliation of inoperable carcinoma of the esophagus and gastroesophageal junction. *Am J Gastroenterol* 1995;**90**:2140–2.

46. Knyrim K, Wagner HJ, Bethge N, Keymling M, Vakil N. A controlled trial of an expansile metal stent for palliation of esophageal obstruction due to inoperable cancer. *N Engl J Med* 1993;**329**:1302–7.

47. Vakil N, Bethge N. Metal stents for malignant esophagela obstruction. *Am J Gastroenterol* 1996;**91**:2471–6.

48. Nelson EB, Silvis SE, Ansel HJ. Management of a tracheoesophageal fistula with a silicone-covered self-expanding metal stent. *Gastrointest Endosc* 1994;**40**: 497–500.

49. Nelson DB, Axelrad AM, Fleischer DE *et al.* Silicone covered Wallstent prototypes for palliation of malignant esophageal obstruction and digestive respiratory fistulas. *Gastrointest Endosc* 1997;**45**:31–7.

50. Kozarek RA, Raltz S, Brugge W *et al.* Prospective multicenter trial of esophageal Z-stent placement for malignant dysphagia and tracheo-esophageal fistula. *Gastrointest Endosc* 1996;**44**:562–7.

51. Wengrower D, Fiorini A, Valero J *et al.* Esophacoil: long-term results in 81 patients. *Gastrointest Endosc* 1998;**48**:172–9.

52. Vakil N, Perrachia A, Segalin A *et al.* Update: final results: randomized control trial of covered expandable metal stent in malignant esophageal obstruction. *Am J Gastroenterol* 2001;**96**:1791–6.

53. Kozarek RA, Raltz S, Marcon N *et al.* Use of the 25 mm flanged esophageal Z-stent for malignant dysphagia: a prospective multicenter trial. *Gastrointest Endosc* 1997; **46**:156–60.

54. Zinopoulos D, Dimitroulopoulos D, Moschandrea I *et al.* Natural course of inoperable esophageal cancer treated with metallic expandable stents: quality of life and cost-effectiveness analysis. *J Gastroenterol Hepatol* 2004;**19**:1397–402.

55. Bethge N, Sommer A, Vakil N. Treatment of esophageal fistulas with a new polyurethane-covered, self-expanding mesh stent: a prospective study. *Am J Gastroenterol* 1995;**90**:2143–6.

56. Neuhaus H, Hoffman W, Dittler HJ, Niedermeyer HP, Classen M. Implantation of self-expanding esophageal stents for palliation of malignant dysphagia. *Endoscopy* 1992;**24**:405–10.

57. Watkinson AF, Ellul J, Entwisle K *et al.* Esophageal carcinoma: initial results of palliative treatment with covered self-expanding endoprostheses. *Radiology* 1995; **195**:821–7.

58. Axelrad AM, Fleischer DE, Kozarek RA *et al.* US multicenter experience with coated Wallstents for palliation of malignant esophageal stricture and pulmonary fistulae [abstract]. *Gastrointest Endosc* 1995;**41**:345.

59. Schaer J, Katon RM, Ivancev H *et al.* Treatment of malignant esophageal obstruction with silicone-coated metallic self-expanding stents. *Gastrointest Endosc* 1995; **27**:495–500.

60. Ell C, May A, Hahn EG. Gianturco Z-stents in the palliative treatment of malignant esophageal obstrcution and esophago-tracheal fistulas. *Endoscopy* 1995;**27**: 495–500.

61. May A, Selmaier M, Hochberg J *et al.* Memory metal stents for palliation of malignant obstruction of the esophagus and cardia. *Gut* 1995;**37**:309–13.

62. May A, Hahn EG, Ell C. Self-expanding metal stents for palliation of malignant obstruction in the upper gastrointestinal tract. *J Clin Gastroenterol* 1996;**22**: 261–6.

63. Axelrad AM, Fleischer DE, Gomes M. Nitinol coil esophageal prosthesis: advantages of removable self-expanding metallic stents. *Gastrointest Endosc* 1996; **43**:155–60.

64. Wengrower D, Fiorini A, Valero J *et al.* EsophaCoil: long-term results in 81 patients. *Gastrointest Endosc* 1998;**48**:376–82.

65. Schoefl R, Winkelbauer F, Haefner M *et al.* Two cases of fractured esophageal nitinol stents. *Endoscopy* 1996;**28**: 518–20.

66. Kozarek RA, Ball TJ, Brandabur JJ *et al.* Expandable versus conventional esophageal prostheses: easier insertion may not preclude subsequent stent-related problems. *Gastrointest Endosc* 1996;**43**:204–8.

67. Kinsman KJ, DeGregorio BT, Katon RM *et al.* Prior radiation and chemotherapy increase the risk of life-threatening complications after insertion of metallic stents for esophagogastric malignancy. *Gastrointest Endosc* 1996;**43**:196–203.

68. Raijman I, Lalor E, Marcon NE. Photodynamic therapy for tumor ingrowth through an expandable esophageal stent. *Gastrointest Endosc* 1995;**41**:73–4.

69. Dasgupta A, Jain P, Sandur S *et al.* Airway complications of esophageal self-expandable metallic stent. *Gastrointest Endosc* 1998;**47**:532–4.

70. Weigert N, Neuhas H, Rosch T *et al.* Treatment of esophagorespiratory fistulas with silicone-coated self-expanding metal stents. *Gastrointest Endosc* 1995;**41**: 490–6.

71. Nelson DB, Axelrad AM, Fleischer DE *et al.* Silicone-covered Wallstent prototypes for palliation of malignant esophageal obstruction and digestive–respiratory fistulas. *Gastrointest Endosc* 1997;**45**:31–7.

Index

Entries in **bold** refer to tables, entries in *italics* refer to figures; please also note that all entries refer to Barrett's esophagus unless otherwise stated.